ANTIBIOTICS: ASSESSMENT OF ANTIMICROBIAL ACTIVITY AND RESISTANCE

A complete list of titles in the Society for Applied Bacteriology Technical Series appears at the end of this volume.

THE SOCIETY FOR APPLIED BACTERIOLOGY
TECHNICAL SERIES NO. 18

ANTIBIOTICS: ASSESSMENT OF ANTIMICROBIAL ACTIVITY AND RESISTANCE

Edited by

A. DENVER RUSSELL

The Welsh School of Pharmacy, UWIST, Cardiff, UK

AND

LOUIS B. QUESNEL

Department of Bacteriology and Virology,
University of Manchester, Manchester, UK

1983

ACADEMIC PRESS
A Subsidiary of Harcourt Brace Jovanovich, Publishers

LONDON · NEW YORK
PARIS · SAN DIEGO · SAN FRANCISCO · SÃO PAULO
SYDNEY · TOKYO · TORONTO

ACADEMIC PRESS INC. (LONDON) LTD
24/28 OVAL ROAD
LONDON NW1 7DX

U.S. Edition Published by
ACADEMIC PRESS INC.
111 FIFTH AVENUE
NEW YORK, NEW YORK 10003

British Library Cataloguing in Publication Data
Antibiotics.—(The Society for Applied Bacteriology
Technical Series ISSN 0300–9610; 18)
1. Antibiotics 2. Structure-activity
relationship (Pharmacology)
I. Russell, A. D. II. Quesnel, L. B.
III. Series
615′.329 RM267

ISBN 0–12–604480–5

LCCCN 82–73221

Typeset by Bath Typesetting Ltd., Bath
and printed in Great Britain by
St. Edmundsbury Press, Bury St. Edmunds, Suffolk

Contributors

P. R. Ball, *Pall Biomedical Ltd., Portsmouth PO1 3PD, UK*

M. L. Bates, *Food Science Division, MAFF, ARC Food Research Institute, Colney Lane, Norwich NR4 7UA, UK*

Angela S. Beale, *Beecham Pharmaceuticals Research Division, Chemotherapeutic Research Centre, Brockham Park, Betchworth RH3 7AJ, UK*

M. G. Boulton, *Microbial Biochemistry Department, Glaxo Group Research Ltd., Greenford UB6 0HE, UK*

A. S. Breeze, *Department of Pharmacy, Heriot-Watt University, 79 Grassmarket, Edinburgh EH1 2HJ, UK*

D. F. Broad, *Department of Chemical and Biochemical Engineering, University College, Torrington Place, London WC1, UK*

M. R. W. Brown, *Microbiology Research Group, Department of Pharmacy, University of Aston in Birmingham, Birmingham B4 7ET, UK*

I. Chopra, *Department of Microbiology, Medical School, University of Bristol, Bristol BS8 1TD, UK*

K. Coleman, *Beecham Pharmaceuticals Research Division, Chemotherapeutic Research Centre, Brockham Park, Betchworth RH3 7AJ, UK*

Janet E. L. Corry, *Food Science Division, MAFF, 65 Romney Street, London SW1P 3RD, UK*

R. M. Cozens, *Ciba-Geigy, Pharma Research, Basle CH4002, Switzerland*

S. P. Denyer, *Department of Pharmacy, University of Nottingham, Nottingham NG7 2RD, UK*

T. Farmer, *Beecham Pharmaceuticals Research Division, Chemotherapeutic Research Centre, Brockham Park, Betchworth RH3 7AJ, UK*

J. A. Frost, *Division of Enteric Pathogens, Central Public Health Laboratory, Colindale Avenue, London NW9 5HT, UK*

D. M. Gibson, *MAFF, Torry Research Station, 135 Abbey Road, Aberdeen AB9 8DG, UK*

P. B. Harper, *Chemotherapy Department, Microbiology Division, Glaxo Group Research, Greenford UB6 0HE, UK*

Carol Hince, *Area Pathology Laboratory, Caernarvon and Anglesey Hospital, Bangor, Gwynedd LL5 2HW, UK*

G. Hobbs, *MAFF, Torry Research Station, 135 Abbey Road, Aberdeen AB9 8DG, UK*

JUDITH HOLT, *Chemotherapy Department, Microbiology Division, Glaxo Group Research, Greenford UB6 0HE, UK*

ELIZABETH T. HOUANG, *Microbiology Department, Chelsea Hospital for Women, London SW3 6LT, UK*

A. J. HOWARD, *Area Pathology Laboratory, Caernarvon and Anglesey Hospital, Bangor, Gwynedd LL5 2HW, UK*

W. B. HUGO, *Department of Pharmacy, University of Nottingham, Nottingham NG7 2RD, UK*

PAMELA A. HUNTER, *Beecham Pharmaceuticals Research Division, Chemotherapeutic Research Centre, Brockham Park, Betchworth RH3 7AJ, UK*

MARTINE JAMES, *Chemotherapy Department, Microbiology Division, Glaxo Group Research, Greenford UB6 0HE, UK*

R. M. M. KLEMPERER, *Microbiology Research Group, Department of Pharmacy, University of Aston in Birmingham, Birmingham B4 7ET, UK*

A. H. LINTON, *Department of Microbiology, Medical School, University of Bristol, Bristol BS8 1TD, UK*

A. F. LOTT, *Microbiology Subdivision, Laboratory of the Government Chemist, Cornwall House, Stamford Street, London SE1 9NQ, UK*

A. MUNRO, *Department of Medical Microbiology, St. Bartholomew's Hospital, West Smithfield, London EC1A 7BE, UK*

D. C. ORR, *Microbial Biochemistry Department, Glaxo Group Research, Greenford UB6 0HE, UK*

I. PHILLIPS, *Department of Microbiology, St. Thomas's Hospital Medical School, London SE1 7EH, UK*

S. J. PLESTED, *Chemotherapy Department, Microbiology Division, Glaxo Group Research, Greenford UB6 0HE, UK*

I. A. PORTER, *Regional Laboratory, City Hospital, Aberdeen, UK*

L. B. QUESNEL, *Department of Bacteriology and Virology, University of Manchester, Stopford Building, Oxford Road, Manchester M13 9PT, UK*

C. READING, *Beecham Pharmaceuticals Research Division, Chemotherapeutic Research Centre, Brockham Park, Betchworth RH3 7AJ, UK*

D. S. REEVES, *Department of Medical Microbiology, Southmead General Hospital, Westbury-on-Trym, Bristol BS10 5NB, UK*

T. M. S. REID, *Regional Laboratory, City Hospital, Aberdeen, UK*

B. ROWE, *Division of Enteric Pathogens, Central Public Health Laboratory, Colindale Avenue, London NW9 5HT, UK*

A. D. RUSSELL, *Welsh School of Pharmacy, University of Wales Institute of Science and Technology, King Edward VII Avenue, Cardiff CF1 3NU, UK*

S. W. SHALES, *QMC Industrial Research Ltd., London E1 4AA, UK*

K. P. SHANNON, *Department of Microbiology, St. Thomas's Hospital Medical School, London SE1 7EH, UK*

M. R. Sharma, *Food Science Division, MAFF, 65 Romney Street, London SW1P 3RD, UK*

Elizabeth J. Shaw, *Department of Medical Microbiology St. Bartholomew's Hospital, West Smithfield, London EC1A 7BE, UK*

Ann M. Simpson, *Department of Pharmacy, Heriot-Watt University, 79 Grassmarket, Edinburgh EH1 2HJ, UK*

I. N. Simpson, *Chemotherapy Department, Microbiology Division, Glaxo Group Research, Greenford UB6 0HE, UK*

D. S. Smith, *Department of Medical Microbiology, St. Bartholomew's Hospital, West Smithfield, London EC1A 7BE, UK*

J. T. Smith, *Microbiology Section, Department of Pharmaceutics, School of Pharmacy, University of London, Brunswick Square, London WC1, UK*

R. Sutherland, *Beecham Pharmaceutics Research Division, Chemotherapeutic Research Centre, Brockham Park, Betchworth RH3 7AJ, UK*

E. J. Threlfall, *Division of Enteric Pathogens, Central Public Health Laboratory, Colindale Avenue, London NW9 5HT, UK*

D. R. Vaughan, *Microbiology Subdivision, Laboratory of the Government Chemist, Cornwall House, Stamford Street, London SE1 9NQ, UK*

Linda R. Ward, *Division of Enteric Pathogens, Central Public Health Laboratory, Colindale Avenue, London NW9 5HT, UK*

P. Ridgway Watt, *Beecham Pharmaceuticals Research Division, Chemotherapeutic Research Centre, Brockham Park, Betchworth RH3 7AJ, UK*

L. O. White, *Department of Medical Microbiology, Southmead General Hospital, Westbury-on-Trym, Bristol BS10 5NB, UK*

G. A. Willshaw, *Divison of Enteric Pathogens, Central Public Health Laboratory, Colindale Avenue, London NW9 5HT, UK*

W. J. Wood, *Regional Laboratory, City Hospital, Aberdeen, UK*

Preface

This volume, number 18 in the Society for Applied Bacteriology Technical Series, is based on the demonstrations given at a Demonstration Meeting of the Society held at the Welsh School of Pharmacy, University of Wales Institute of Science and Technology, Cardiff, on 23 September 1981.

The advent of antibiotics has had an enormous impact on the treatment of infectious diseases, but there is an adverse side: partly due to the sometimes indiscriminate use of these drugs, micro-organisms capable of resisting the effects of antibiotic action continue to increase in numbers and kind. Improved knowledge of the nature of this resistance coupled with chemical modification of antibiotic molecules have resulted in the introduction of a number of useful, new chemotherapeutic agents. Whereas some of these have a broad spectrum of activity, the present insights into the determinants of resistance and the biochemistry of antibiotic 'target molecules' in different species have enabled drug molecules to be tailored to perform specific antibacterial roles. This volume aims to give an explanation of how some of these insights have been obtained and of the ways in which their relevance and application in clinical, pharmaceutical and public health contexts can be routinely monitored and assessed.

This volume brings together contributions from more than fifty microbiologists from pharmaceutical companies, university departments of microbiology, medical microbiology and pharmacy, public health laboratories, hospital laboratories and food and government establishments. It contains theoretical and practical information on a variety of techniques and will, it is hoped, prove to be a useful reference work for all those who are engaged in chemotherapeutic work.

We wish especially to thank all those who presented demonstrations at the meeting, our co-organizer (Dr Janet Corry), as well as Professor P. S. J. Spencer and technical staff of the Welsh School of Pharmacy for their invaluable help and advice in the staging of the demonstration.

Financial assistance from Beecham Pharmaceuticals Ltd., CIBA-Geigy Ltd. and Glaxo Research Holdings is greatefully acknowledged.

January 1983

A. D. Russell
L. B. Quesnel

Contents

Introduction

L. B. Quesnel

Department of Bacteriology and Virology,
University of Manchester, Manchester, UK

A. D. Russell

Welsh School of Pharmacy,
University of Wales Institute of Science and Technology,
Cardiff, UK

Historical

An antibiotic was originally defined as a substance produced by one micro-organism that inhibits the growth of other micro-organisms. This definition is no longer strictly accurate because some antibiotics have now been produced synthetically (e.g. chloramphenicol) or semi-synthetically (e.g. several penicillins, cephalosporins). Thus, the term antibiotic is now considered as referring to a substance produced by a micro-organism or to a similar substance that, in low concentrations, inhibits the growth of micro-organisms.

While the fundamental concepts of chemotherapy and the early impetus towards its successful achievement were due largely to the efforts of Paul Erlich at the beginning of this century, modern antibiotic development began with the chance observation by Fleming in 1928 that a contaminating *Penicillium* would produce a substance that was lytic to staphylococci. Subsequent studies by Florey, Chain, Abraham and their colleagues at Oxford, and the American pharmaceutical industry, eventually resulted in the isolation and characterization of the pure, active constituent, penicillin. (A detailed account is provided by Selwyn 1980.) There followed extensive investigations both in Europe and the United States, into antibiotic substances produced from moulds, streptomycetes and other bacteria. *Streptomyces* spp. in particular, have yielded many important antibiotics;

ANTIBIOTICS
ISBN 0 12 604480 5

streptomycin, the original tetracyclines, chloramphenicol, erythromycin, novobiocin and kanamycin, among others, were all isolated in the 1940s and 1950s. The original *Cephalosporium* mould which provided the starting point for the development of the cephalosporin antibiotics was isolated from the sea by Brotzu, at the sewage outfall off Cagliari in Sardinia, as early as 1945.

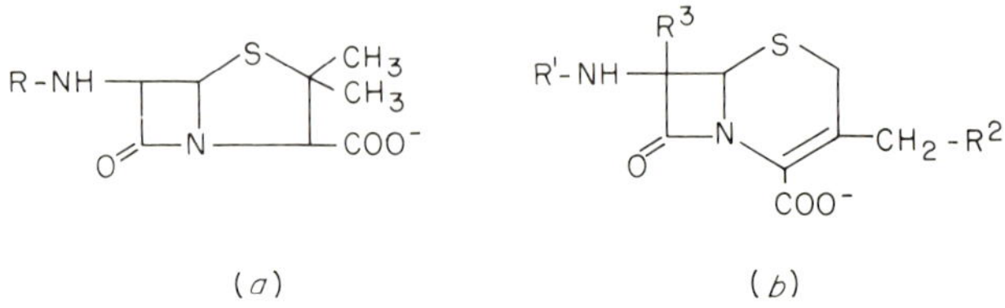

FIG. 1. β-lactam antibiotics. (*a*) General structure of penicillins (in 6-amino-penicillanic acid, R = H). (*b*) General structure of cephalosporins (in 7-amino-cephalosporanic acid, R^1 = H, R^2 = –O.CO.CH_3 and R^3 = H).

By 1960 both the penicillin nucleus, 6-aminopenicillanic acid (6-APA, Fig. 1*a*) and the cephalosporin nucleus, 7-aminocephalosporanic acid (7-ACA, Fig. 1*b*) had been isolated and the ability to substitute various side-chains in place of the original naturally occurring ones, has led to the production of large numbers of semi-synthetic β-lactam antibiotics of immense importance.

In recent years a resurgence of interest in β-lactam antibiotics has resulted in the development of cephamycins (7α-methoxy-cephalosporins), clavams, oxacephems, carbapenems, monobactams and a number of other groups.

Targets for Antibiotic Action

It is, as yet, seldom possible that examination of chemical structure alone permits any conclusions regarding the activity of a particular antimicrobial, or the range of organisms against which it may be effective, and a bewildering variety of chemical molecules has been shown to have such properties. Some 7000 antibiotics have been recognized and no simple classification of chemical types is possible, although a number of well-recognized classes of drugs feature among the relatively small fraction of these compounds which are of proven therapeutic value.

For convenience we will outline some of these with a summary of their known modes of action on the basis of their biochemical targets in the cell. More extensive discussions can be found in a number of recent publications (Selwyn 1980; Franklin & Snow 1981; Garrod *et al.* 1981; Gale *et al.* 1981).

Inhibitors of Cell Wall Synthesis

The stages in the biosynthesis of wall peptidoglycan, together with the sites of action of β-lactam antibiotics, vancomycin, bacitracin, phosphonomycin, alafosfalin, tunicamycin, ristocetin and cycloserine are presented in Fig. 2. D-Cycloserine is a competitive inhibitor of both alanine racemase and synthetase enzymes, vancomycin binds specifically to the D-ala-D-ala group on the peptide chain of a membrane-bound intermediate, and bacitracin to polyprenyl pyrophosphatase, inhibiting the reactivation of the phospholipid carrier molecule for polymer units.

The most recently synthesized inhibitors of wall synthesis are the phosphonopeptides, L-ala-L-ala-P (alafosfalin) and the tri-ala-P being the most active, the former primarily against Gram negative organisms. These drugs have low toxicity and may be useful therapeutics of the future.

β-Lactam antibiotics

There are now several different types of β-lactam antibiotics with proven or potential value as antibacterial agents (Brown 1981).

Penicillins

Pride of place must still go to the penicillin sub-group (Fig. 1*a*, with varying side-chain R). Included in this group are

(a) narrow spectrum, β-lactamase labile penicillins (benzylpenicillin, phenoxymethylpenicillin) with specific activity against Gram positive bacteria;
(b) β-lactamase-stable, narrow spectrum drugs such as methicillin (orally inactive) and cloxacillin and flucloxacillin (both orally active);
(c) broad-spectrum, β-lactamase labile penicillins (ampicillin, amoxycillin) which are inactive against *Pseudomonas aeruginosa*;
(d) broad-spectrum, β-lactamase labile drugs (e.g. carbenicillin) including activity against *Ps. aeruginosa*;
(e) pro-drugs, i.e. antibiotics that are themselves inactive but are hydrolysed *in vivo* to give the active drug;
(f) substituted ampicillins (R = $C_6H_5.CH_2(NH_2).CO$), e.g. piperacillin, mezlocillin and azlocillin, which combine the properties of ampicillin and carbenicillin

Cephalosporins

Cephalosporins have two side-chains, viz. R^1 (at 7) and R^2 (at 3) as depicted in Fig. 1*b*. In addition, the cephamycins (methoxycephalosporins) have a methoxy, $-OCH_3$, group at 7α (R^3) which markedly increases stability to β-lactamases (O'Callaghan 1980).

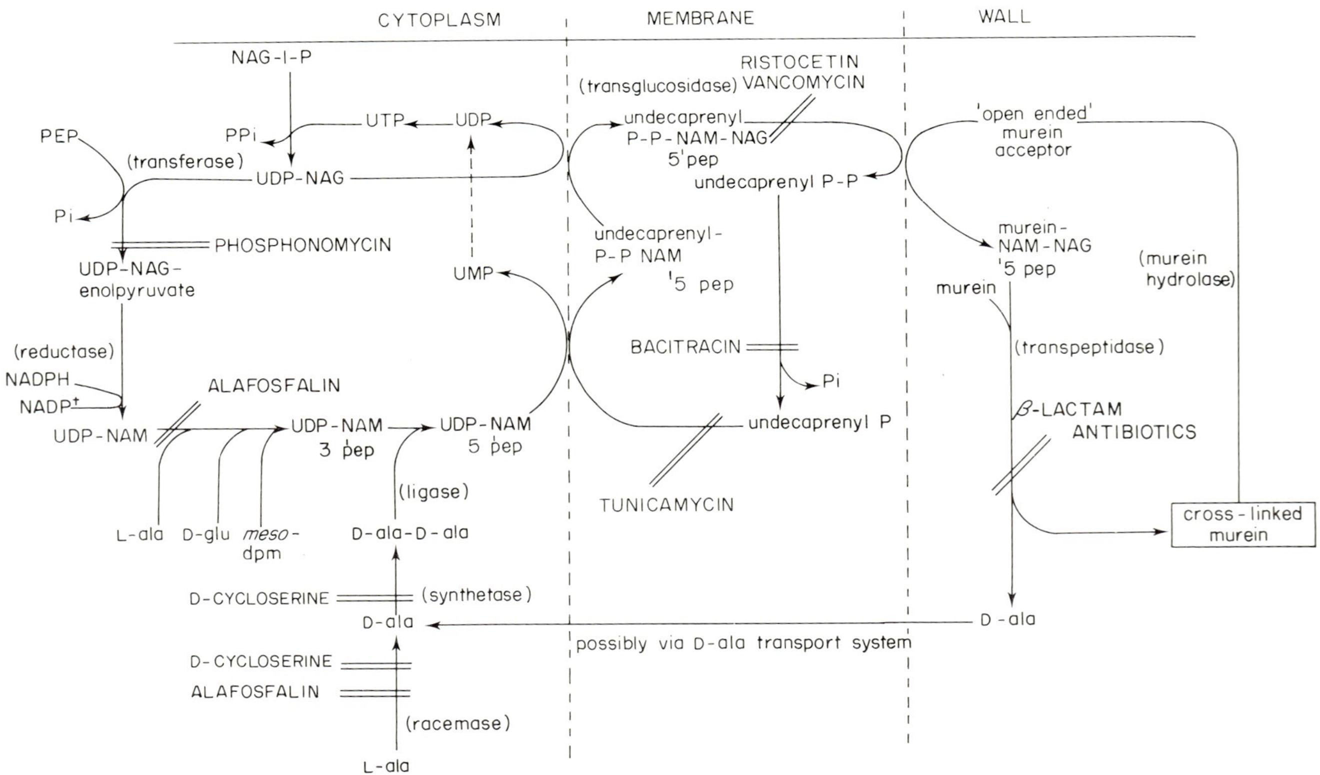

FIG. 2. Peptidyoglycan (murein) synthesis (in *Escherichia coli*) and the effects of antibiotics. NAG, *N*-acetylglucosamine; PEP, phosphoenolpyruvate; NAM, *N*-acetylmuramic acid.

Some of the "first generation" cephalosporins (cephaloridine, cephalothin) are very susceptible to β-lactamases produced by Gram negative bacteria, whereas the newer members, especially cefotaxime, are highly resistant.

Δ^3-Cephalosporins (based on Fig. 1*b*) are highly active antibacterials but alteration of the position of the double bond in the dihydrothiazine ring, to give Δ^2-cephalosporins, gives an inactive molecule.

Cephalosporins with an ester grouping at R^2 are susceptible to human esterases and are esterified to less active compounds.

Clavams

Replacement of the S atom of the thiazolidine ring by oxygen leads to a reduction in antibacterial activity. However, clavulanic acid (Fig. 3*a*) an oxapenicillin with no side-chain, is an important new inhibitor of Richmond & Sykes (1973) Types II, III, IV and V β-lactamases (Cole 1980: see Reading & Farmer, pp. 141–159).

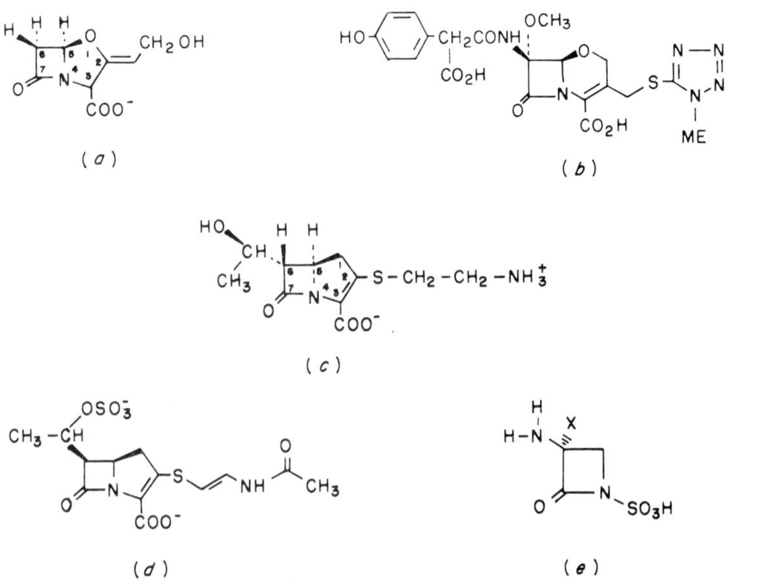

FIG. 3. Some newer types of β-lactam antibiotics. (*a*) Clavulanic acid. (*b*) Moxalactam. (*c*) Thienamycin. (*d*) Olivanic acid. (*e*) 3-Aminobactamic acid.

Oxacephems

Moxalactam (Fig. 3*b*) is a highly active 1-oxacephalosporin derived semi-synthetically from penicillin, and has oxygen at position 1 in place of S.

This would tend to make it less chemically stable and more enzyme labile; however, the presence of the 7α-methoxy group, as in cefoxitin, stabilizes the molecule.

Carbapenems

In these, the sulphur of the thiazolidine ring has been replaced by carbon and a double bond introduced at C_2—C_3. Important members of the 1-carbapenems are the olivanic acids (general structure, Fig. 3*d*) which act as competitive inhibitors of β-lactamases and are also broad-spectrum antibiotics in their own right. Another 1-carbapenem, thienamycin (Fig. 3*c*) is also a broad-spectrum antibiotic but is a poor β-lactamase inhibitor.

Monobactams

The monobactams are a new group of β-lactam antibiotics chemically based on 3-aminomonobactamic acid (3-AMA; Fig. 3*e*). They have been isolated from various species of bacteria (Imada *et al.* 1981; Sykes *et al.* 1981) and one member, Azthreonam, has been shown to be highly active against Gram negative but not Gram positive bacteria.

Mechanism of action

β-lactam antibiotics prevent transpeptidation between peptidoglycan chains. These drugs have, in fact, been shown to inhibit multiple penicillin-sensitive enzymes. These are diffiicult to purify and it is much easier in practice to measure binding of ^{14}C-benzylpenicillin to membrane proteins, known as penicillin-binding proteins (PBPs). At least seven of these are known in *Escherichia coli* of which PBPs 1, 2 and 3 appear to be the most important and are the lethal targets (transpeptidases) of drug action. PBPs 4, 5 and 6 have been associated with carboxypeptidase action. Cephaloridine binds predominantly to PBP1, mecillinam solely to PBP2 and ampicillin mainly to PBP3. Boulton & Orr (pp. 161–181) describe methods of measuring β-lactam binding to PBPs. Only three PBPs have been identified in *Neisseria gonorrhoeae* and four in *Staphylococcus aureus*, of which PBPs 2 and 3 are the probable killing targets.

Membrane-active Agents

Several agents are known to cause damage to the cytoplasmic membrane of micro-organisms. Polyenic antibiotics (e.g. amphotericin B) bind specifically to membrane sterols in fungi and are thus without effect on bacteria. The polymyxins disrupt the cytoplasmic membrane of susceptible Gram negative bacteria, although they also affect the outer membrane of the cell envelope (Brown 1975).

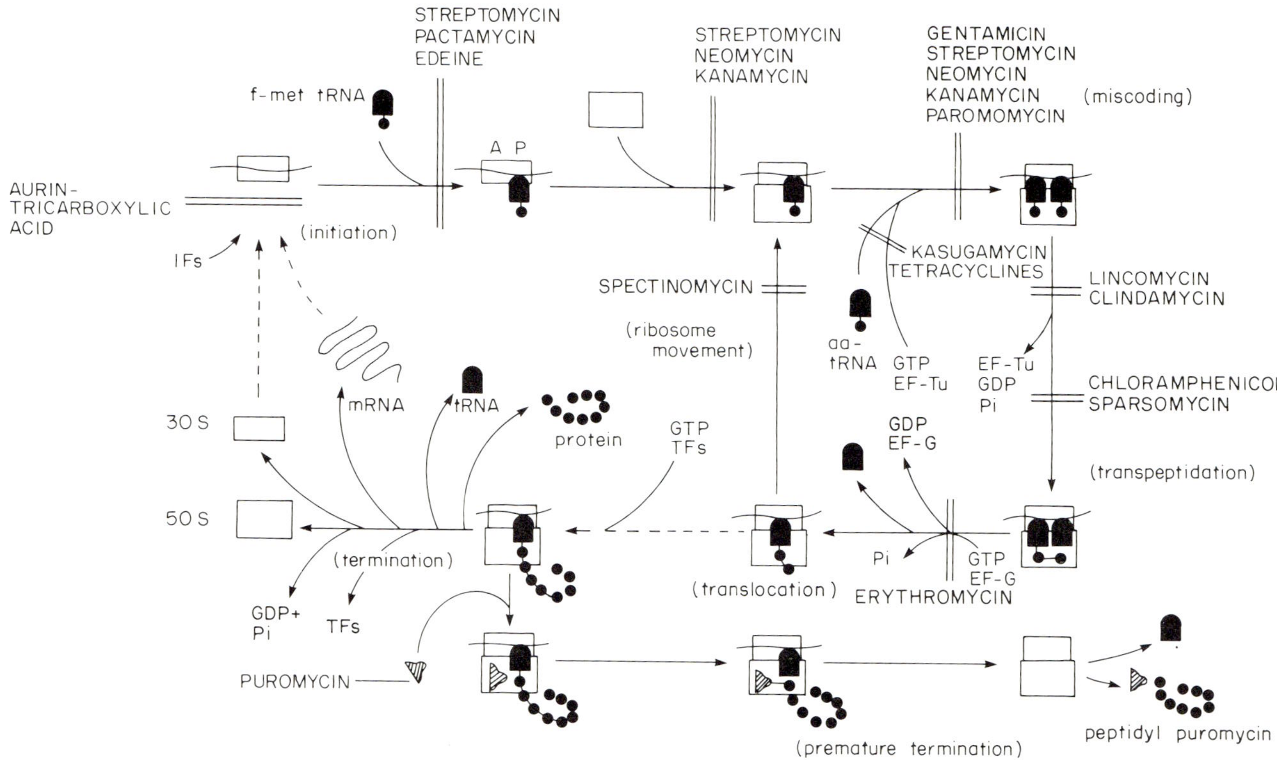

FIG. 4. Protein synthesis and the effect of inhibitors.

Other inhibitors of ribosome function

Several other antibiotics of clinical importance act to inhibit protein synthesis, notably the macrolides (e.g. erythromycin, oleandomycin), lincomycins (lincomycin, clindamycin), chloramphenicol and fusidic acid. All of these have as their primary site of action the 50S ribosomal subunit.

Inhibitors of Nucleic Acid Synthesis

Rifampicin binds specifically to the β-subunit of bacterial RNA polymerase inhibiting attachment to a promotor site. Actinomycin D, by binding strongly to helical double-stranded DNA, inhibits the function of DNA-dependent RNA polymerase. Covalent linking occurs between mitomycin C and DNA such that cross-links are formed between complementary strands of DNA. The synthetic drug nalidixic acid is an inhibitor of DNA synthesis (DNA gyrase A) but recent studies point to a multiplicity of effects (Crumplin *et al.* 1980). Novobiocin inhibits DNA gyrase B, an enzyme that introduces negative super-helical turns into covalently closed circular double-stranded DNA (Staudenbauer 1975).

Inhibitors of Metabolic Function

Folate inhibitors

Most bacteria are capable of synthesizing dihydrofolic acid from its components, i.e. *p*-aminobenzoic acid (PAB; 4-aminobenzoic acid), pteridine and glutamic acid. Dihydrofolate itself plays no important part in bacterial metabolism. It is, however, reduced by the enzyme dihydrofolate reductase (DHFR) to tetrahydrofolic acid which is involved in the production of methionine, purines, thymine, constituents of nucleic acids, etc.

Sulphanilamide (Fig. 7) was the first widely used chemotherapeutic agent. It was shown by Trefouël *et al.* (1935), to be the active component released in the body upon breakdown of Prontosil, introduced in 1935 by Domagk. Sulphanilamide, and the many active modifications which comprise the sulphonamide family of drugs, is a competitive inhibitor of dihydropteroate synthetase, the enzyme condensing pteridine and PAB. The sulphonamides have no action on preformed folate so that the inhibition of growth is delayed and their action is bacteristatic. As a group they have widely differing pharmacological properties and some are comparatively toxic; the most useful clinically have pK values around physiological pH (Williams 1974).

Some diaminopyrimidine derivatives exhibit high specificity for particular dihydrofolate reductase enzymes and the most active antibacterial compounds synthesized have been trimethoprim (Fig. 7) and, to a lesser extent, tetroxoprim, while pyrimethamine is specifically antiprotozoal (Burchall 1979).

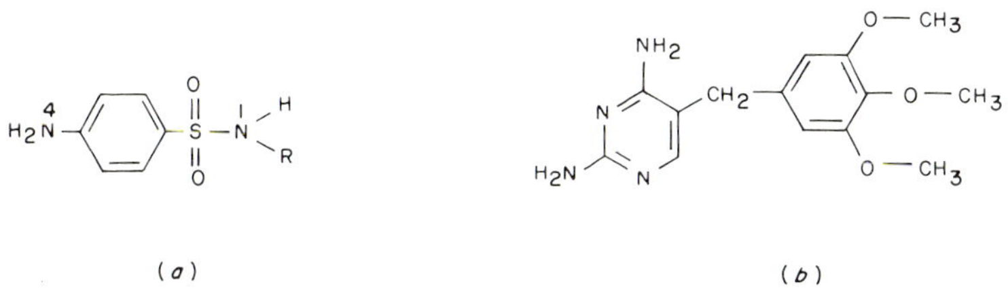

FIG. 7. (*a*) The structure of sulphonamides (in sulphanilamide, R=H). (*b*) Trimethoprim.

Since the sulphonamides and trimethoprim inhibit sequential stages in folate metabolism (see Fig. 8) it seemed logical to use a combination of a sulphonamide (sulphamethoxazole) and the diaminopyrimidine. However, much criticism has been directed at the clinical use of this mixture (see, for example, Lacey 1979) and trimethoprim is now often used alone.

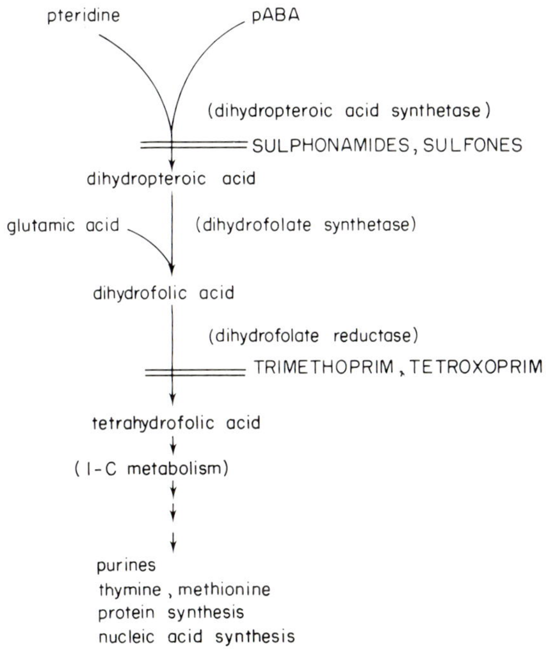

FIG. 8. Stages in, and inhibition of, folic acid biosynthesis.

Broad & Smith (pp. 245–263) give a comprehensive account of the methods of studying inhibitors of bacterial folate metabolism.

Transferable Resistance

Resistance to antibiotics may be transferred from cell to cell by three main mechanisms: (1) transformation, (2) transduction and (3) conjugation.

While gene transfer by transformation is of comparatively minor importance in the development and spread of drug resistance, transduction mediated by bacteriophages promotes the spread of both chromosomally and plasmid-borne resistance genes. It is the mechanism common to staphylococci, and is also found among Gram negative organisms.

Multiple drug resistance and the block transfer of such resistances was first observed in Japan during dysentry epidemics in the 1950s and the mechanism of transmissibility was first proposed simultaneously but independently by Akiba *et al.* (1960) and Ochiai *et al.* (1959). Transferable drug resistance is now an important clinical problem that undoubtedly has been accelerated by the widespread (and often injudicious) use of antibiotics.

In conjugative transfer cell to cell contact is essential. In the streptococci plasmid transfers take place either at high frequency or low frequency depending upon the production by recipients of "sex pheromones" which induce in the donor the synthesis of a mating factor of clumping-inducing agent (CIA) which promotes aggregation (Clewell 1981). In the Enterobacteriaceae conjugative plasmid transfer appears to depend on the presence of a plasmid-borne *tra* gene complex which confers fertility upon the donor cell associated with the ability to produce specific sex pili of several different types. (Resistance transfer factor (RTF) should not be used for the *tra* complex since many conjugative plasmids are not associated, and need not be associated, with drug resistance.) On the other hand some drug-resistance plasmids may not be conjugative and for transfer of these resistances it is necessary that the cell be superinfected with a second plasmid which is conjugative and can therefore mobilize the first (Falkow 1975).

The whole problem of drug resistance was further complicated by the discovery that genes conferring antibotic resistance could jump from one location to another within DNA strands or from chromosome to plasmid or vice versa (Hedges & Jacob 1974; Cohen 1976).

In vitro methods of studying transferable drug resistance are described by Frost *et al.* (pp. 265–284) and the use of phage typing and plasmid characterization in the epidemiology of multiresistant *Salmonella typhimurium* by Threlfall *et al.* (pp. 285–297).

Bacterial Resistance to Antibiotics

Bacterial resistance to antibiotics has long been a problem and will continue to be so for the foreseeable future, although the design of new antibiotics, such as β-lactamase inhibitors (Cole 1980) will still be an important part of effective defence mechanisms.

Resistance can arise in several different ways and some of these will be considered in more detail here.

Inactivation or modification

Probably the best known example of resistance concerns the inactivation of penicillin by β-lactamase, as a result of which there is opening of the β-lactam ring (Fig. 1*a*) of the antibiotic. Some penicillins are resistant to such inactivation. Cephalosporins susceptible to β-lactamases are converted to the corresponding cephalosporoic acid with loss of the substituent R^2 (except in cephalexin, where $R^2 = H$) and subsequent degradation of the molecule. Several cephalosporins are inactivated by some β-lactamases produced by Gram negative bacteria, whereas others (e.g. cefoxitin, cefotaxime) are highly resistant.

Some bacteria produce enzymes (reviewed by Davies & Smith 1978) that can modify aminoglycoside antibiotics (e.g. in Fig. 5) and the detection of such strains is described by Shannon & Phillips (pp. 183–198). Not all of the antibiotic is modified, however, and drug remaining in the external environment is unchanged. It seems possible that either the modified antibiotic is not transported to its primary site of action at the ribosome or alternatively that the modified drug prevents uptake of the unmodified compound (Bryan & van den Elzen 1977).

Chloramphenicol is inactivated by some bacteria and the resistance gene is frequently plasmid borne. Strains of *Staph. aureus* produce an inducible enzyme, chloramphenicol acetyltransferase, whereas in resistant Gram negative bacteria this is constitutive (Shaw 1971*a*, *b*).

Extraction and purification of antibiotic-destroying enzymes is described by Broad & Smith (pp. 93–110). Plested *et al.* (pp. 111–126) explain methods for detecting and identifying β-lactamases and Holt *et al.* (pp. 127–139) discuss the techniques for studying the effects of cell-free β-lactamases on β-lactam antibiotics.

Impermeability

The composition of the cell envelope affects the activity of antibiotics and other antibacterial agents (Brown 1975). This is particularly true with Gram negative bacteria, and Nikaido & Nakae (1979) have described outer membrane peptidoglycan-associated proteins (porins) which are involved in the production of non-specific pores, thereby forming a major pathway for the diffusion of hydrophilic substances of low molecular weight. Cephaloridine, which readily penetrates Gram negative cells, has a diminished passage through the outer membrane of porin-deficient mutants of *Salm. typhimurium*. Hydrophobic molecules are unable to gain entry via these porins (see Russell 1982, for a detailed account).

Mechanisms of resistance to tetracyclines have yet to be fully elucidated. There is no inactivation of the antibiotics but tetracycline-resistant R^+ strains of Gram negative bacteria synthesize 'resistance proteins', located in the outer or inner membrane that reduce drug uptake and, in some instances, promote efflux of antibiotic from resistant cells (Chopra *et al.* 1981).

Methods of studying bacterial resistance to tetracycline are considered by Chopra *et al.* (pp. 223–243) and Cozens *et al.* (pp. 61–75) describe how cell envelope composition can influence antibiotic activity.

Changes in target sites or enzymes

Alteration in target site is known to be one mechanism for bacterial resistance to antibiotics. Thus, resistance to streptomycin and erythromycin has arisen as a consequence of changes in the relevant ribosomal binding site, i.e. 30S and 50S, respectively (Franklin & Snow 1981). Changes in penicillin-sensitive enzymes (PSEs linked to PBPs) may be responsible for different sensitivities to β-lactams (Spratt 1980). One method of trimethoprim resistance results from production by the bacterial cell of an altered dihydrofolate reductase (Smith 1979).

Tolerance

Tolerance of an organism to β-lactam antibiotics is a resistance to the irreversible effects of these drugs and appears to be associated with defective autolysin activity (Tomasz 1979).

Measurement of Antibiotic Activity

There are several methods of measuring the activity of antibiotics. One of the easiest is to use sensitivity discs and the relationship between diameters of zone inhibition to minimum inhibitory concentration (MIC) is discussed by Linton (pp. 19–30). MIC values are usually obtained by serial dilution of antibiotic in liquid media or on agar, but it should be noted that the actual values may vary with the composition of the culture medium

(Houang *et al.*, pp. 31–48), with the size of the inoculum and, in the case of the aminoglycosides the presence of oxygen. When combined antibiotic activity is being measured, the fractional inhibitory concentrations (FIC) are derived (Beale & Sutherland, pp. 299–315). MIC values of antifungal agents can be determined in a similar manner, although problems can arise when testing imidazole antifungals. Among the newer methods for determining sensitivities is the utilization of conductance measurements described by Porter *et al.* (pp. 49–60).

The lethal effects of antibiotics can be assessed by determining minimum bactericidal concentrations (MBC values) or by counting the numbers of survivors at specified time intervals. A neutralizing (inactivating) agent should be used wherever possible (Russell *et al.* 1979).

Some antibiotics, notably some β-lactam antibiotics, induce lysis of growing cells and this can readily be followed by measuring changes in turbidity. A multi-channel biophotometer (Coleman *et al.*, pp. 317–330) is particularly useful in this context.

All of the above methods employ whole bacterial or fungal cells. They can provide useful information on the level of activity of an antibiotic, on its lethal effects and whether or not it induces lysis. They do not, however, necessarily demonstrate the nature of the inhibitory or lethal effect and for this more delicate techniques must be carried out. In recent years, specific effects of antibiotics on enzyme systems have been noted, e.g. chloramphenicol inhibits peptidyl synthetase involved in protein synthesis, and novobiocin and nalidixic acid have inhibitory activity on DNA gyrase (Franklin & Snow 1981). Likewise, the action of β-lactam antibiotics on penicillin-sensitive enzymes (PSEs) is increasingly being studied by the binding of these antibiotics to penicillin binding proteins (PBPs). Specific binding to one or more of the most important PBPs (1, 2 and 3) has been demonstrated (Boulton & Orr pp. 161–181) and this is of importance in explaining the differing effects of members of this group.

Some β-lactam antibiotics can act as β-lactamase inhibitors (see "β-Lactam antibiotics", p. 3). This can readily be demonstrated by their effect in preventing hydrolysis by a β-lactamase of a susceptible β-lactam substrate with, for example, a spectrophotometric technique (Reading & Farmer, pp. 141–159).

Antibiotic Assay

The classical method of assaying antibiotics is the agar zone diffusion technique (Linton, pp. 19–30), in which there is a linear relationship between the response and the $\log_{10}$ dose. This technique is still widely used but suffers from the disadvantage that it is unsatisfactory when results are needed rapidly, although it can be speeded up by the use of a heavy inoculum.

The blood levels of patients receiving antibiotics such as gentamicin must be monitored at regular intervals to ensure that there is no accumulation of the drug, and thus rapid methods are necessary in such instances. An enzymatic assay for gentamicin is rapid and makes use of the fact that some bacteria are resistant to it (and possibly to other aminoglycoside antibiotics also) because they can synthesize specific enzymes that modify the antibiotic (White & Reeves, pp. 199–210).

Another rapid type of method of assaying gentamicin involves immunoassay (Shaw 1979). In radioimmunoassay, the procedure uses ^{125}I as the chosen isotope label, although the labelling of gentamicin is carried out by first coupling the antibiotic to another species and then iodinating the attached reagent. In fluoroimmunoassay (Shaw *et al.*, pp. 211–221) a non-isotopic label, fluorescein, is used since this is easily conjugated to gentamicin; in the simplest technique, the quenching fluorescence procedure, the fluorescence of the fluorescein-labelled drug is quenched on binding of antibody to gentamicin. The extent of antibody quenching provides an estimate of the amount of gentamicin present.

Sterility Testing of Antibiotics

Although there has long been controversy about the need in general for carrying out sterility tests on sterilized pharmaceutical products, a sterility test will, in fact, serve as a final check on a sterilization process and should always be done with products prepared aseptically. Antibiotics are widely used parenterally as such, or by their inclusion (intravenous additives) in intravenous infusions and there are instances where it is necessary to know whether sterile products containing them are free from contaminating micro-organisms. One way of carrying out a sterility test on an antibiotic is by membrane filtration, followed by washing of the membrane *in situ* to remove antibiotic and then culturing it in an appropriate medium. Another is to use an inactivating agent, e.g. a specific β-lactamase for a penicillin or cephalosporin. Breeze & Simpson (pp. 339–348) discuss the various methods available, and describe a new procedure for testing aminoglycoside antibiotics which is based on a drug-modifying enzyme system.

In another context, the principles of sterility testing (inactivation or removal of an antibiotic) ideally should be applied whenever the lethal effect of an antibiotic is being studied in order to ensure that no inhibitory concentration of drug is incorporated into recovery agar used for the determination of numbers of survivors.

Detection and Identification of Antibiotics

Instances occur where it is necessary not only to detect, but also to identify, antibiotics present in animal tissues, in animal feeding stuffs and in milk. Lott & Vaughan (pp. 331–338) have devised a high voltage electrophoretic technique for identifying antibiotics and Corry *et al.* (pp. 349–373) describe methods for detecting antibiotic residues.

References

Akiba, T., Koyama, K., Ishiki, Y., Kimura, S. & Fukushima, T. 1960 On the mechanism of the development of multiple drug-resistant clones of Shigella. *Japanese Journal of Microbiology* **4,** 219.

Brown, A. G. 1981 New naturally occurring β-lactam antibiotics. *Journal of Antimicrobial Chemotherapy* **7,** 15–48.

Brown, M. R. W. 1975 The role of the cell envelope in resistance. In *Resistance of Pseudomonas aeruginosa* ed. Brown, M. R. W., pp. 71–107. London: John Wiley & Sons.

Bryan, L. E. & van den Elzen, H. M. 1977 Effects of membrane-energy mutations and cations on streptomycin and gentamicin accumulation by bacteria. A model for entry of streptomycin and gentamicin in susceptible and resistant bacteria. *Antimicrobial Agents and Chemotherapy* **12,** 163–177.

Burchall, J. J. 1979 The development of the diaminopyrimidines. *Journal of Antimicrobial Chemotherapy* **5** (Supplement B), 3–14.

Chopra, I., Howe, T. G. B., Linton, A. H., Linton, K. B., Richmond, M. H. & Speller, D. C. E. 1981 The tetracyclines: prospects at the beginning of the 1980s. *Journal of Antimicrobial Chemotherapy* **8,** 5–21.

Clewell, D. B. 1981 Plasmids, drug resistance and gene transfer in the genus *Streptococcus. Microbiological Reviews* **45,** 409–436.

Cohen, S. N. 1976 Transposable genetic elements and plasmid evolution. *Nature, London* **263,** 731–738.

Cole, M. 1980 'β-Lactams' as β-lactamase inhibitors. *Philosophical Transactions of the Royal Society of London* **B289,** 207–223.

Crumplin, G. C., Midgley, J. M. & Smith, J. T. 1980 Mechanisms of action of nalidixic acid and its congeners. In *Topics in Antibiotic Chemistry* ed. Sammes, P. G., Vol. 3, pp. 9–38. Chichester: Ellis Horwood.

Davies, J. & Smith, D. I. 1978 Plasmid-determined resistance to antimicrobial agents. *Annual Review of Microbiology* **32,** 469–518.

Falkow, S. 1975. *Infectious Multiple Drug Resistance.* London: Pion Limited.

Franklin, T. J. & Snow, G. A. 1981 *Biochemistry of Antimicrobial Action* 3rd edn. London: Chapman and Hall.

Gale, E. F., Cundliffe, E., Reynolds, P. E., Richmond, M. H. & Waring, M. J. 1981 *The Molecular Basis of Antibiotic Action* 2nd. edn. London: John Wiley & Sons.

Garrod, L. P., Lambert, H. P. & O'Grady, F. 1981 *Antibiotic and Chemotherapy* 5th edn. London: Churchill Livingstone.

Harold, F. M., Altendore, K. H. & Hirata, H. 1974 Probing membrane transport mechanisms with ionophores. *Annals of the New York Academy of Sciences* **235,** 149–160.

Hedges, R. W. & Jacob, A. E. 1974 Transposition of ampicillin resistance from RP4 to other replicons. *Molecular and General Genetics* **132,** 31–40.

IMADA, A., KITANO, K., KINTAKA, K., MUROI, M. &. ASAI, M. 1981 Sulfazecin and isosulfazecin, novel β-lactam antibiotics of bacterial origin. *Nature, London* **289,** 590–591.

LACEY, R. W. 1979 Mechanism of action of trimethoprim and sulphonamides: relevance to synergy *in vivo*. *Journal of Antimicrobial Chemotherapy* **5** (Supplement B), 75–83.

NIKAIDO, H. & NAKAE, N. 1979 The outer membrane of Gram-negative bacteria. *Advances in Microbial Physiology* **20,** 163–250.

NOVICK, R. P. 1980 Plasmids. *Scientific American* **243,** 76–90.

O'CALLAGHAN, C. H. 1980 Structure–activity relations and β-lactamase resistance. *Philosophical Transactions of the Royal Society of London* **B289,** 197–205.

OCHIAI, K., YAMANAKA, T., KIMURA, K. & SAWADA, O. 1959 Inheritance of drug resistance (and its transfer) between *Shigella* and *E. coli* strains. *Nihon Iji Shimpo* **1861,** 34 (in Japanese).

RICHMOND, M. H. & SYKES, R. B. 1973 The β-lactamases of Gram-negative bacteria *Advances in Microbial Physiology* **9,** 31–88.

RUSSELL, A. D. 1982 Modification of the bacterial cell envelope and enhancement of antibiotic susceptibility. In *The Control of Antibiotic-resistant Bacteria* ed. Stuart-Harris, C. H. and Harris, D. M., Beecham Research Colloquium No. 4. London and New York: Academic Press.

RUSSELL, A. D., AHONKHAI, I. & ROGERS, D. T. 1979 Microbiological applications of the inactivation of antibiotics and other antimicrobial agents. *Journal of Applied Bacteriology* **46,** 207–245.

SELWYN, S. 1980 *The Beta-lactam Antibiotics*. London: Hodder and Stoughton.

SHAW, E. 1979 Immunoassays for antibiotics. *Journal of Antimicrobial Chemotherapy* **5,** 625–628.

SHAW, W. V. 1971*a* Comparative enzymology of chloramphenicol resistance. *Annals of the New York Academy of Science* **182,** 234–242.

SHAW, W. V. 1971*b* Biochemical mechanisms of transferable drug resistance. *Advances in Pharmacology and Chemotherapy* **9,** 131–172.

SMITH, J. T. 1979 Some biochemical mechanisms of antibiotics acting together on bacterial folate metabolism. In *Antibiotic Interactions* ed. Williams, J. D., Beecham Research Colloquium No. 1, pp. 87–98. London & New York: Academic Press.

SPRATT, B. G. 1980 Biochemical and genetical approaches to the mechanism of action of penicillin. *Philosophical Transactions of the Royal Society of London* **B289,** 273–283.

STAUDENBAUER, W. L. 1975 Novobiocin—a specific inhibitor of semiconservative DNA replication in permeabilized *Escherichia coli* cells. *Journal of Molecular Biology* **96,** 201–205.

SYKES, R. B., CIMARUSTI, C. M., BONNER, D. P., BUSH, K., FLOYD, D. M., GEORGOPAPADAKOU, N. H., KOSTER, W. H., LIU, W. C., PARKER, W. L., PRINCIPE, P. A., RATHNUM, M. L., SLUSARCHYK, W. A., TREJO, W. H. & WELLS, J. S. 1981 Monocyclic β-lactam antibiotics produced by bacteria. *Nature, London* **291,** 489–491.

TOMASZ, A. 1979. The mechanism of the irreversible antimicrobial effects of penicillins: how the β-lactam antibiotics kill and lyse bacteria. *Annual Review of Microbiology*, **33,** 113–137.

TREFOUËL, J., NITTI, F. & BOVET, D. 1935 Activity of *p*-amino phenylsulfamide (sulphonamide) on experimental streptococcal infections of the mouse and the rabbit. *Comptes rendus de la société de biologie* **120,** 756–758.

WILLIAMS, J. D. (1974) The sulphonamides. *British Journal of Hospital Medicine* **12,** 722–730

Theory of Antibiotic Inhibition Zone Formation, Disc Sensitivity Methods and MIC Determinations

A. H. LINTON

Department of Microbiology, Medical School, University of Bristol, Bristol, UK

Determinations of susceptibility or resistance of clinical isolates to antibiotics, and the microbiological assay of antibiotic solutions using standard strains of proven susceptibility, are widely used in clinical bacteriology and other disciplines. Yet, all too often, these tests are performed with little appreciation of the basic physical and biological principles involved in the various systems, systems which are readily influenced by many factors inherent in the techniques. In this paper the theory underlying the formation of inhibition zones is first considered; this is followed by guidance on the practice of sensitivity testing.

Theory of Antibiotic Inhibition Zone Formation

Since the Oxford workers (Abraham *et al.* 1941) applied the agar diffusion technique to the assay of antibiotics, the method has been widely used. An understanding of the theory underlying this test has been deduced from assay procedures, mainly using the tube technique of Mitcheson & Spicer (1949), which allows accurate temperature control and this will be described. Essentially, however, the basic conclusions apply equally to plate assay techniques and susceptibility testing. In either test the size of inhibition zones in seeded agar plates is the criterion of assessment. Zone size is the consequence of two dynamic systems proceeding simultaneously. The first is diffusion of the antibiotic from a confined source and the second, growth of the test organism. The position of the zone edge in an agar gel is fixed at a point in time when specific criteria in the two systems are fulfilled independently. Each is first considered separately and then as it impinges on the other. For a fuller, mathematical treatment the references quoted should be consulted, especially Cooper (1963).

ANTIBIOTICS
ISBN 0 12 604480 5

Diffusion of the antibiotic

Using an established formula for the diffusion of neutral particles in gases, Cooper & Woodman (1946) demonstrated its application to the diffusion of antibiotics through agar gels. The formula may be written:

$$X^2 = 4\,DT\,2{\cdot}3\,(\log m_0 - \log m')$$

in which $X =$ the distance between the source of the antibiotic and the edge of the zone of inhibition (i.e. the zone size); $D =$ the diffusion coefficient of the antibiotic; $T =$ the time taken for the zone to be fixed; $m_0 =$ the antibiotic concentration at source; $m' =$ the critical concentration of the antibiotic which inhibits the test organism under conditions of diffusion.

Diffusion coefficient

An antibiotic diffuses into an agar gel from a point source at a constant rate depending on the chemical and physical properties of the gel and the ionic charge on diffusing molecules. Two factors significantly affect this constant. (1) Temperature. Forces which bring about diffusion of molecules are proportional to the absolute temperature. Most microbiological assays are carried out under uniform temperature conditions and the diffusion coefficient for a given antibiotic is likely to be relatively constant. However, should the assay plates be held for part of the time at a different temperature (e.g. to allow pre-diffusion of the antibiotic) or at a higher temperature (e.g. using thermophiles as the test organism) a different diffusion coefficient will apply for the same antibiotic during the altered temperature period and correspondingly the slope of the assay curve will be different. (2) Viscosity of the solvent. The charge on the solvent molecules sets up a resistance to the diffusing molecules and therefore reduces the rate of diffusion. Most assays use water as solvent but other solvents may strongly influence the diffusion coefficient. If other substances are dissolved in the antibiotic solution (e.g. sugars) this too will have an effect on the diffusion coefficient.

The concentration of antibiotic diffusing from a reservoir and the size of the zone of inhibition (X)

The antibiotic concentration and the size of the inhibition zone are both dependent on each other. Under *standard* conditions the size of the zone is directly related to the concentration of the antibiotic being used. High concentrations at source drive an inhibitory concentration (m') of the antibiotic further out into the agar in time T (see below). This results in large zones being produced. Low concentrations do not drive the inhibitory concentration so far out into the agar and the zones are correspondingly smaller (Fig. 1). Where the difference between m_0 and m' is large the concentration gradient is steep and the zone edge tends to be crisp: where they are similar the resultant shallow concentration gradient may result in diffuse zone edges.

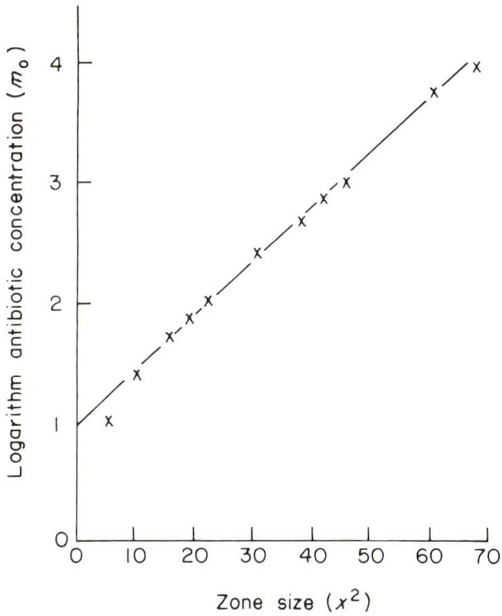

FIG. 1. The relationship between inhibition zone sizes (mm) and log of the concentrations (μg/ml) of antibiotic. A straight line is obtained by plotting the square of the zone of inhibition (i.e. the distance from the antibiotic source to the zone edge). Data with streptomycin and *Klebsiella pneumoniae* as test organism at 35°C. The point of intersection on the concentration axis is the critical minimum inhibitory concentration (m') for this combination of antibiotic and test organism.

Under the normal conditions of assay, m_0 may be considered to be constant throughout the period T. However, in disc susceptibility tests, the concentration of antibiotic at source is not known. The disc is impregnated with a known *amount* of the drug but this dissolves in an *unknown volume* of water in the sensitivity agar. Hence the concentration cannot be determined and, for this reason, it is not possible to relate directly the size of zones produced by solutions of known concentrations with discs of known amounts.

The critical inhibitory concentration of the antibiotic (m' *and MIC*)

For each antibiotic there is a minimum concentration (m') diffusing from the reservoir which inhibits each test organism under conditions of diffusion. This is constant for each organism: it can be determined by extrapolation and, being independent of many factors such as temperature of incubation (Fig. 2*a*) and inoculum size, is one of the most accurate determinations of sensitivity.

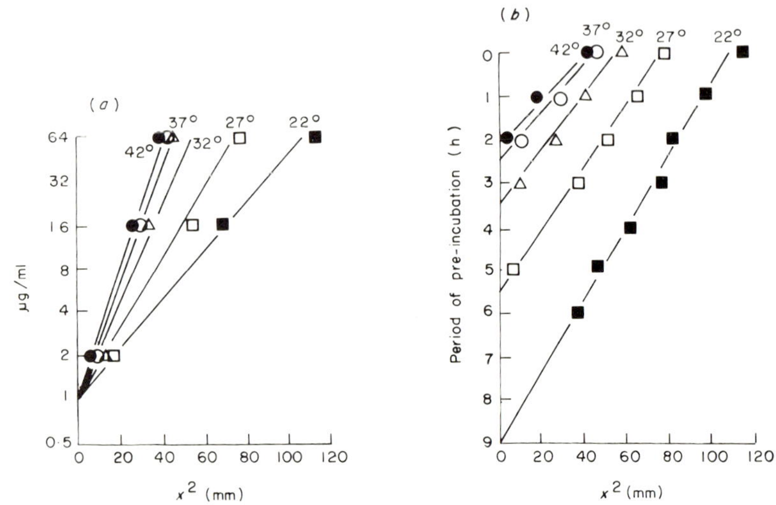

FIG. 2. Determinations of the critical inhibitory concentration (m') (*a*) and the time (T) taken for inhibition zones to be formed at different temperatures (*b*), with streptomycin and *Staphylococcus aureus* as test organism (Cooper & Gillespie 1952). Experimental points: ● 42°C; ○ 37°C; △ 32°C; □ 27°C; ■ 22°C.
(*a*) The relation of X^2 (zone sizes) to log concentration of streptomycin (64, 16 and 2 μg/ml were used) for different temperatures and without pre-incubation. Theoretical lines were calculated using the formula on p. 20; values of the diffusion coefficient (D) were calculated from values of the viscosity of water for each temperature together with experimental values of X^2 and T values from (*b*).
(*b*) The influence of temperature on T is shown by the results of pre-incubation with one concentration of streptomycin (64 μg/ml). The theoretical lines use the calculated values of D for the different temperatures and a constant value for m' taken from (*a*). Experimental points demonstrate good agreement with the theoretical lines in both figures.

Invariably the m' value is 2 to 4 times greater than the minimum inhibitory concentration (MIC) for the same organism. The methods by which each is determined, however, are instrinsically different. MICs are determined by exposing the organism directly to the antibiotic at different concentrations from time zero: the m' value is the inhibitory concentration of the antibiotic reaching the growing organism with time by diffusion.

The time (T) required for the zone edge to be formed

Usually zones are measured after at least overnight incubation. The zone edge, however, is fixed very much earlier, usually after a few hours from time zero (Fig. 3). Thereafter the test organism grows up outside the zone to render the edge of the zone visible and measurable. The critical time (T) is the time required for the critical inhibitory concentration (m') to reach the position in the agar where the zone edge will be formed. This coincides with a certain density of bacteria considered below: see also pages 25 and 26.

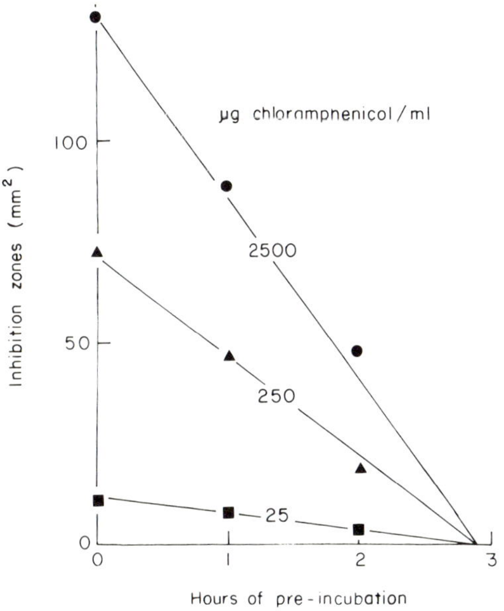

FIG. 3. Determination of the value of T (i.e. the time taken for zones of inhibition to be formed) using a range of concentrations of chloramphenicol (2500, 250 and 25 μg/ml) and a standard inoculum of *Staphylococcus aureus* as test organism. The test was set up at 36°C. Series of seeded agar tubes were incubated for defined periods of time before adding the antibiotic. The extrapolated curves of the experimental points for each concentration intersect the axis at time T.

Growth of the test organism

The time T is also the time required for the inoculum to reach a certain bacterial density by growth. From the moment of incubation the inoculum on a seeded agar plate follows the normal laws of growth. After an initial lag phase, the inoculum moves fairly rapidly into a log phase of growth having a relatively constant doubling time. The time taken to reach the critical density will be dependent on many factors, including the biological nature of the organism under test, and particularly its doubling time, the nutritional status of the medium, the temperature of incubation and the size of the inoculum used. With dense inocula the time required to reach this critical density will be much shorter than with a light inoculum. Also, if very dense inocula are used, no zones of inhibition will be obtained even with high concentrations of antibiotics (Fig. 4). This illustrates the fundamental difference between diffusion and incorporation methods of sensitivity testing.

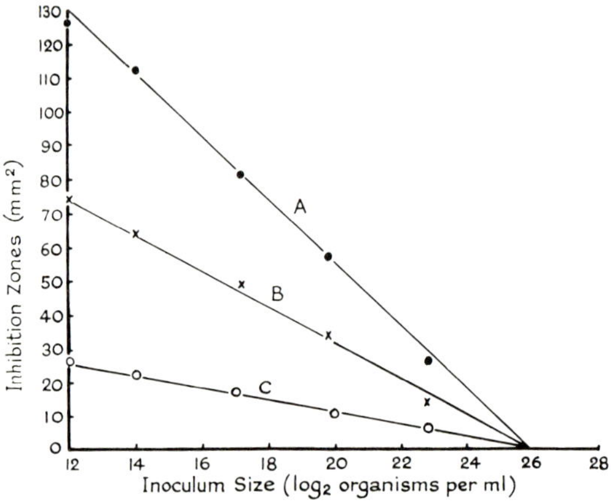

FIG. 4. The influence of inoculum size on inhibition zones. The data are for *Klebsiella pneumoniae* as test organism and with three concentrations of streptomycin (1000, 100 and 10 μg/ml: A, B, C respectively); the test was carried out at 35°C. The denser the inoculum, the smaller the zone sizes until, with an inoculum of $\log_2 = 26$ and greater, no zones were produced (after Linton 1958).

Diffusion and growth considered together

Diffusion of the antibiotic and growth of the test organism proceed simultaneously and the zone edge is formed when criteria in both systems coincide. The time (T) taken for the zone to form is determined when the critical inhibitory concentration of the antibiotic (m') reaches *for the first time* a critical density of bacteria which has grown up from the inoculum. The interaction of these two dynamic systems is demonstrated in Fig. 5. With standard inocula, during the early hours of incubation all organisms in the area of the plate which eventually will be within the zone are inhibited by the critical inhibitory concentration of the antibiotic diffusing out from the antibiotic source. As time proceeds, the test organism further out in the plate grows into an ever increasing density. Eventually the inhibitory concentration reaches a density of cells which is sufficiently large to absorb antibiotic in its immediate vicinity thereby lowering the concentration to a level which is no longer inhibitory. Thereafter, as the test organism grows exponentially, the density of bacteria maintains the diffusing antibiotic at a sub-inhibitory level and the test organism grows uninhibited to become visible and measurable.

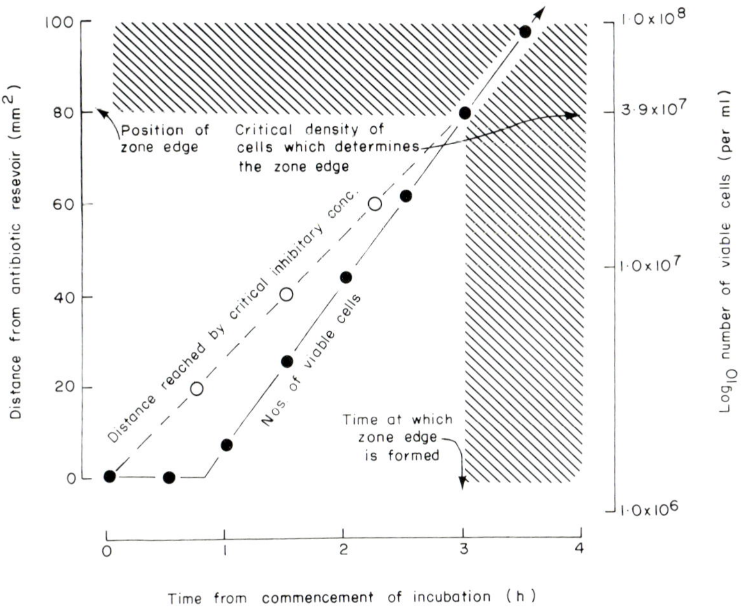

FIG. 5. Graphical representation of inhibition zone edge formation. The plots are based on experimental data with streptomycin and *Staphylococcus aureus* using the tube technique of Mitcheson & Spicer (1949): inoculum $1{\cdot}26 \times 10^6$ organisms/ml; temperature of incubation, 35°C; critical inhibitory concentration, 1·8 μg/ml. This is an oversimplified attempt to relate diffusion of the antibiotic and growth of the test organism. The distance in the agar reached by diffusion from the reservoir with time is related to the bacterial density which is increasing throughout the same period. The zone edge is formed where the critical inhibitory concentration (m') arrives in the agar coincident with a critical density of viable bacteria having arisen by growth. All bacteria inside the zone are inhibited; those outside the zone continue to propagate exponentially as incubation proceeds and eventually grow up to produce visible growth which demarcates the zone edge (after Linton 1961).

Sometimes pre-diffusion of the antibiotic is practised with slowly diffusing antibiotics; where this is done the commencement of growth of the test organism is delayed. Under these conditions the time at which the zone is formed will be the sum of the period of pre-diffusion and the time taken for the test organism to reach a critical bacterial density. The longer time invariably results in larger zones but it must be stressed that the test is not thereby made more sensitive since the minimum inhibitory concentration is constant. Where plates are pre-incubated before diffusion is commenced, the time taken for the bacterial mass to grow relative to diffusion of the antibiotic will be shorter than normal and consequently the zones will be smaller. If the plates are pre-incubated beyond time *T* before adding the antibiotic, no zones are formed irrespective of the sensitivity of the organism (Figs 2*b*, 3).

Agar Diffusion Susceptibility Test

The paper disc susceptibility test has been used by microbiologists for over three decades and many variations in technique and interpretation have been introduced (Balows 1974). Factors which influence the agar diffusion assay technique, already considered, also have a profound effect on the disc sensitivity test, and failure to standardize or control the many variables commonly introduces errors. Rather than describe one established technique, therefore, consideration will be given to ways by which the basic technique may be standardized and controlled. Where these recommendations are practised the test generates reliable and reproducible data for typical organisms.

Medium

The choice of medium must be based on a number of criteria. It must be able to support rapid growth of regular clinical isolates, produce clearly defined zones of inhibition, consist of a standard nutritional formula which is routinely reproducible and, in most laboratories, be free of sulphonamide antagonists so that this drug may be included in the range of antibacterials used. The widely used Kirby–Bauer technique (see Bauer *et al.* 1966) requires the use of Mueller–Hinton agar: to overcome certain disadvantages of this medium other formulations have been created, e.g. Sensitest Agar (Oxoid, CM 409) and the semisynthetic Iso-sensitest Agar (Oxoid, CM 471). The latter is reported to be satisfactory for sulphonamide sensitivity testing but we have achieved more consistent results by the addition of 1% lysed horse blood.

It is important to maintain the medium between pH 7·2 and 7·4. Zones of inhibition with tetracycline increase as the pH is lowered; the opposite is the case with streptomycin, lincomycin and erythromycin. The pH of a poured plate can easily be checked using a surface electrode.

A standard volume of medium should be dispensed into each Petri dish (e.g. 25 ml into a 9-cm plate) and stored between 2 and 8°C for not longer than 7 days. Prior to use, the plates should be dried in an incubator until no surface moisture remains.

Inoculum

The sensitivity test is qualitatively useful for a wide range of organisms but the quantitative interpretation based on zone size, can be made reliably only with rapidly growing bacteria (including staphylococci, Enterobacteriaceae and *Pseudomonas* spp. etc.) and not with fastidious, slow growing organisms or anaerobes.

Pure cultures must always be used to avoid mixtures of different biological kind and of mixed sensitivity. Four or five well-isolated colonies of the same morphological type should be picked into 4 ml of nutrient broth, preferably of the same nutrient formula as the sensitivity agar being used. After incubation at 35°C, the inoculum is prepared by diluting to a density comparable to a standard opacity tube or by using photometric equipment such as the nephelometer or absorptiometer. Alternatively, by culturing the broth culture overnight the maximum viable population is attained which is constant for each species. This should be diluted 1/50 to form a standard inoculum.

The freshly prepared suspension is shaken and a small cotton wool swab dipped into the inoculum, excess fluid removed by rotating against the side of the tube and the swab spread over the entire plate. This is repeated twice, the plate being rotated 60° each time. The lid is replaced and time allowed for the inoculum to be absorbed. After incubation the surface should be evenly covered by a confluent or nearly confluent growth.

Direct plating of clinical material for sensitivity testing should never be practised since it is not possible to control either the inoculum size or the purity of the test organism. The most this test can provide is an indication of the presence of resistant organisms but artefacts due to the interaction of organisms are possible.

Antibiotic discs

Discs are commercially available with the necessary quality controls built into their manufacture. However, each laboratory should regularly check the potency of their stock by testing samples from each batch against standard strains of known sensitivity. To maintain potency, stocks should be held at −64°C in sealed containers containing silica gel. An adequate supply for day to day use should be transferred to the 4°C refrigerator. At the time of setting up the test, the sealed container should be removed from the refrigerator and time allowed for it to warm up to room temperature before opening to avoid condensation of moisture on the discs. Discs are removed aseptically with sterile forceps and pressed against the seeded agar surface of the test plate in an arrangement which allows sufficient distance between discs for the inhibition zone to be entire and avoids placing antibiotics adjacent to each other if they exhibit antagonism or synergism.

The choice of antibiotics to be used and their potency must be decided in the light of the biological nature of the organism under test. A suggested list is given (Table 1). Some laboratories consider that where broad spectrum antibiotics are used, discs of higher potency should be used with Gram negative organisms than with Gram positive ones.

TABLE 1

Potency of discs (μg) useful in routine sensitivity testing

	Staphylococcus aureus	Enterobacteriaceae	*Pseudomonas aeruginosa*
Ampicillin	2	25	—
Benzylpenicillin	1·5	—	—
Carbenicillin	—	100	100
Cephaloridine	5	25	—
Chloramphenicol	10	50	50
Cloxacillin	5	—	—
Colistin sulphate	—	10	10
Co-trimoxazole	25	25	—
Erythromycin	10	—	—
Gentamicin	10	10	10
Kanamycin	5	30	—
Methicillin	10	—	—
Nalidixic acid*	—	30	—
Neomycin	10	—	—
Nitrofurantoin*	—	200	—
Polymyxin B	—	300	300
Streptomycin	10	25	—
Sulphafurazole*	—	500	—
Tetracycline	10	50	—

* Only with micro-organisms recovered from urinary tract infections.

Incubation

Plates should be incubated aerobically, with ample spacing to allow rapid and even warming of all plates. Overstocking of incubators should be avoided. Increased CO_2 must not be added to the atmosphere since this lowers the pH of the medium. The incubation temperature is normally 35°C; other temperatures may be chosen where the optimum temperature for growth of the test organism is higher or lower, or where the activity of the antibiotic varies with temperature.

Measurement of inhibition zones

Under well controlled, standard conditions the zone size is directly related to the sensitivity of the test organism for discs of specified potency. Accurate measurement of zone diameter, using callipers or template, can be used as a definitive assessment of sensitivity on a comparable basis, i.e. against zones obtained under identical conditions with standard strains of known sensitivity and of average growth characteristics.

Minimum Inhibitory Concentration

The most commonly used technique for the quantitative estimate of the sensitivity of organisms or the assay of antibiotic in fluids, is by dilution of the antibiotic solution in the growth medium and determination of the minimum concentration (MIC) which inhibits growth of the test organism. This test has certain advantages over the diffusion technique. The antibiotic is incorporated in the test medium and no diffusion is required, hence antibiotics of large molecular size can be tested by this method. The test can also be used with a wide range of organisms, including anaerobes, and yields a direct measure of the inhibitory concentration. Against these a number of disadvantages must be considered. The method is technically more exacting, both in time and accuracy; much of this is now reduced by automation of the dilution series. The dilution steps may render the end point difficult to read; if close together, as in doubling dilutions, growth of a diminishing degree over a number of tubes may result; if too wide apart, as in decimal dilutions, a margin of error may be experienced since the end point falls between two widely spaced levels of concentration. In contrast, the disc diffusion test presents a concentration gradient which avoids stepwise levels of concentration. The MIC test is also more prone to contamination, especially in the broth dilution technique, and a single contaminant, if resistant, may grow up and occlude the end point of the test organism. Further, should the inoculum include organisms of differing sensitivity the test will measure the sensitivity of the most resistant members of the population. Another disadvantage lies in the fact that dilute solutions of antibiotics, either in broth or in agar plates, may lose their potency with time during incubation.

Despite these disadvantages it is possible to obtain reliable estimates of sensitivity if the test is carefully managed. As with disc sensitivity tests it is necessary to standardize the media and to use standard inoculum, often ten times less dense than for disc tests. Should the organism produce antagonistic enzymes, such as β-lactamase, small inocula will have least influence on the end point.

Correlation between MIC and Zone Size Determinations

Ericsson & Sherris (1971) produced standard regression lines in which they related MIC determinations for different organisms with their corresponding zone sizes observed by the disc diffusion test, with the same antibiotic. They claimed that since under carefully controlled conditions it is possible to obtain highly reproducible results by the disc diffusion method, this test should be adopted and the corresponding MIC be read by reference to the standard regression lines. This value may be obtained by reading the zone size on the axis and extrapolating to the corresponding MIC value of the abscissa (x-axis).

References

ABRAHAM, E. P., CHAIN, E., FLETCHER, C. M., FLOREY, H. W., GARDNER, A. D., HEATLEY, N. G. & JENNINGS, M. A. 1941 Further observations on penicillin. *Lancet* **ii,** 177–188.

BALOWS, A. ed. 1974 *Current Techniques for Antibiotic Susceptibility Testing.* Illinois, USA: Charles Thomas.

BAUER, A. W., KIRBY, W. M. M., SHERRIS, J. C. & TURCK, M. 1966 Antibiotic susceptibility testing by a standardized single disc method. *American Journal of Clinical Pathology* **45,** 493–496.

COOPER, K. E. 1963 The theory of antibiotic inhibition zones. In *Analytical Microbiology* ed. Kavanagh, F., pp. 1–86. New York & London: Academic Press.

COOPER, K. E. & GILLESPIE, W. A. 1952 The influence of temperature on streptomycin inhibition zones in agar cultures. *Journal of General Microbiology* **7,** 1–7.

COOPER, K. E. & WOODMAN, D. 1946 The diffusion of antiseptics through agar gels with special reference to the agar cup assay method of estimating the activity of penicillin. *Journal of Pathology and Bacteriology* **58,** 75–84.

ERICSSON, H. M. & SHERRIS, J. C. 1971 Antibiotic sensitivity testing: report of an international collaborative study. *Acta Pathologica et Microbiologica Scandinavica* Section B, Supplement No. 217.

LINTON, A. H. 1958 Influence of inoculum size on antibiotic assays by the agar diffusion technique with special reference to *Klebsiella pneumoniae* and streptomycin. *Journal of Bacteriology* **76,** 94–103.

LINTON, A. H. 1961 Interpreting antibiotic sensitivity tests. *Journal of Medical Laboratory Technology* **18,** 1–20.

MITCHESON, D. A. & SPICER, C. C. 1949. A method of estimating streptomycin in serum and other body fluids by diffusion through agar enclosed in glass tubes. *Journal of General Microbiology* **3,** 184–203.

The Effect of Composition of Culture Media on MIC Values of Antibiotics

ELIZABETH T. HOUANG

Microbiology Department, Chelsea Hospital For Women, London, UK

CAROL HINCE AND A. J. HOWARD

Area Pathology Laboratory, Caernarvon and Anglesey Hospital, Bangor, Gwynedd, UK

The quantitative expression of antimicrobial activity of many antibiotics may be markedly influenced by the composition of the culture medium utilized in undertaking the test. In addition, general factors such as pH, incubation atmosphere and protein concentration may also affect the susceptibility of a given bacterial species. This paper seeks to review these effects and discuss measures that can be taken to standardize tests of this kind.

Influence of Organic Compounds on Antimicrobial Susceptibility

Pyrimidines and related substances

Sulphonamides and trimethoprim

Both agents act by inhibiting bacterial folate synthesis, sulphonamides by competing with *para*-aminobenzoic acid (1,4-aminobenzoic acid) for incorporation into dihydropteroate, and trimethoprim by blocking the conversion of dihydrofolate to tetrahydrofolate. It was recognized early in the development of sulphonamides that composition of the medium had a profound effect on the antibacterial activity of these drugs. This was particularly related to the presence of peptones which were inhibitory to their action. The specific antagonist was not recognized at first but Koch &

ANTIBIOTICS
ISBN 0 12 604480 5

Burchall (1971) produced evidence to suggest it was thymidine. This compound also reverses the activity of trimethoprim (Table 1).

TABLE 1

The influence of thymidine on the susceptibility of a strain of* Haemophilus influenzae *to trimethoprim*

Concentration of thymidine (mg/l)	MIC (mg/l)
0	0·1
0·5	1·0
5	10
50	100

* Medium: DST Agar (Oxoid) supplemented with haemin (10 mg/l) and NAD (10 mg/l).

TABLE 2

The influence of different concentrations of lysed horse blood on the activity of trimethoprim against a strain of Haemophilus influenzae *when tested on five commercial media*

% Lysed blood	Oxoid Isosensitest Agar	Oxoid DST Agar	Southern Group Nutrient Agar	Oxoid Tryptone Soya Agar	Oxoid Columbia Agar
0	+	+	−	−	−
0·25	+	+	−	−	−
1	+	+	+	−	−
2	+	+	+	−	−
4	+	+	+	−	−
5	+	+	+	−	−
10	+	+	+	+	−
15	+	+	+	+	−

+, Zone of inhibition > 20 mm diam. around a 1·2 μg trimethoprim disc.
−, No zone of inhibition.

Harper & Cawston (1945) demonstrated that the inhibition of sulphonamide activity by bacteriological culture media could be reversed by the addition of lysed horse blood (the Harper–Cawston factor, HCF) and it was later shown that such addition had a similar effect on the activity of trimethoprim. Ferone *et al.* (1975) identified HCF as thymidine phosphorylase. This enzyme acts by converting thymidine to thymine which in contrast to the former compound is poorly utilized by most bacterial species. Occasionally organisms are encountered (e.g. *Streptococcus faecalis*) which can efficiently utilize thymine. For these organisms thymidine-containing media are not markedly improved by lysed horse blood. The amount of lysed horse blood required to inactivate sulphonamide/trimethoprim inhibitors in a given culture medium depends on the concentration of antagonists present. Media containing high concentrations of thymidine cannot be rendered suitable for sulphonamide or trimethoprim testing however much lysed horse blood is added (Table 2).

The trimethoprim antagonism exhibited by some media can also be reversed by the addition of uridine (Amyes & Smith 1978; Table 3).

TABLE 3
The activity of trimethoprim against a strain of Escherichia coli *in the presence or absence of uridine*

Type of agar	MIC (mg/l) of trimethoprim in agar containing uridine at (mg/l) 0	10	100
DM	1·25	1·25	1·25
DM + VC + Ad + Th 10 mg/l	80	1·25	1·25
DM + VC + Ad + Td 1 mg/l	80	40	20
Isosensitest	1·25	1·25	1·25
Oxoid Tryptone Soya	20	10	1·25

DM, Davis–Mingioli minimal medium; VC, Vitamin-free casamino acids; Ad, adenine; Th, thymine; Td, thymidine.
From Amyes & Smith (1978).

Commercially available sensitivity test media suitable for testing sulphonamides and trimethoprim contain low concentrations of thymidine and are now generally supplemented with uridine.

5-*Fluorocytosine* (*flucytosine*)

5-Fluorocytosine is an antifungal agent which is deaminated by sensitive organisms to 5-fluorouracil. This is then incorporated into *t*RNA resulting in the synthesis of non-functional proteins. The incorporation of 5-fluorocytosine into RNA is, however, less efficient than that of cytosine and consequently the presence of exogenous cytosine (and also uridine, but not cytidine, uracil, thymine or thymidine) results in antagonism of the compound (Hoeprich & Finn 1972).

The MIC of 5-fluorocytosine for *Candida albicans* ranges from 2·3 mg/l when tested on yeast nitrogen base agar (YNB) to 3550 mg/l on brain–heart infusion agar (BHI); it is 11·6 mg/l on synthetic amino acid medium fungal (SAAMF) and 310 mg/l on Sabouraud glucose agar (SAB). Neither SAAMF nor YNB contains pyrimidines or pyrimidine derivatives.

It is thus a reasonable assumption that the reduction of antifungal activity in complex, undefined media is attributable to the presence of such compounds. As neither pyrimidines nor pyrimidine nucleosides are present in detectable quantities in the extracellular fluids of man (Bendich 1955), media free of these antagonists should be used to predict the outcome of therapy.

Amino acids and peptides

D-*Cycloserine*

D-Cycloserine is a structural analogue of D-alanine (Fig. 1) and acts as a competitive antagonist of D-alanine in bacterial cell wall synthesis. More specifically the antibiotic inhibits alanine racemase and D-alanyl-D-alanine synthetase. These enzymes catalyse the conversion of L-alanine to D-alanine and D-alanine to D-alanyl-D-alanine prior to its incorporation into a uridine nucleotide cell wall precursor.

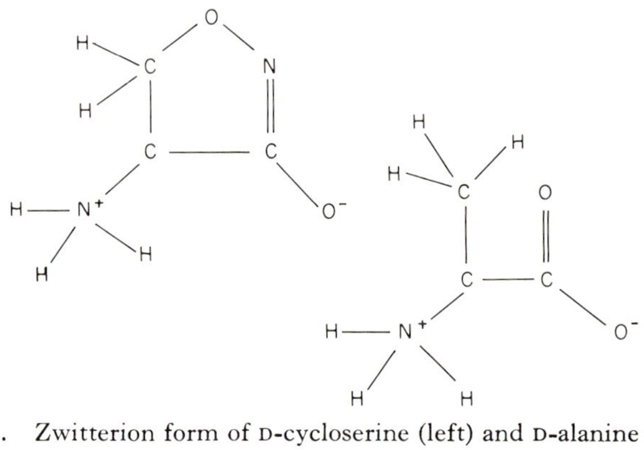

FIG. 1. Zwitterion form of D-cycloserine (left) and D-alanine (right).

Alanine in bacteriological culture media will reverse the inhibitory activity of D-cycloserine (Shockman 1959; Zygmunt 1962; Hoeprich 1963). This is illustrated in Table 4 which demonstrates that it is the D-isomer of alanine which is the best reversal agent.

Alanine is present in most bacteriological culture media so that D-cycloserine is generally ineffective in the usual susceptibility tests. D-Alanine is absent in the blood and body fluids of humans and thus a synthetic alanine-free medium must be used for antimicrobial sensitivity testing. A satisfactory medium is described by Hoeprich (1963).

TABLE 4
The reversal by alanine of D*-cycloserine-induced growth inhibition of* Escherichia coli *and* Staphylococcus aureus

Alanine	Reversal (%) of growth inhibition of *E. coli*	*Staph. aureus*
DL	52	50
L	3	1
D	90	90

D-Cycloserine concentration, $6{\cdot}54 \times 10^{-4}$ mol/l; alanine concentration, $14{\cdot}88 \times 10^{-4}$ mol/l; molar ratio of antagonist/metabolite: 0·44.
From Zygmunt (1962).

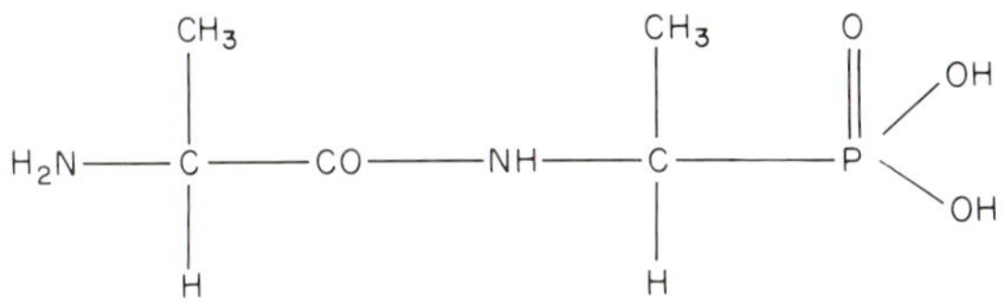

FIG. 2. Structure of the phosphonodipeptide antibacterial agent, L-Ala-L-Ala (p) (Alaphosphin, Alafosfalin).

Phosphonopeptides

Alaphosphin (Alafosfalin) is a structural analogue of L-alanyl-L-alanine (Fig. 2) which selectively inhibits cell wall biosynthesis in bacteria (Allen *et al.* 1979; Atherton *et al.* 1979*a*, *b*). The compound acts primarily by inhibiting alanine racemase. Although the dipeptide exhibits high activity against a wide variety of bacteria when tested using minimal media, the antibacterial effect is abolished by the use of complex media such as DST (Oxoid), Isosensitest (Oxoid) and Mueller–Hinton (MH) (Oxoid). The constituents reversing the inhibitory activity of alaphosphin have been shown to be amino acids and peptides, especially D-alanine and L-alanyl-L-alanine (Table 5).

The effect of protein in culture media

The degree of protein binding of an antibiotic must be taken into account when the activity of a compound is evaluated in the context of clinical usage. However, in antibiotic susceptibility testing, the protein content of media used is usually insufficient to markedly influence results even for highly protein bound compounds. This is illustrated in Table 6 where the MIC of flucloxacillin (protein binding 94·7%) (Craig & Byungse Suh 1980),

TABLE 5
The effect of amino acid, peptide and peptone additions on the activity of alaphosphin in defined agar

	MIC (mg/litre) of alaphosphin in a defined agar containing				
	No addition	L-ala (2 m mol/l)	D-ala (2 m mol/l)	L-ala-L-ala (2 m mol/l)	Peptone (1 g/l)
E. coli NCIB 8879	0·25	1	128	128	8
K. aerogenes KA1	0·25	1	128	128	16
Enterobacter sp. 1398	1	8	128	128	32
Strep. faecalis FS5	1	2	128	128	16
Staph. aureus NCTC 8625	16	16	32	128	64

ala, alanine.
From Allen *et al.* (1979).

for a β-lactamase-producing strain of *Staphylococcus aureus* has been determined on media containing three different concentrations of horse serum. An eight-fold rise in minimum inhibitory concentration (MIC) occurs when serum concentration is increased from 0 to 95%. The addition of serum to a final concentration of 5% is usually sufficient for the requirements of organisms dependent on this factor for growth.

TABLE 6
Effect of serum on the activity in broth of flucloxacillin against a β-lactamase-producing strain of Staphylococcus aureus

Final concn. (%) of serum	MIC (mg/l) of flucloxacillin
0	0·15
5	0·3
95	1·25

Influence of Inorganic Ions on Antimicrobial Activity

Divalent cations

The concentration of divalent cations, particularly Ca^{2+} and Mg^{2+} in culture media will affect the susceptibility of strains of various pseudomonads to tetracycline, aminoglycosides and polymyxin B (D'Amato *et al.* 1975; Garrod & Waterworth 1969; Gilbert *et al.* 1971). The relative influence of increasing cation concentration in different *Pseudomonas* species is illustrated in Table 7.

TABLE 7

Increase in MIC of antibiotics by addition of both Ca^{2+} (87 mg/l) and Mg^{2+} (37 mg/l) to Mueller–Hinton (MH) broth

Species	Increase in MIC (-fold) of (relative to MH broth without added cations)		
	Tetracycline	Gentamicin	Polymyxin B
Pseudomonas aeruginosa	32	128	32
Ps. fluorescens	16	0	64
Ps. putida	4	0	32
Ps. pseudomallei	8	2	0
Ps. cepacia	8	0	0
Ps. stutzeri	16	64	32
Ps. putrefaciens	16	64	16
Ps. maltophilia	8	16	64
Ps. diminuta	≥8	2	16
Ps. testosteroni	8	4	4
Ps. alcaligenes	4	4	0
Ps. pseudoalcaligenes	4	16	8
Ps. acidovorans	16	4	8

From D'Amato *et al.* (1975).

The mechanism by which divalent cations exert this effect is not fully understood. It appears that Ca^{2+} and Mg^{2+} are important in stabilizing the surface structures of these bacteria (Repaske 1958). Following the incorporation of these ions into the cell envelope it is possible that it then becomes less permeable to aminoglycosides and other compounds (Zimelis & Jackson 1973). Alternatively the cations may compete with gentamicin for binding on or in the cell (Ramirez-Ronda *et al.* 1975). Metallic cations may also inactivate some antibiotics, particularly tetracyclines, by chelation (Weinberg 1957).

In commercially prepared media, considerable variation may exist in Ca^{2+} and Mg^{2+} content in batches from different manufacturers and in different batches from the same manufacturers (Table 8) (Gilbert *et al.* 1971; Reller *et al.* 1974). The concentrations of three other divalent cations (Zn^{2+}, Ca^{2+} and Fe^{2+}) may also vary from manufacturer to manufacturer as much as 4-fold in the case of zinc (mean, 0·662 mg/l; range, 0·285–1·22 mg/l), 10-fold for copper (mean, 0·141 mg/l; range, 0·068–0·665 mg/l) and 8-fold for iron (mean, 1·587 mg/l; range, 0·551–4·03 mg/l) (Washington *et al.* 1978). There is a need to standardize Mg^{2+} and Ca^{2+} content of media if consistent and reliable results are to be obtained for antibiotic testing of *Pseudomonas* species. All batches of media should be shown to produce acceptable results with control strains of *Ps. aeruginosa* before they are accepted as suitable for use.

TABLE 8
Total concentrations of Mg^{2+} and Ca^{2+} in normal serum and commercial batches of Mueller–Hinton (MH) medium

Medium (no. batches tested)	Concentration (mg/l)* of Mg^{2+}	Ca^{2+}
MH broth		
BBL (5)	3·0 ± 0·8	10·8 ± 10·4
Difco (5)	4·2 ± 1·0	15·0 ± 10·5
MH agar		
BBL (6)	16·7 ± 2·9	50·8 ± 19·7
Difco (7)	26·3 ± 7·5	70·7 ± 16·6
Pfizer (10)	17·8 ± 7·5	46·8 ± 5·6
Human serum (60)	21·7 ± 1·2	98·0 ± 2·5

* Mean ± SD.
From Reller *et al.* (1974).

Monovalent ions

Gentamicin

Variation in the ionic strength of a medium produces marked changes in the activity of aminoglycosides against Gram negative rods; the lower the ionic strength, the more effective the drug. This is illustrated in Table 9 where it can be seen that quantitative differences in the activity of gentamicin could be detected when tested against three bacterial species using different media. The nutrient broth used was found to have less Na^+ and Cl^- and a lower ionic strength than MH broth. Supplementing nutrient broth with NaCl resulted in susceptibilities equivalent to those obtained in MH medium (Beggs & Andrews 1976; Medeiros *et al.* 1971).

Mecillinam

Mecillinam acts by inhibiting a shape-determining protein (penicillin binding protein 2 of *Escherichia coli*) resulting in the production of ovoid and then large round cells (Spratt 1977). The large cells are stable in media of high osmolality and conductivity, resulting in large discrepancies in susceptibility studies carried out in media differing in these respects (Neu 1976). Mecillinam may also be unstable in media with a high osmolality which may contribute to the decrease in activity seen under these conditions (Neu 1976).

TABLE 9

Effect of sodium chloride on the antibacterial activity of gentamicin

Organism	NaCl added (m mol/l)	MIC (mg/litre) of gentamicin in	
		Nutrient broth	MH broth
Ps. aeruginosa	0	0·06	1·0
	174	1·0	Nt
Serratia marcescens	0	0·06	1·0
	174	0·5	Nt
E. coli	0	0·007	0·25
	174	0 5	Nt

Nt, not tested.
Adapted from Medeiros *et al.* (1971).

Effect of pH and Incubation Atmosphere on Antimicrobial Activity

The commonly used antibiotics can be divided into three groups according to the effect of pH on their antimicrobial activity (see Table 10).

TABLE 10

Effect of pH on antimicrobial activity of antibiotics

Little affected	Less active in acid medium	Less active in alkaline medium
Penicillin	Aminoglycosides	Tetracyclines
Chloramphenicol	Lincomycin	Methicillin
Polymyxins	Erythromycin group	Cloxacillin
Vancomycin	Cephaloridine	Fucidin

From Garrod *et al.* (1973).

A small variation in the pH of the medium may affect the MICs significantly. For example, Hansen *et al.* (1981) showed that a shift in the initial pH from 7·0 to 7·2 changed the MICs of erythromycin for 90% of strains of *Bacteroides fragilis* studied from 32 to 1 mg/l (Table 11). Activity of this antibiotic is so enhanced in alkaline medium that its use together with an alkalizing agent has been suggested in the treatment of urinary tract infections due to Gram negative bacilli (Zinner *et al.* 1971). The increased activity of clindamycin at alkaline pH is less dramatic, and does not extend to Gram negative bacilli (Sabath & Toftegaard 1974).

TABLE 11

Effects of the pH of the medium on the activity of erythromycin against Bacteroides fragilis *group (25 strains) on Wilkins–Chalgren agar*

Initial pH	Final pH	MIC (mg/l)* Range	for % of strains 50	90
7·0	6·8	16–256	32	32
7·2	7·0	0·12–2·0	0·5	1·0
7·4	7·3	0·12–0·5	0·25	0·25
7·6	7·4	0·12–0·5	0·12	0·25

*After incubation for 48 h in GasPak jars.
Modified from Hanson *et al.* (1981).

The effect of pH on the activity of the aminoglycoside streptomycin, was noted as early as 1946 (Abraham & Duthie 1946). The enhanced activity of aminoglycosides at alkaline pH covers both Gram negative bacilli and Gram positive cocci (Table 12).

TABLE 12

Effect of pH on gentamicin activity in heart infusion agar incubated aerobically

Organism	No. of strains	Median MIC (mg/l) at pH 5	5·2	5·5	6·5	7·4	8·5
Klebsiella spp.	13	125		62	7	2	0·5
Proteus spp.	5	175		150	12	6	0·7
Staph. aureus	36		25	12·5		0·19	0·09

Modified from Sabath & Toftegaard (1974).

It is not clear how pH affects the antimicrobial activity of these antibiotics although it has been suggested that the change in pH either alters the charge in the cell surface affecting binding or permeability of the drug, or that hydronium ions compete with basic drugs for a receptor (Abraham & Duthie 1946).

Many factors, for example medium composition, incubation atmosphere and bacterial growth, have all been shown to contribute to changes in the pH of bacterial culture media during incubation. Such changes may be associated with variations in antimicrobial activity consistent with the effects described above.

Effect of medium composition on pH

During incubation, the pH of the medium may be changed as a result of bacterial metabolism, especially if the medium contains fermentable carbohydrate. This is illustrated by data from Barry (1976) who used a semi-micro electrode and a pH meter attached to a continuous reading apparatus, to monitor the pH changes over the first 24 h of incubation following the inoculation of a standard strain of *E. coli* into five different broth media (Fig. 3). By the sixth hour of incubation, a drop in pH of at least 1·5 units was seen in media containing glucose. Synthetic amino acid medium which contained two effective organic buffers (Tris and MOPS) and trypticase soy broth without glucose showed little variation in pH during incubation.

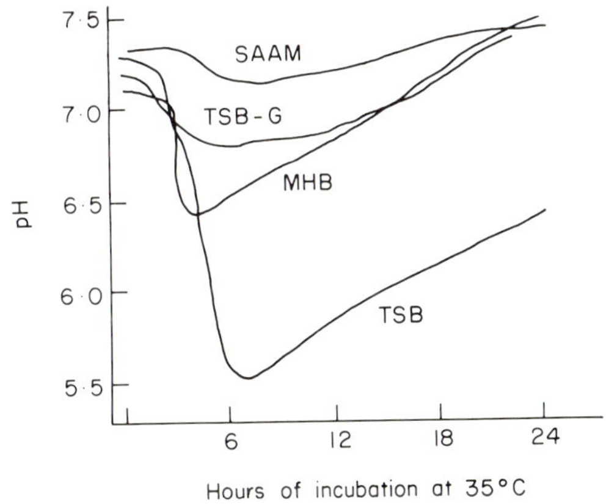

FIG. 3. Shift in pH of different media during growth of *Escherichia coli*. SAAM, synthetic amino acid medium; TSB-G, trypticase soy broth without glucose; TSB, trypticase soy broth; MHB, Mueller–Hinton broth. From Barry (1976).

Table 13 shows the influence of additional glucose on the activity of aminoglycosides and tetracycline against a strain of *E. coli* when tested in Peptone Water (Oxoid).

TABLE 13

The influence of different concentrations of glucose on the activity of aminoglycosides and tetracycline against a strain of Escherichia coli

Glucose (%) added to peptone water	MIC (mg/l)			
	Tobramycin	Gentamicin	Amikacin	Tetracycline
0	0·25	0·25	0·5	8
10	1	0·5	1	4
20	2	2	2	2

Effect of atmosphere

Atmospheric conditions during incubation affect the pH of the medium and the growth and metabolism of the bacterial culture.

This was investigated by Rosenblatt & Schoenknecht (1972) who measured the pH changes and colony sizes following inoculation of MH agar with *E. coli* and incubation in a variety of different atmospheres (Fig. 4).

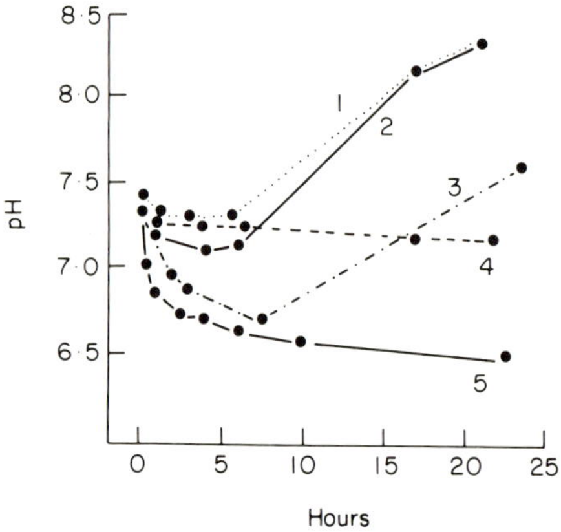

FIG. 4. Shift in pH of MH blood agar plates inoculated with *Escherichia coli* and incubated under different atmospheric conditions. 1, aerobic (no CO_2); 2, aerobic; 3, aerobic + 5–7% CO_2; 4, anaerobic (no CO_2); 5, anaerobic + 5–7% CO_2. From Rosenblatt & Schoenknecht (1972).

During the first 1–2 h of incubation, there was a small decrease in pH of 0·1 to 0·2 units in all atmospheres used. This could be related to a change from room temperature to 37°C. The fall in pH continued over the first 6–7 h in plates incubated in conditions with additional CO_2. The late rise in pH seen in plates incubated in both the aerobic ($-CO_2$) and aerobic ($+$ 5–7% CO_2) conditions is probably due to microbial growth and metabolism, especially the deamination of amino acids, since peptones or hydrolysates of casein are the principal nutrients in MH agar. Uninoculated plates used as controls and incubated under similar conditions produced the same early medium pH change without the later pH rise. This terminal alkalinization of medium was also not seen in inoculated plates incubated anaerobically with or without CO_2. Under such conditions, the growth of *E. coli* was poor with smaller colonies. The metabolism of sugar by *E. coli* produces more acid in anaerobic than aerobic conditions.

In clinical microbiology, plates for sensitivity testing are usually incubated under conditions which promote the optimal growth of the bacterial strain under investigation. Thus, anaerobes are incubated in O_2-free conditions with 5–10% CO_2 and micro-aerophilic organisms are sometimes incubated in air with 5–10% CO_2. Different atmospheric conditions of this kind may result in variation in the activity of antibiotics. Ingham *et al.* (1970) showed that the MICs of erythromycin and lincomycin hydrochloride for *B. fragilis* were 4–32 times higher when grown in H_2 + 10% CO_2 than the values obtained when the strains were grown in pure H_2. This reduction of activity in hypercapnic conditions did not apply equally to all organisms studied. It was most marked with *B. fragilis*, nearly as marked with *Haemophilus influenzae* and *Clostridium tertium* but much less apparent with the Oxford staphylococcus, a Group A streptococcus, and *Strep. faecalis*. 7-Chloro-lincomycin and rifamycin B diethylamide, to which the strains of *B. fragilis* were uniformly sensitive, were not significantly affected by the additional CO_2.

Similar findings concerning gentamicin and other aminoglycosides were obtained by Reynolds *et al.* (1976). A 10-fold reduction in the activity of gentamicin was observed with *Staph. aureus* and of 2·5 to 3·5 fold with *E. coli*, *Klebsiella*, *Enterobacter*, *Proteus rettgeri* and *P. morganii*, when the MICs obtained under aerobic conditions with or without the addition of 4% CO_2 were compared.

It is not clear why the reduction in activity of erythromycin and aminoglycosides in the presence of additional CO_2 affects some species more than others. Many bacteria grow better in the presence of 5–10% CO_2, and it may be that this CO_2-related enhanced growth has an effect on the result of sensitivity study in addition to the pH change produced by the CO_2.

The MIC of metronidazole against *Gardnerella vaginalis* varies with

TABLE 14

Effect of anaerobiosis per se *on the MICs of some antibiotics*

Antimicrobial	Medium used (reference)	Organism	MIC ratio $\left(\frac{\text{anaerobic}}{\text{aerobic}}\text{ MIC}\right)$
Aminoglycosides	Sensitest agar (a)	*Staph. aureus*	Up to 20
	Mueller–Hinton agar (b)	*E. coli* *Klebsiella* *Proteus*	2·5–15
Sulphamethoxazole, Trimethroprim	Wellcotest (c)	*Staph. aureus* *Staph. albus* *Proteus* *E. coli*	Up to 100
Cephalothin Cefazolin Cefamandole	Mueller–Hinton agar (b)	*Staph. aureus* *E. coli* *Klebsiella* *Proteus*	1

Modified from: (a) Reynolds *et al.* (1976); (b) Verklin & Mandell (1977); (c) Virtanen (1974).

the incubation conditions. Ralph *et al.* (1979) reported that only 13% of *G. vaginalis* strains were sensitive to 8 mg/l of metronidazole under aerobic conditions but that 48% were sensitive under anaerobic conditions. Recent evidence indicates that the increased activity of metronidazole under anaerobic conditions may be due in part to the activity of the 2-hydroxymethyl metabolite of metronidazole. The MICs of the 2-hydroxymethyl metabolite vary from $\frac{1}{4}$ to $\frac{1}{16}$ of those of metronidazole (Ralph & Amatnieks 1980; Balsdon & Jackson 1981).

Anaerobiosis *per se* may affect the activity of antimicrobials against some facultatively anaerobic organisms. Table 14 shows the effect of anaerobic incubation on the activity of some antibiotics against the bacteria listed. The mechanism of the inhibitory action of anaerobiosis *per se* is unclear. It cannot be fully explained in terms of the pH change which may occur after incubation (Reynolds *et al.* 1976). Anaerobiosis brings about changes in nutritional requirements and metabolic pathways in staphylococci (Lascelles 1974). The uptake and lethality of streptomycin was shown to require respiration (electron transport) (Hancock 1962). This led to the suggestion that molecular oxygen could be necessary for the optimal entrance of aminoglycosides into bacterial cells (Verklin & Mandell 1977). Campbell & Kadner (1980), however, demonstrated that the effect of anaerobiosis was not a specific response to oxygen, but rather to the inhibition of electron transport, as this requirement for electron transport could be supplied by an alternate electron acceptor, e.g. nitrate. The uptake of aminoglycosides by sensitive cells may be divided into three phases (Bryan & van den Elzen 1976; Miller *et al.* 1980): energy-independent binding of the drug to the cell surface, followed by energy-dependent transport process and binding to sensitive ribosomes. The last phase accounts for the most rapid and extensive accumulation of the drug and is responsible for the lethal action of the antibiotics. Anaerobiosis and inhibitors of electron transport do not prevent the initial phase of uptake. Their effect on the energy-dependent phases is freely reversible upon O_2 addition or removal of the inhibitors (Bryan & van den Elzen 1975, 1976). The exact component of the electron transport involved has yet to be identified. It is likely that the partly or fully oxidized state of such a component would be required in the uptake of aminoglycosides (Miller *et al.* 1980; Hancock 1981).

References

Abraham, E. P. & Duthie, E. S. 1946 Effect of pH of the medium on activity of streptomycin and penicillin and other chemotherapeutic substances. *Lancet* **i**, 455–459.

ALLEN, J. G., ATHERTON, F. R., HALL, M. J., HASSALL, C. H., HOLMES, S. W., LAMBERT, R. V., NISBET, L. J. & RINGROSE, P. S. 1979 Phosphonopeptides as antibacterial agents: alaphosphin and related phosphonopeptides. *Antimicrobial Agents and Chemotherapy* **15,** 684–695.

AMYES, S. G. B. & SMITH, J. T. 1978 Trimethoprim antagonists: effect of uridine on laboratory media. *Journal of Antimicrobial Chemotherapy* **4,** 421–429.

ATHERTON, F. R., HALL, M. J., HASSALL, C. H., LAMBERT, R. W. & RINGROSE, P. S. 1979*a* Phosphonopeptides as antibacterial agents: rationale, chemistry and structure activity relationships. *Antimicrobial Agents and Chemotherapy* **15,** 677–683.

ATHERTON, F. R., HALL, M. J., HASSALL, C. H., LAMBERT, R. W., LLOYD, W. J. & RINGROSE, P. S. 1979*b* Phosphonopeptides as antibacterial agents: mechanism of action of alaphosphin. *Antimicrobial Agents and Chemotherapy* **15,** 696–705.

BALSDON, M. J. & JACKSON, D. 1981 Metronidazole metabolite and *Gardnerella vaginalis. Lancet* **i,** 1112.

BARRY, A. L. 1976 *The Antimicrobic Susceptibility Test. Principles and Practices* p. 65. Philadelphia: Lea & Febiger.

BEGGS, W. H. & ANDREWS, F. A. 1976 Role of ionic strength in salt antagonism of aminoglycoside action on *Escherichia coli* and *Pseudomonas aeruginosa. Journal of Infectious Diseases* **134,** 500–504.

BENDICH, A. 1955 Chemistry of purines and pyrimidines. In *The Nucleic Acids* Vol. 1, ed. Chargaff, E. & Davidson, J. V. pp. 81–136. New York & London: Academic Press.

BRYAN, L. E. & VAN DEN ELZEN, H. M. 1975 Gentamicin accumulation by sensitive strains of *Escherichia coli* and *Pseudomonas aeruginosa. Journal of Antibiotics* **28,** 696–703.

BRYAN, L. E. & VAN DEN ELZEN, H. M. 1976 Streptomycin accumulation in susceptible and resistant strains of *Escherichia coli* and *Pseudomonas aeruginosa. Antimicrobial Agents and Chemotherapy* **9,** 928–938.

CAMPBELL, B. D. & KADNER, R. J. 1980 Relation of aerobiosis and ionic strength to the uptake of dihydrostreptomycin in *Escherichia coli. Biochimica et Biophysica Acta* **593,** 1–10.

CRAIG, W. A. & BYUNGSE, SUH. 1980 Protein binding and the antibacterial effects. In *Antibiotics in Laboratory Medicine*, ed. Lorian, V. pp. 265–298. Baltimore: Williams & Wilkins.

D'AMATO, R. F., THORNSBERRY, C., BAKER, C. N. & KIRVEN, L. A. 1975 Effect of calcium and magnesium ions on the susceptibility of Pseudomonas species to tetracycline, gentamicin, polymyxin B and carbenicillin. *Antimicrobial Agents and Chemotherapy* **7,** 596–600.

FERONE, R., BUSHBY, S. R. M., BURCHALL, J. J., MOORE, W. D. & SMITH, D. 1975 Identification of Harper–Cawston factor as thymidine phosphorylase and removal from media of substances interfering with susceptibility testing to sulphonamides and diamino pyrimidines. *Antimicrobial Agents and Chemotherapy* **7,** 91–98.

GARROD, L. P. & WATERWORTH, P. M. 1969 Effect of medium composition on the apparent sensitivity of *Pseudomonas aeruginosa* to gentamicin. *Journal of Clinical Pathology* **22,** 534–538.

GARROD, L. P., LAMBERT, H. P., O'GRADY, F. &. WATERWORTH, P. M. 1973 *Antibiotic and Chemotherapy* 4th edn, p. 493. Edinburgh: Churchill Livingstone.

GILBERT, D. N., KUTSCHER, E., IRELAND, P., BARNETT, J. A. & SANFORD, J. P. 1971 Effect of the concentrations of magnesium and calcium on the in vitro susceptibility of *Pseudomonas aeruginosa* to gentamicin. *Journal of Infectious Diseases* **124** (Supplement), 537–545.

HANCOCK, R. E. W. 1962 Uptake of ^{14}C-streptomycin by some microorganisms and its relation to their streptomycin sensitivity. *Journal of General Microbiology* **28,** 493–501.

HANCOCK, R. E. W. 1981 Aminoglycoside uptake and mode of action, with special reference to streptomycin and gentamicin. I. Antagonists and mutants. *Journal of Antimicrobial Chemotherapy* **8,** 249–276.

HANSEN, S. L., SWOMLEY, P. & DRUSANO, G. 1981 Effect of carbon dioxide and pH on susceptibility of *Bacteroides fragilis* group to erythromycin. *Antimicrobial Agents and Chemotherapy* **19,** 335–336.

HARPER, G. J. & CAWSTON, W. C. 1945 *In vitro* determination of sulphonamide sensitivity of bacteria. *Journal of Pathology and Bacteriology* **57,** 59–66.

HOEPRICH, P. D. 1963 Alanine: cycloserine antagonism. *Archives of Internal Medicine* **112,** 159–168.

HOEPRICH, P. D. & FINN, P. D. 1972 Obfuscation of the activity of antifungal antimicrobics. *Journal of Infectious Diseases* **126,** 353–361.

INGHAM, H. R., SELKON, J. B., CODD, A. A. & HALE, J. H. 1970 The effect of carbon dioxide on the sensitivity of *Bacteroides fragilis* to certain antibiotics in vitro. *Journal of Clinical Pathology* **23,** 254–258.

KOCH, A. E. & BURCHALL, J. J. 1971 Reversal of the antimicrobial activity of trimethoprim by thymidine in commercially prepared media. *Applied Microbiology* **22,** 812–817.

LASCELLES, J. 1974 Anaerobic growth requirement of staphylococci and the enzymes of pyrimidine synthesis. *Annals of the New York Academy of Sciences* **236,** 96–104.

MEDEIROS, A. A., O'BRIEN, T. F., WALKER, W. E. C. & YULUG, N. F. 1971 Effect of salt concentration on the apparent in vitro susceptibility of *Pseudomonas* and other Gram-negative bacilli to gentamicin. *Journal of Infectious Diseases* **124** (Supplement), 859–864.

MILLER, M. H., EDBERG, S. C., MANDEL, L. J., BEHAIR, C. F. & STEIGBIGEL, N. H. 1980 Gentamicin uptake in wild-type and aminoglycoside-resistant small-colony mutants of *Staphylococcus aureus*. *Antimicrobial Agents and Chemotherapy* **18,** 722–729.

NEU, H. C. 1976 Mecillinam, a novel penicillanic acid derivative with unusual activity against Gram-negative bacteria. *Antimicrobial Agents and Chemotherapy* **9,** 793–799.

RALPH, E. D. & AMATNIEKS, Y. E. 1980 Relative susceptibilities of *Gardnerella vaginalis, Neisseria gonorrhoeae* and *Bacteroides fragilis* to metronidazole and its two major matabolites. *Journal of Sexually Transmitted Diseases* **7,** 157–160.

RALPH, E. D., AUSTIN, T. W., PATTISON, F. L. M. & SCHIEVEN, B. C. 1979 Inhibition of *Haemophilus vaginalis* by metronidazole, tetracycline and ampicillin. *Journal of Sexually Transmitted Diseases* **6,** 199.

RAMIREZ-RONDA, C. H., HOLMES, R. K. & SANFORD, J. P. 1975 Effect of divalent cations on binding of aminoglycoside antibiotics to human serum proteins and to bacteria. *Antimicrobial Agents and Chemotherapy* **7,** 239–245.

RELLER, L. B., SCHOENKNECHT, F. D., KENNY, M. A. & SHERRIS, J. C. 1974 Antibiotic susceptibility testing of *Pseudomonas aeruginosa*: election of a control strain and criteria for magnesium and calcium content in media. *Journal of Infectious Diseases* **130,** 454–463.

REPASKE, R. 1958 Lysis of Gram-negative organisms and the role of versene. *Biochimica et biophysica acta* **30,** 225–232.

REYNOLDS, A. V., HAMILTON-MILLER, J. M. T. & BRUMFITT, W. 1976 Diminished effect of gentamicin under anaerobic or hypercapneic conditions. *Lancet* **i,** 447–449.

ROSENBLATT, J. E. & SCHOENKNECHT, F. 1972 Effect of components of anaerobic incubation on antibiotic susceptibility test results. *Antimicrobial Agents and Chemotherapy* **1,** 433–440.

SABATH, L. D. & TOFTEGAARD, I. 1974 Rapid microassays for clindamycin and gentamicin when present together and the effect of pH and of each on the antibacterial activity of the other. *Antimicrobial Agents and Chemotherapy* **6,** 54–59.

SHOCKMAN, G. D. 1959 Reversal of cycloserine inhibition by D-alanine. *Proceedings of the Society of Experimental Biology and Medicine* **101,** 693–695.

SPRATT, B. G. 1977 The mechanism of action of mecillinam. *Journal of Antimicrobial Chemotherapy* **3** (Supplement B), 13–19.

VERKLIN, R. M. JR. & MANDELL, G. L. 1977 Alteration of effectiveness of antibiotics by anaerobiosis. *Journal of Laboratory and Clinical Medicine* **89,** 65–71.

VIRTANEN, S. 1974 Antibacterial activity of sulphamethoxazole and trimethoprim under diminished oxygen tension. *Journal of General Microbiology* **84,** 145–148.

WASHINGTON, J. A., SNYDER, R. J., KOHNER, P. C., WILTSE, C. G., ILSTRUP, D. M. & MCCALL, J. T. 1978 Effect of cation content of agar on the activity of gentamicin, tobramycin and amikacin against *Pseudomonas aeruginosa*. *Journal of Infectious Diseases* **137**, 103–110.

WEINBERG, E. D. 1957 The mutual effects of antimicrobial compounds and metallic cations. *Bacteriological Reviews* **21,** 46–68.

ZIMELIS, V. M. & JACKSON, G. G. 1973 Activity of aminoglycoside antibiotics against *Pseudomonas aeruginosa*: specificity and site of calcium and magnesium antagonism. *Journal of Infectious Diseases* **127,** 663–669.

ZINNER, S. H., SABATH, L. D., CASEY, J. I. & FINLAND, M. 1971 Erythromycin plus alkalinization in treatment of urinary infections due to Gram-negative bacilli. *Lancet* **i,** 1267.

ZYGMUNT, W. A. 1962 Reversal of D-cycloserine inhibition of bacterial growth of alanine. *Journal* of *Bacteriology* **84,** 154–157.

Conductance Measurements for Determining Antibiotic Sensitivity

I. A. PORTER, T. M. S. REID AND W. J. WOOD

Regional Laboratory, City Hospital, Aberdeen, UK

D. M. GIBSON AND G. HOBBS

MAFF, Torry Research Station, 135 Abbey Road, Aberdeen, UK

There have been many ideas proposed for automating or mechanizing the routine procedures of clinical microbiology, but few devices have reached commercial production or widespread use. Many physical and chemical principles have been examined, one of the first being measurement of the changes in the electrical properties of bacterial cultures described by Stewart (1899). He made measurements of the AC resistance of broth cultures and showed that, as various putrefactive and pathogenic bacteria grew in blood or artificial media, the curves of the changes in conductivity with time were parallel to those of the number of bacteria. He proposed (Stewart 1898, 1899) that such an approach could be used as a measure of bacterial activity. He also indicated that the assays were reproducible and specific, so that by comparing the conductivity curves obtained by the growth of different bacteria in a range of media a scheme for the detection and identification of cultures might be possible. The change in the resistance of cultures was ascribed to the effects of bacterial metabolism, in that macromolecules, such as proteins, which are poor charge carriers are converted to low molecular weight charged metabolites. Thus, by 1900, Stewart had the essentials of a method for measuring bacterial growth based on the electrical properties of the culture.

The technique was virtually neglected except for the occasional research paper, e.g. Baernstein (1928); Allison *et al.* (1938) until the early 1970s, when two distinct developments occurred culminating in two instruments,

ANTIBIOTICS
ISBN 0 12 604480 5

one described by Ur & Brown (1975), the other by Cady (1975), at the First International Symposium on Rapid Methods and Automation held in 1973. Both instruments compare the impedance of a sample with that of a control broth held in small specially constructed electrode cells, at frequent time intervals. They are much more sensitive than Stewart's apparatus, make frequent measurements and automatically display the results on chart recorders. The published data help to establish the technique confirming earlier work on the possibilities for detecting and identifying bacterial growth. The prime advantage over traditional methods is the speed of response, positive results being available in about one-third of the usual time. As Ur & Brown (1975) pointed out, the sensitivity of the methods allows for very early detection of activity in a culture. Thus many common pathogens at 10^5/ml are detected within 2 h and their susceptibility to a range of antibiotics may be established within a few hours.

In 1978, an instrument with improved precision and sensitivity was described by Richards *et al.* which also automated data collection and handling of up to 128 samples simultaneously. There were two main differences from the earlier instruments. Firstly, the conductance or resistance alone, rather than overall impedance, was measured by means of a phase-sensitive demodulator system using platinum electrodes. The authors showed that only the resistive component of impedance followed bacterial growth; hence, elimination of the capacitive component should lead to increased sensitivity. Much of the capacitance is due to polarization at the electrodes and this is greatly reduced by the use of platinum in their construction. Secondly, the incubation temperature was closely controlled by using water baths rather than air or metal block incubators. Control of the temperature of the sample is the main parameter limiting the sensitivity of such electrical measurements, since the temperature coefficient of resistance of common bacteriological media is 1·67%/°C and the overall change caused by bacterial growth is *ca.* 2%. By controlling the temperature of the sample to within a millidegree, Richards *et al.* (1978) improved the sensitivity of their instruments by a factor of 10 compared with previous models which gives an earlier detection of growth. Purpose-built water baths and temperature controllers were necessary for this. With such control, it is not necessary to balance each sample against a reference. The instrument, in effect, connects each sample in turn to a measuring device at regular time intervals, converts the demodulator output to a digital form, and presents it to a computer or microprocessor.

There is now sufficient evidence to show that the parameters measured by the three instruments already mentioned are an adequate measure of bacterial growth. The ease and precision with which each instrument will detect and measure growth will depend on its ability to separate changes due to spurious effects such as temperature fluctuations, electrode polarization and other electronic noise, from that due to bacterial activity. This becomes increasingly important where the numbers of bacteria in the sample are low. The time taken to detect growth or change in conductance/impedance is inversely proportional to the logarithm of the numbers in the sample, i.e. the fewer the bacteria present the longer they take to multiply to give a measurable response. Thus, the more sensitive the instrument the less time taken for detection of growth and to confirm the lack of growth.

The use of impedance measurements to determine the sensitivities of cultures to antibiotics has been described (Cady 1975; Ur & Brown 1975; Colvin & Sherris 1977). In the present work conductance equipment rather than impedance instruments has been used for this purpose and the results have been compared with those obtained by using the existing routine procedures.

As might be expected, inhibition of growth in culture caused by an antibiotic can be deduced soon after growth in a control has been detected; and the same considerations apply regarding the resolution of the measurements as discussed above.

Materials and Methods

Equipment

Some of the preliminary work was carried out using the prototype instruments described by Richards *et al.* (1978), but most of the work to be described was carried out using equipment developed from them by Malthus Instruments Limited (see Fig. 1).

The samples are held in standard glass ampoules fitted with a reusable platinum electrode (Fig. 2). Eight ampoules are clipped into a rack which is plugged into the water bath to make the electrical connections to the instrument. The microcomputer controls the operations as well as holding, displaying and analysing the data. The presence of samples is sensed automatically and their conductance measured every 5 or 10 min. The computer display screen shows whenever a conductance change of more than a given preselected value has occurred and at the end of the experiment (usually 6·3 h at present) all the data for each sample can be seen either graphically as conductance change (G_B) against time or numerically. Figures were prepared from the traces produced by an XY plotter. The y axis was set at 100 μS (the unit of conductance being the siemen, S) so that the plateau shown by the control samples represents saturation of the output. Such a scale was chosen to allow better resolution of the results of samples treated with antibiotics.

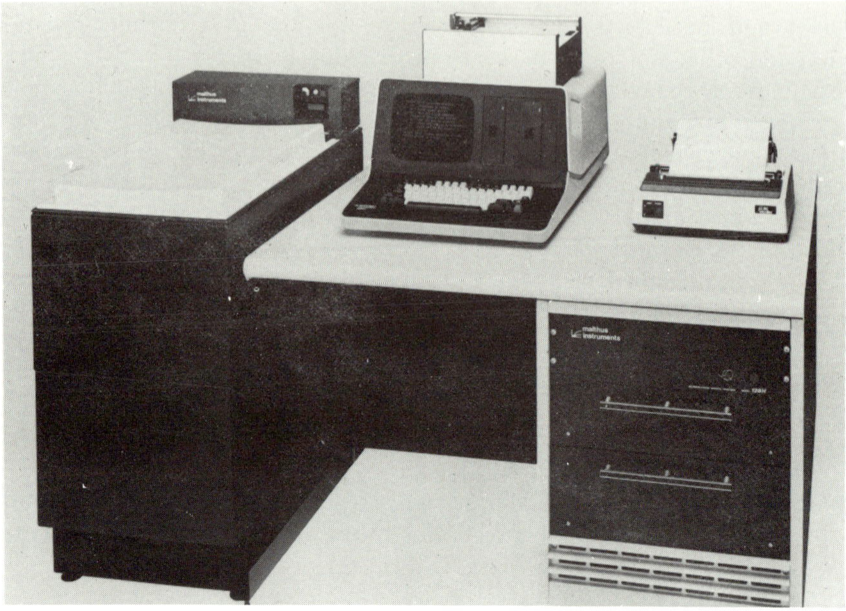

FIG. 1. Conductance measuring equipment ('Malthus') provided by Malthus Instruments Ltd, William Clowes Street, Burslem, Stoke-on-Trent ST6 3AT. The water bath containing the ampoules is on the left.

Routine bacteriology

The Laboratory at the City Hospital, Aberdeen, receives clinical specimens from hospitals and from general practitioners in the Grampian region. About 200 urine samples are processed daily of which *ca.* 20% contain significant numbers of bacteria ($\geqslant 10^5$/ml). Isolates from these samples are then examined for their sensitivity to a range of antibiotics. The routine procedure currently in use at this laboratory is the disc diffusion assay carried out on Oxoid Isosensitest agar. The test organism is suspended in Bacto Tryptose broth to give a density known to produce a semi-confluent growth in 18 h when inoculated on to the plates. The antibiotics used and the disc contents can be seen in Table 1. To determine minimum inhibitory concentrations (MICs), doubling dilutions of antibiotic are made in 1-ml amounts of Mueller–Hinton (MH) broth. The test organism is suspended in Bacto Tryptose broth and the suspension adjusted by comparison with turbidity standards so that the final density in the assay tubes is 10^6 organisms/ml. The broths are then incubated overnight at 37°C and the MIC read as the lowest concentration of antibiotic which inhibited growth of the test organism.

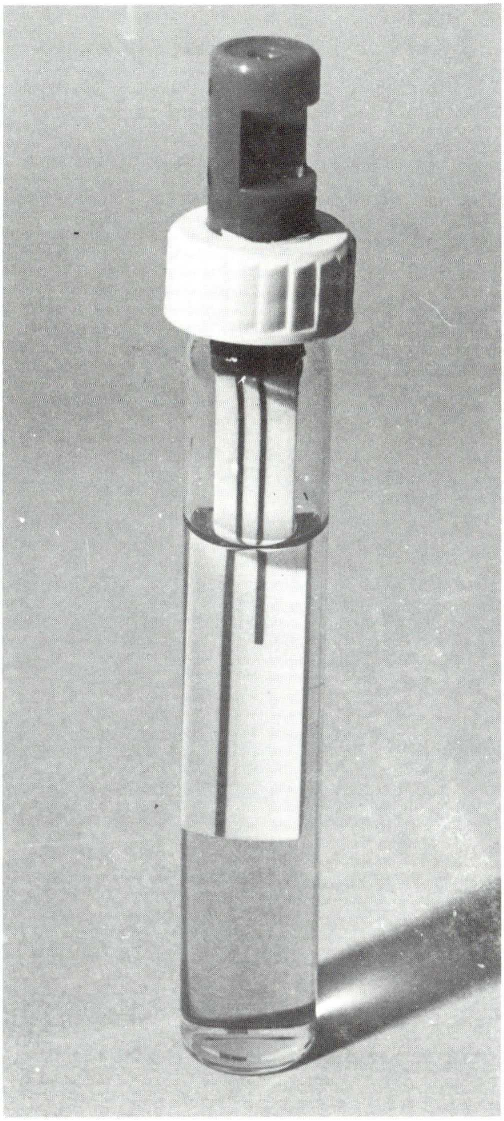

FIG. 2. Ampoule with electrode assembly.

Development of Malthus protocol

Escherichia coli (ATCC 25922) is used routinely for quality control purposes in the laboratory, and was used as test organism for the development of this method and as a control throughout the work.

Inoculum size

As with disc methods, the inoculum size is of importance for the proper interpretation of the results. The time taken for detection of growth is inversely proportional to the logarithm of the inoculum number (Richards *et al.* 1978). With most strains of *E. coli* including ATCC 25922, an inoculum of 10^8/ml was detected immediately whereas an inoculum of 10^0 took *ca.* 7–8 h. Detection is defined as the time taken for an increase in conductance of 10 μS (see Richards *et al.* 1978) compared with an un-inoculated control, which invariably gives a flat baseline.

The effect of varying the inoculum density was studied using a constant concentration of each of the antibiotics under test. Tubes containing 10 ml of MH broth were inoculated with a series of dilutions of a suspension of *E. coli* (ATCC 25922) in Bacto Tryptose broth. The results of a typical experiment using gentamicin (1·6 μg/ml) are shown in Fig. 3. It can be seen that an inoculum of 10^6/ml permits early detection not only of bacterial growth but also of the inhibitory effect of those agents to which the organism is sensitive. In addition, the concentration of 10^6/ml is in keeping with the number of organisms present in the urine of a patient with clinically significant urinary tract infection. Indeed the Malthus technique can be used as a rapid screening method for identifying urine samples with significant bacteriuria ($\geqslant 10^5$ organisms/ml).

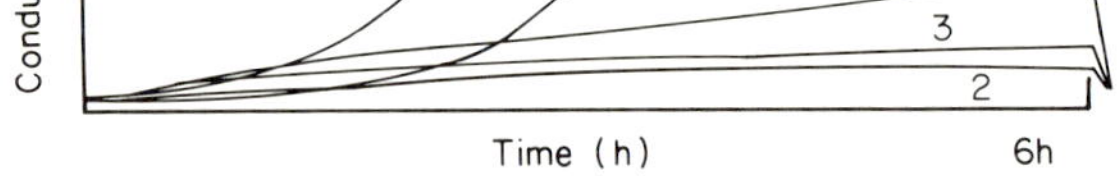

FIG. 3. Effect of the inoculum size (N) on conductance change (G_B) in the presence of gentamicin (1·6 μg/ml). 1: N = 10^6/ml, no gentamicin; 2: N = 10^2/ml; 3: N = 10^4/ml; 4: N = 10^6/ml; 5: N = 10^8/ml.

Antibiotic concentration

Assays were performed using doubling dilutions of the antibiotics under test (Table 1) and a typical result is shown in Fig. 4. Disc assays and MIC tests in MH broth were set up in parallel. Standard concentrations of the antibiotics were chosen which on preliminary testing appeared to give good

TABLE 1

Antibiotics studied—disc contents, breakpoint concentration, concentrations used in Malthus and clinically achievable urinary concentrations

Antibiotic	(a) Disc content (μg)	(b) Breakpoint concentration (μg/ml)	(c) Concentration in conductance assay (μg/ml)	(d) Clinically achievable urine levels in healthy subjects (μ/ml)
Cotrimoxazole	25	64	64	50–200
Nalidixic acid	30	32	32	50–500
Nitrofurantoin	200	64	6·4	250–500
Ampicillin	25	32	32	200–> 1000
Cefuroxime	30	30	60	500–1000
Gentamicin	10	16	1·6	30–70
Tetracycline	30	32	10	10–40

correlation with the results of overnight disc diffusion assays and allowed analysis of the characteristics of the antibiotic-induced growth suppression, if any, after continuous monitoring for 6·3 h. The concentrations chosen are shown in Table 1. Using the Malthus system it is not only possible to demonstrate suppression of growth but also to establish the characteristics of the suppressive effect, viz. the bactericidal rate, the duration of the suppression and length of exposure required to achieve an observable effect.

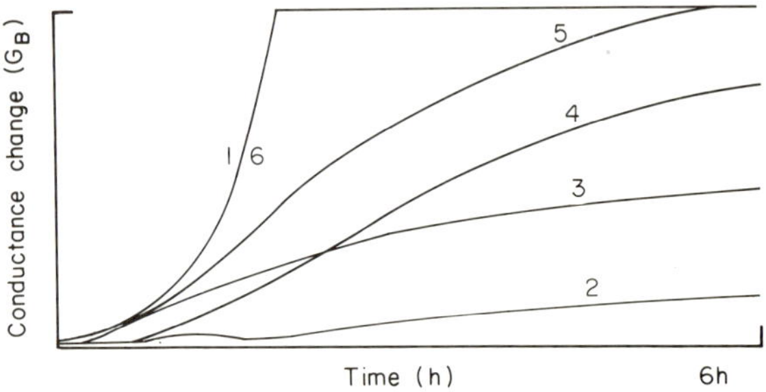

FIG. 4. Effect of antibiotic concentration on conductance change (G_B). 1: Control (no antibiotic); 2: ampicillin 160 μg/ml; 3: 80 μg/ml; 4: 40 μg/ml; 5: 20 μg/ml; 6: 10 μg/ml.

The major differences in concentration from those recommended for breakpoint assay were noted for nitrofurantoin, gentamicin and tetracycline, where the concentration had to be reduced from 64 to 6·4 μg/ml, from 16 to 1·6 μg/ml and from 32 to 10 μg/ml, respectively, to permit demonstration of growth and its subsequent inhibition by antibiotic.

Results

Some typical results are shown in Fig. 5*a*, *b* and *c*. The data are clear cut and easy to interpret. In a series of 462 tests, there were 13 discrepancies between the results of the disc diffusion tests and the conductance measurements. Eight of these involved cotrimoxazole and in each case the organism was reported as resistant on disc testing but sensitive in the Malthus assay. MIC determinations were performed in MH broth and in all instances the MIC was equal to or marginally less than the breakpoint figure used in the Malthus system. When the disc diffusion test was repeated with a lower inoculum density the organisms were considered

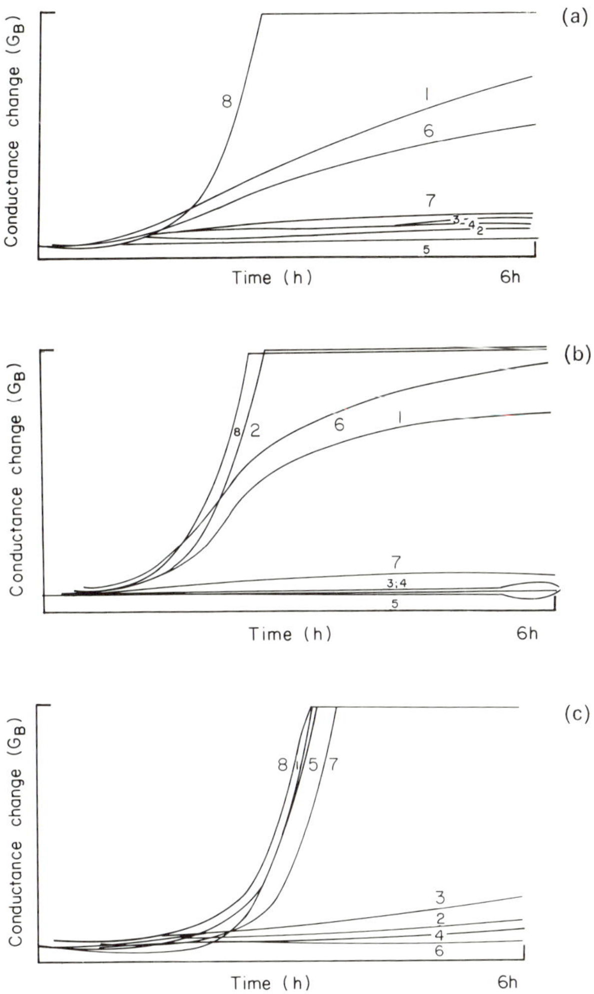

FIG. 5*a*, *b*, *c*. Typical plots obtained with urinary cultures set up in MH broths with the antibiotics at the concentrations shown in Table 1, column (c). 1: Ampicillin; 2: nalidixic acid; 3: nitrofurantoin; 4: gentamicin; 5: Cotrimoxazole; 6: cefuroxime; 7: tetracycline; 8: control.

sensitive. One strain of *Klebsiella aerogenes* appeared sensitive to ampicillin in the Malthus system but resistant on disc testing. On repeating the Malthus test the organism was considered to be resistant. The MIC for ampicillin was greater than 32 but less than 64 μg/ml.

One strain of *E. coli* was resistant on disc testing and to concentrations of

1·6 and 3·2 μg/ml of nitrofurantoin in the Malthus test but sensitive to 6·4 μg/ml which was the concentration adopted in the Malthus system. Two strains of *E. coli* were sensitive to the 30 μg disc but resistant when tested against 60 μg/ml cefuroxime in the Malthus test. They were, however, sensitive to 100 μg/ml. On the other hand, a strain of *Streptococcus faecalis* was resistant to cefuroxime on disc testing but sensitive in the Malthus test.

Discussion

The Malthus system can be used in antibiotic sensitivity testing by the breakpoint dilution method. In order to establish the value of the Malthus system for antibiotic sensitivity testing it is necessary to compare its results with those obtained in the traditional disc diffusion test. One must recognize, however, that the latter well-established method is subject to many errors and pitfalls in interpretation and standardization which make absolute comparisons difficult and in certain circumstances misleading. In an attempt to overcome these problems many laboratories, including our own, are changing to breakpoint dilution methods for sensitivity testing which can be easily automated.

By adjusting the inoculum density and the concentration of antibiotic it is possible to obtain results in 2–3 h using the Malthus system which are comparable with those obtained by overnight disc diffusion tests. Such discrepancies as were observed involved organisms with MIC values close to the single breakpoint concentration chosen for the Malthus system. There is great debate as to whether single or multiple breakpoint concentrations should be used in sensitivity testing. If two breakpoint concentrations were used such organisms would probably fall into the intermediate category, i.e. lying between full sensitivity and resistance. While the Malthus system is well suited to testing multiple breakpoint concentrations it may be unnecessary to resort to this manoeuvre if the single breakpoint concentration is chosen with care to reflect the clinically achievable concentration in the tissues, or in this case the urine. It would then be possible not only to improve the reliability of antibiotic sensitivity testing but also to issue an all-or-none sensitive or resistant report which is what the clinician desires. The choice of appropriate breakpoint concentrations is thus of considerable importance.

If one were to use the antibiotic at the clinically attainable concentration (Table 1) and an inoculum density commensurate with that found in a urinary tract infection (e.g. *E. coli* $> 10^5$/ml) it is arguable that the results obtained would be more relevant to the clinical management of the patient. These results would doubtless show a poorer correlation with those obtained using the overnight disc diffusion test since one recognized method of improving the correlation between rapid and overnight broth dilution MICs is to reduce the antibiotic concentration used in the rapid test (Thornsberry *et al.* 1975) as we have demonstrated with certain antibiotics in the Malthus system (see Table 1).

It is known that MIC values may increase with duration of incubation particularly where β-lactamase-producing strains are involved (Lampe *et al.* 1975). The speed with which Malthus tests are read (< 3h) as compared to the overnight incubation of disc diffusion tests may contribute to differences in the results obtained with β-lactam antibiotics.

Various factors appear to influence the speed with which an antibiotic sensitivity can be obtained using the Malthus system. The lower the inoculum density the longer it takes to detect growth and consequently inhibition of growth by an antibiotic. As the inoculum density increases the time taken to detect growth decreases. Furthermore the time taken to inhibit growth by an antibiotic is also decreased unless very small amounts of antibiotic are used. If a high concentration of antibiotic is used growth may be totally suppressed.

Growth curves which lie between the steeply rising control and total inhibition of growth may represent either a sublethal concentration of bactericidal antibiotic or a purely bacteriostatic effect. It is possible that in the former a prolonged lag phase with subsequent bacterial multiplication would be noted whereas in the latter the effect of the bacteriostatic antibiotic is to induce a slowing of the metabolism manifested in a prolongation of generation time and a slow linear growth curve. This may well be an over-simplification since different antibiotics vary greatly in their mode of action. In effect, once a difference of more than 10 μS exists between the control and experimental curves, sensitivity is assumed by means of either of the above mechanisms.

Older methods of sensitivity testing have relied on overnight reading of results. The aim of rapid, mechanized and automated techniques such as the Malthus test system is to provide results within hours and, if possible, within the course of a working day. Clinically useful sensitivity reports in the Malthus system with the organisms studied can be produced in 2–3 h.

Automation not only provides earlier detection but in addition eliminates considerable technical manipulation and visual assessment of endpoint, both potential sources of error. By modifying the basic computer software it is possible to tailor the Malthus system to meet the individual requirements of microbiology laboratories. Thus the computer can be programmed to detect significant changes, e.g. differences of 10 μS between the growth curves obtained in the tubes containing antibiotic and the controls, and to produce a printout of these results in terms of sensitivity or resistance of the test organism to the antibiotics used. Information regarding the patient and source of the organism can be incorporated into the printout and the data stored for subsequent analysis.

In summary the Malthus system can be used as a rapid and sensitive method for antibiotic sensitivity testing. It is capable of producing antibiotic sensitivity reports to the clinician within 3 h thus facilitating the initiation of specific therapy with the appropriate antibiotic.

References

ALLISON, J. B., ANDERSON, J. A. & COLE, W. H. 1938 The method of electrical conductivity in studies on bacterial metabolism. *Journal of Bacteriology* **36,** 571–586.

BAERNSTEIN, H. D. 1928 The conductivity method and proteolysis. II. An interpretation of the conductivity changes. *Journal of Biological Chemistry* **78,** 481–493.

CADY, P. 1975 Rapid automated bacterial identification by impedance measurement. In *New Approaches to the Identification of Microorganisms* ed. Heden, C. G. & Illéni, T. pp. 74–99. London: Wiley.

COLVIN, H. J. & SHERRIS, J. C. 1977 Electrical impedance measurements in the reading and monitoring of broth dilution susceptibility tests. *Antimicrobial Agents and Chemotherapy* **12,** 61–66.

LAMPE, M. F., AITKEN, C. L., DENNIS, P. G., FORSYTHE, P. S., PATRICK, K. E., SCHOENKNECHT, F. D. & SHERRIS, J. C. 1975 Relationship of early readings of minimal inhibitory concentrations to the results of overnight tests. *Antimicrobial Agents and Chemotherapy* **8,** 429–433.

RICHARDS, J. C. S., JASON, A. C., HOBBS, G., GIBSON, D. M. & CHRISTIE, R. H. 1978 Electronic measurement of bacterial growth. *Journal of Physics, E; Scientific Instruments* **11,** 560–568.

STEWART, G. N. 1898 Experiments on molecular concentration and electrical conductivity. *British Medical Journal* **2,** 778.

STEWART, G. N. 1899 The changes produced by the growth of bacteria in the molecular concentration and electrical conductivity of culture media. *Journal of Experimental Medicine* **4,** 235–247.

THORNSBERRY, C., GAVAN, T. L., SHERRIS, J. C., BALOWS, A., MATSEN, J. M., SABATH, L. D., SCHOENKNECHT, F., THRUPP, L. D. & WASHINGTON, J. A. II 1975 Laboratory evaluation of a rapid automated susceptibility testing system. Report of a collaborative study. *Antimicrobial Agents and Chemotherapy* **7,** 466–480.

UR, A. & BROWN, D. F. J. 1975 Monitoring of bacterial activity by impedance measurements. In *New Approaches to the Identification of Microorganisms* ed. Heden, C. G. & Illéni, T. pp. 61–71. London: Wiley.

The Influence of Cell Envelope Composition on Antibiotic Activity

R. M. Cozens,* R. M. M. Klemperer and M. R. W. Brown

Microbiology Research Group, Department of Pharmacy, University of Aston in Birmingham, Gosta Green, Birmingham, UK

The bacterial cell envelope is a complex organelle interposed between the cytoplasm and the environment, serving both to protect the cell and to regulate the uptake of essential nutrients into it. As the environment continually changes, so does the cell envelope in response. Whether an antibiotic acts at a site within the envelope, or traverses the envelope to reach a target within the cell, changes in the cell envelope may alter its effective concentration and therefore the apparent sensitivity of the cell.

Gram positive and Gram negative envelopes differ considerably. However, there is increasing evidence that both groups are commonly covered with regularly arranged protein sub-units (S-layer). A barrier role seems probable (Sleytr 1978) but the precise function of these proteins remains speculative.

The Gram positive cell envelope has a relatively simple structure (Reaveley & Burge 1972; Costerton 1977; Krause 1977; Rogers *et al.* 1978) as shown in Fig. 1. Variation in the limiting nutrient or the growth rate is associated with variation in the composition of the envelope (Ellwood & Tempest 1972) and this has been linked to changes in resistance both to drugs and lysozyme (Gilbert & Brown 1980). In addition, staphylococci depleted of lipids by growth in biotin-deficient conditions become more sensitive to benzylpenicillin and tetracycline (Hugo & Davidson 1973).

The structure of the Gram negative envelope has been elucidated in considerable detail in recent years (Costerton 1977; Nikaido & Nakae 1979; Osborn & Wu 1980) and is outlined in Fig. 2. A compartmental model (Fig. 3) indicates possible routes of drug entry, which will be

*Present address: Ciba-Geigy, Pharma Research, Basle, CH 4002, Switzerland.

ANTIBIOTICS
ISBN 0 12 604480 5

affected by the compound's hydrophilicity, molecular size and electric charge (Brown *et al.* 1979; Nikaido & Nakae 1979).

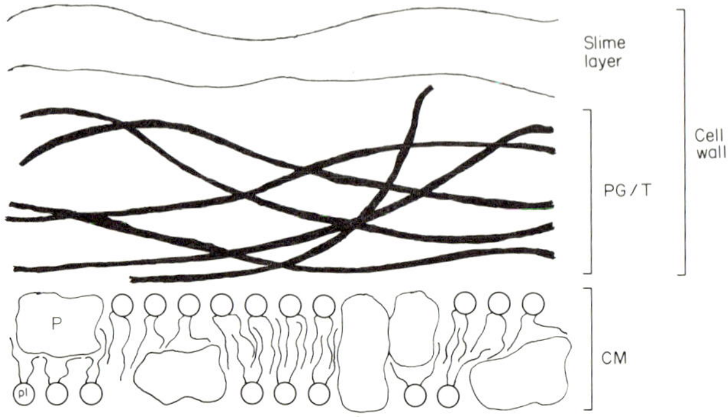

FIG. 1. Diagrammatic representation of the Gram positive cell envelope. pl, phospholipid; P, protein; CM cytoplasmic membrane; PG/T, peptidoglycan/ teichoic and teichuronic acid polymers.

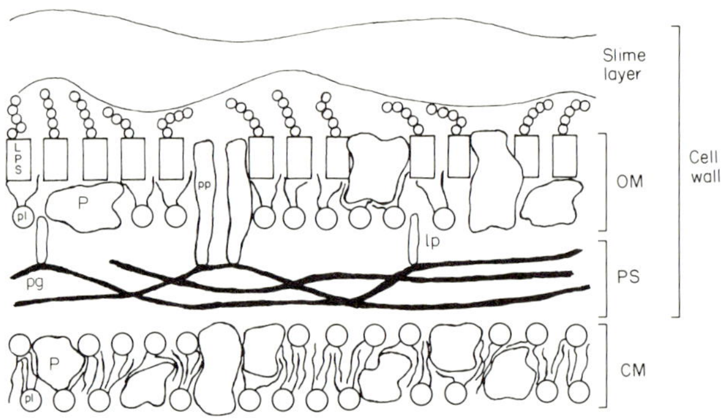

FIG. 2. Diagrammatic representation of the Gram negative cell envelope. LPS, lipopolysaccharide; pl, phospholipid; P, protein; lp, lipoprotein; pp, porin protein; pg, peptidoglycan; OM, outer membrane; CM, cytoplasmic membrane; PS, periplasmic space. The periplasmic space contains the peptidoglycan and some enzymes.

A mainly hydrophilic pathway through the outer membrane consists of protein-framed pores with size exclusion limits and with some degree of specificity (van Alphen *et al.* 1978; Nikaido 1979). The hydrophobic route is by diffusion through the outer membrane and exists most fully in deep rough mutants of enteric bacteria, when the almost impenetrable close-stacked lipopolysaccharide (LPS) is largely replaced by more mobile phospholipid (Nikaido 1979). There is evidence that the periplasm and the cytoplasm are iso-osmotic and that an electrical potential exists across the outer membrane (Stock *et al.* 1977). This potential may possibly contribute to a regulation of pore closing (Schindler & Rosenbusch 1978).

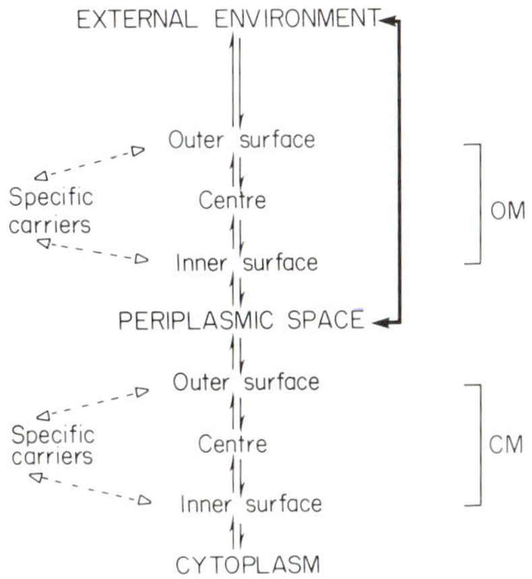

FIG. 3. A compartmental model describing drug disposition in Gram negative bacteria. OM, outer membrane; CM, cytoplasmic membrane; ◁ - - - - ▷, transport by specific carrier proteins; ⇌, diffusion and partitioning; ◀——▶, diffusion through hydrophilic pores. The idea of continuity between the external environment and the periplasm via pores must be considered in the light of evidence that cytoplasm and periplasm are iso-osmotic (Stock *et al.*, 1977).

The inherent thermodynamic instability of the outer membrane means that small perturbations may lead to large changes. In particular, the electrostatic repulsion between negatively charged groups is a cause of instability, which may be minimized by the addition of Mg^{2+} (Nikaido & Nakae 1979). Variations in osmolarity, within the range common in bacteriological media, affect porin composition of *Escherichia coli* (van Alphen & Lugtenberg 1977), as do the sugar content and the growth temperature (Lugtenberg *et al.* 1976). The addition of maltose to the medium induces the formation of a porin-like protein (Braun & Krieger-Brauer 1977). Similarly, in the inner membrane, most transport systems are inducible and the enzymic composition varies markedly with the conditions of growth (Braun 1978). Quantitative changes in the slime-layer with various media are well known (Brown *et al.* 1969; Sutherland 1979) and high cation concentrations stimulate the production of a fibrillar glycocalyx by cystic fibrosis strains of *Pseudomonas aeruginosa* (Costerton *et al.* 1979). Nutrient depletion, as cells pass from the exponential phase to the stationary phase, leads to a variety of envelope changes which have been linked with changes in resistance (Brown, 1977; Kenward *et al.* 1979;

Klemperer *et al.* 1980). Growth rate has also been found to be an important parameter affecting both envelope composition and drug penetration (Gilbert & Brown 1978).

The purpose of antibiotic assay is usually to determine concentrations effective *in vivo*. Little is known about the micro-environment in most infections, but nutritional immunity is an important component of the body defences (Weinberg 1978). Iron limitation of growth has special significance *in vivo* (Griffiths *et al.* 1980) and bacterial doubling times may be very long, measured in hours rather than minutes (Meynell & Subbiah 1963; Eudy & Burroughs 1973). It therefore seems unlikely that traditional nutrient broth cultures will be the best models for the *in vivo* situation and it may well be that slow-growing iron-limited cultures are more relevant for many purposes (Brown 1977).

Because many changes occur at the same time in response to a particular environment, it is usually difficult to identify which is the most important determinant of resistance. *Ps. aeruginosa* becomes resistant to the cationic antibiotics gentamicin and polymyxin when depleted of Mg^{2+} and at the same time forms large amounts of outer membrane protein H1. Resistant mutants also form this protein, which is thought may protect a binding site for cations (Nicas & Hancock 1980). One binding site, at least for polymyxin, may be neutral and anionic phospholipids (Teuber & Bader 1976). When *Ps. fluorescens* is depleted of phosphate it becomes resistant to polymyxin and these phospholipids are gradually replaced by a positively charged ornithine-amide lipid (Dorrer & Teuber 1977), which does not bind to polymyxin (Teuber & Miller 1977). Phosphate-depleted *Ps. aeruginosa* also becomes resistant to polymyxin, whether grown in batch culture or a chemostat. In this case, phospholipids are replaced by neutral lipids and fatty acids (M. Noy, pers. comm.). The reduction in cell envelope phosphorus content in chemostat-grown *Ps. aeruginosa* has also been linked to gentamicin resistance (Dean *et al.* 1976).

The permeability of the Gram negative outer membrane to nutrients is attributed to the protein pores, which change with changing conditions (Nikaido & Nakae 1979; Lugtenberg *et al.* 1976). It seems likely that the increased permeability of cells grown at high dilution rates will contribute to their increased sensitivity to hydrophilic antibiotics, such as gentamicin (Dean *et al.* 1976) and carbenicillin (Ombaka, 1980). Carbenicillin is thought to enter *E. coli* specifically through the *ompF* porin (Harder *et al.* 1981). The amount of this porin varies with different conditions, particularly osmolarity. As the concentration of saline is increased, the amount of porin decreases; in normal saline only about one-third as much is formed as in dilute media (van Alphen & Lugtenberg 1977).

Preparation of Defined Cells

Nutrient depletion in batch culture

At constant pH and temperature, growth rate is dependent upon the concentration of nutrients (Monod 1949). It can therefore be assumed that the onset of a slowing of the growth rate at the end of the exponential phase corresponds to the onset of the depletion of a particular nutrient. When all other ingredients are in excess, then cell mass at this point is proportional to the initial concentration of that nutrient. From a series of growth curves using different nutrient concentrations, a medium can be constructed which can be varied to permit depletion of any named ingredient, with all others in known excess (Table 1). On entering the stationary phase following exhaustion of an essential nutrient, the cell will begin to make an envelope appropriate to that particular depletion. The change is gradual and the longer the cells are 'stationary', the greater may be the change in properties (Klemperer 1976–77).

TABLE 1

Nutrient requirements for three Gram negative strains

Nutrient	Concentration (mmol/l) required for exponential aerobic growth to optical density = 1·0 (420 nm)		
	*Escherichia coli**	*Escherichia coli†*	*Proteus mirabilis‡*
Glucose	2·5	2·8	3·0
NH_4^+	1·85	1·75	5·0
K^+	0·026	0·042	0·035
Mg^{2+}	0·013	0·025	0·015
Fe^{2+}	0	0·0001	0
SO_4^{2-}	0·026	0·019	0·05
PO_4^{3-}	0·17	0·56	17·0

To determine requirement for each nutrient, all other nutrients were present in excess, approximately × 10.
* *E. coli* K12 W3110, buffered with 25 mmol/l 3-(*N*-morpholino) propane sulphonate (MOPS) pH 7·2 (Klemperer *et al.* 1979*b*).
† *E. coli* K12 W3110, containing R-plasmid RP1, buffered as * (Klemperer *et al.* 1979*b*).
‡ *P. mirabilis* NCTC 5887, buffered with 25 mmol/l MOPS pH 7·0 (Al-Dujaili 1979).

Method

(1) Using absorbance as an indicator of cell mass, prepare a series of growth curves for each ingredient.

(2) Plot the relation of absorbance at the onset of depletion to concentration of added nutrient.
(3) Calculate the concentration of each nutrient required to give a known absorbance and choose appropriate combinations of salts to permit depletion of one substance at the required absorbance with all other ingredients in excess (Klemperer *et al.* 1979*b*).

Nutrient limitation in continuous culture

Unlike a batch culture, which is a closed system in which the environment is gradually modified by the cells until it can no longer support rapid growth, a continuous culture is an open system in which the continual input of new medium and the removal of spent medium and cells maintain the cells growing in steady-state conditions.

Growth in a chemostat, in which the growth rate is determined by the dilution rate (D = rate of inflow of medium/volume of culture vessel), can be described by constants derived from batch culture (Herbert *et al.* 1956).

It can be calculated that in steady state conditions

$$\text{cell mass } (\bar{x}) = Y\left\{S_{\text{R}} - K_{\text{S}}\left(\frac{D}{\mu_{\text{m}} - D}\right)\right\},$$

where Y = yield constant, i.e. weight of cells formed/weight of substrate used; S_{R}^{-} = substrate concentration in the medium reservoir; K_{S} = saturation constant; μ_{m} = maximum specific growth rate. Y can be calculated from the graphs determined by batch culture and K_{S} and μ_{m} from a reciprocal plot of growth rate upon nutrient concentration.

Dilution rates can be varied theoretically from 0 (= batch culture) to μ_{m}. When $D > \mu_{\text{m}}$, cells are washed out faster than they can grow. Loss of substrate in the outflow is, in practice, negligible up to a high dilution rate and the theoretical yield (i.e. efficiency of utilization) is therefore nearly constant until the wash-out point is reached. However, cell properties may vary with growth rate and different limitations and this may be reflected in the yield (Tempest 1970).

Apparatus for continuous culture does not need to be sophisticated. A culture vessel with a side-arm for the culture outflow and some means of aeration can provide useful results. A simple system which can be made by any glass-blower has been described by Gilbert & Stuart (1977).

Measurement of Resistance

Effect of resuspending medium on resistance

Having obtained defined cells, the problem arises as to how to compare them under standard conditions. Cells depleted in batch culture may be tested for resistance *in situ*. This minimizes damage to cells, which may occur during handling and as a result of change of environment (Farwell & Brown 1971). Furthermore, the extent of damage due to physical stress, such as osmotic shock, may vary with envelope properties (Kenward & Brown 1978).

In many cases it is desirable to resuspend cells before testing. In batch culture, cell products liberated during growth, which may include cell wall polymers (Rothfield & Pearlman-Kothencz 1969), and which will vary with the depleting nutrient, may interfere with the assay of resistance. In continuous culture there is always a slight excess of the limiting substrate present (because growth rate is limited by the dilution rate) and cells harvested from continuous culture must either be exposed to the test antibiotic at once or be resuspended in a non-growth-supporting medium, so that they retain the characteristics of chemostat growth. The resuspending medium should be chosen to avoid large changes in pH or osmolarity, to reduce the risk of cell damage. Furthermore, the constitution of the medium may affect the action of the antibiotic (Zimelis & Jackson 1973; Klemperer *et al.* 1979*a*).

Assay of resistance

The effects of cell envelope variation on resistance have been analysed extensively using polymyxin, an antibiotic with a disinfectant-like action, which acts on non-growing cells (Finch & Brown 1975; Kenward *et al.* 1979). Most antibiotics act only on growing cells, and over a prolonged period of time cell envelopes would be expected to assume the characters of those associated with cells growing at a rate determined by the antibiotic. However, nutrient-depleted cells may retain their envelope characteristics for several generations (Brown & Melling 1969) and it has been found that differently defined cells show different sensitivities to a variety of antibiotics, presumably reflecting the cell wall permeabilities at the time of addition of the antibiotic (Dean *et al.* 1976; Ombaka 1980).

The flow chart shown in Fig. 4 indicates possible methods of test.

Cell Envelope Composition

Preparation of envelope fractions

Cell envelopes can be prepared by enzyme digestion of crude envelope preparations (Gray & Wilkinson, 1965), obtained by breaking cells using a variety of physical and chemical techniques. These methods may lead to a loss of some constituents, but until recently were the only ones available for the study of many types of cell.

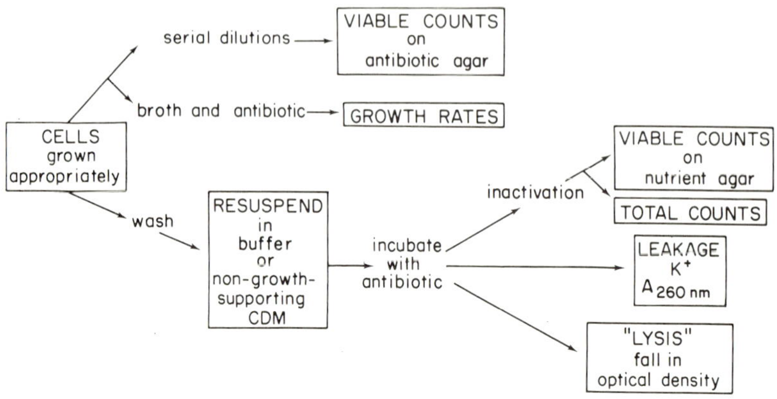

FIG. 4. Flow diagram showing possible methods of testing the effect of phenotypic variation on resistance to antibiotics. CDM, chemically defined medium.

Outer and cytoplasmic membranes from several Gram negative species have been separated by differential centrifugation on sucrose gradients (Osborn *et al.* 1972; Miura & Mizushima 1968; Hasin *et al.* 1975; Booth & Curtis 1977; Mizuno & Kageyama 1978; Hancock & Nikaido 1978) using cells growing in logarithmic phase in complex media.

Membranes change their characters with changing conditions, and when close in density are difficult to separate. Cozens & Brown (1981) have improved the resolution of this method and separated the outer and cytoplasmic membranes from both stationary phase and slow-growing chemostat cultures of *Ps. aeruginosa.*

Outer membranes may also be studied following the selective solubilization of the cytoplasmic membrane with detergents such as sarkosyl. This technique has been used to investigate protein composition (Filip *et al.* 1973; Schnaitmann 1971), and attempts are being made in this laboratory to apply the method to other membrane components.

Chemical analysis

Lipids may be readily extracted with chloroform : methanol (Bligh & Dyer 1959; Brown & Watkins 1970), and can be fractionated using organic solvents (Brown & Watkins 1970). The fractions can be assayed quantitatively by thin-layer chromatography. Phospholipids can be separated and their fatty acid content assayed by gas chromatography (McGarrity & Armstrong 1975).

Lipopolysaccharide (LPS) is present only in the outer membrane of Gram negative bacteria. In most species, it contains a unique sugar acid, 2-keto 3-deoxyoctonic acid (KDO). Determination of KDO by a colour reaction with thiobarbituric acid (Weissbach & Hurwitz 1959; Osborn *et al.* 1972) will give an indication of the LPS content.

Metal cations can be assayed by atomic absorption spectroscopy following digestion of membranes with boiling concentrated nitric acid and dissolution of the resulting 'ash' in concentrated hydrochloric acid (Kenward *et al.* 1979).

Extracellular material (e.g. slime) is most easily assayed gravimetrically, following precipitation from culture supernatants by the use of organic solvents (Ombaka 1980).

Protein content may be determined colorimetrically with Folin–Ciocalteu reagent as described by Lowry *et al.* (1951). Separation of proteins of differing molecular size can be carried out by polyacrylamide gel electrophoresis in the presence of sodium dodecyl sulphate (SDS–PAGE). We have found that the acrylamide concentration of 14% w/v used for *E. coli* (Lugtenberg *et al.* 1975) also produces good resolution of the major outer membrane proteins of *Ps. aeruginosa.*

Quantitative analysis of these proteins may be accomplished by densitometry of stained gels.

Antibiotics and Body Defence Mechanisms

The action of antibiotics on bacteria, especially on their envelopes, may influence the efficiency of body defence mechanisms. Thus polymyxin enhances the activity of lysozyme (Warren *et al.* 1957) and complement (Pruul & Reynolds 1972). Phagocytosis and intracellular killing may be either enhanced or antagonized (Alexander & Good 1968; Nishida *et al.* 1976; Pruul & McDonald 1979; Zak & Kradolfer 1979; Finch 1980; McDonald *et al.* 1981; Root *et al.* 1981). Adhesion of bacteria to tissue may also be enhanced or antagonized by antibiotics (Vosbeck *et al.* 1979; Sugarman, 1980).

There is much recent evidence that adhesion and engulfment occur mainly because of the difference in the surface free energies of phagocyte and particle (van Oss 1978). Correlations have been found between the surface hydrophobicity of bacteria and the degree to which they are engulfed by phagocytes. Specific surface components of both Gram positive (Miörner *et al.* 1980) and Gram negative (Stendahl *et al.* 1979) bacteria contribute to surface hydrophobicity. It is also influenced by iron limitation of growth (Magnussen *et al.* 1979). Furthermore, antibiotics may increase or decrease the surface hydrophobicity of bacteria and so alter the rate of engulfment (van Oss 1978). Tissue adhesion by bacteria is influenced by hydrophobicity in some cases (Carruthers & Anderson 1979; Gerson 1980).

Techniques for measuring surface hydrophobicity are relatively simple. The contact angle made with saline drops and layers of bacteria or phagocytes can be measured with a telescope attached to a goniometer (van Oss *et al.* 1975; van Oss 1978). The critical interfacial tension for spreading on cell layers has been determined from contact angles of a series of polymeric droplets from aqueous two-phase systems of dextrans and poly(ethylene glycol) (Schürch *et al.* 1981). Contact angles have also been calculated by measuring drop diameters (Dahlgren & Sunqvist 1981). Partitioning of bacteria in aqueous two-polymer phase systems has also been used to measure surface hydrophobicity (Stendahl *et al.* 1979). A rapid quantitative assay for hydrophobicity involves measuring the relative affinity of cells for liquid hydrocarbons or an aqueous phase (Rosenberg *et al.* 1980). Hydrophobic interaction chromatography has been used recently to screen bacteria for surface properties (Dahlbäck *et al.* 1981).

References

AL-DUJAILI, D. A. 1979 The effect of nutrient limitation on the drug resistance of *Proteus* species. Ph.D. Thesis, University of Aston in Birmingham.

ALEXANDER, J. W. & GOOD, R. A. 1968 Effect of antibiotics on the bactericidal activity of human leukocytes. *Journal of Laboratory and Clinical Medicine* **71,** 971–983.

BLIGH, E. G. & DYER, W. J. 1959 A rapid method of total lipid extraction and purification. *Canadian Journal of Biochemistry and Physiology* **37,** 911–917.

BOOTH, B. R. & CURTIS, N. A. C. 1977 Separation of the cytoplasmic and outer membrane of *Pseudomonas aeruginosa* PAO1. *Biochemical and Biophysical Research Communications* **74,** 1168–1176.

BRAUN, V. 1978 Structure–function relationships of the Gram-negative bacterial cell envelope. In *Relations between Structure and Function in the Prokaryotic Cell,* ed. Stanier, R. Y., Rogers, H. J. and Wood, B. J. pp. 111–138. Society for General Microbiology Symposium 28. Cambridge: Cambridge University Press.

BRAUN, V. & KRIEGER-BRAUER, H. J. 1977 Interrelationship of the phage λ receptor protein and maltose transport in mutants of *Escherichia coli* K-12. *Biochimica et Biophysica Acta* **469,** 89–98.

BROWN, M. R. W. 1977 Nutrient depletion and antibiotic susceptibility. *Journal of Antimicrobial Chemotherapy* **3,** 198–201.

BROWN, M. R. W. & MELLING, J. 1969 Role of divalent cations in the action of polymyxin B and EDTA on *Pseudomonas aeruginosa*. *Journal of General Microbiology* **59,** 263–274.

BROWN, M. R. W. & WATKINS, W. 1970 Low magnesium and phospholipid content of cell walls of *Pseudomonas aeruginosa* resistant to polymyxin. *Nature, London* **227,** 1360–1361.

BROWN, M. R. W., SCOTT-FOSTER, J. H. & CLAMP, J. R. 1969 Composition of *Pseudomonas aeruginosa* slime. *Biochemical Journal* **112,** 521–525.

BROWN, M. R. W., GILBERT, P. & KLEMPERER, R. M. M. 1979 Influence of the bacterial cell envelope on combined antibiotic action. In *Antibiotic Interactions*, ed. Williams, J. D. pp. 72–76. London & New York: Academic Press.

CARRUTHERS, M. M. & ANDERSON, B. 1979 Inhibition by polyanions of adherence by Kanagawa positive *Vibrio parahaemolyticus:* A physico-chemical effect. *Journal of Infectious Diseases* **140,** 119–122.

COSTERTON, J. W. 1977 Cell envelope as a barrier to antibiotics. In *Microbiology*, ed. Schlessinger, D. pp. 151–157. Washington: American Society for Microbiology.

COSTERTON, J. W., BROWN, M. R. W. & STURGESS, J. M. 1979 The cell envelope: its role in infection. In *Pseudomonas aeruginosa: Clinical manifestations and Current Therapy*, ed. Doggett, R. G. pp. 41–62. London & New York: Academic Press.

COZENS, R. M. & BROWN, M. R. W. 1981 Separation of outer and cytoplasmic membranes from stationary phase and chemostat cultures of *Pseudomonas aeruginosa. Society for General Microbiology Quarterly* **8,** 131.

DAHLBÄCK, B., HERMANSSON, M., KJELLEBERG, S. & NORKRANS, B. 1981 The hydrophobicity of bacteria—an important factor in their initial adhesion at the air–water interface. *Archives of Microbiology* **128,** 267–270.

DAHLGREN, C. & SUNQVIST, T. 1981 Phagocytosis and hydrophobicity: a method of calculating contact angles based on the diameter of sessile drops. *Journal of Immunological Methods* **40,** 171–179.

DEAN, A. C. R., ELLWOOD, D. C., MELLING, J. & ROBINSON, A. 1976 The action of antibacterial agents on bacteria grown in continuous culture. In *Continuous Culture 6: Applications and New Fields*, ed. Dean, A. C. R., Ellwood, D. C., Evans, C. G. T. and Melling, J. pp. 251–261. Chichester: Ellis Horwood.

DORRER, E. & TEUBER, M. 1977 Induction of polymyxin resistance in *Pseudomonas fluorescens* by phosphate limitation. *Archives of Microbiology* **114,** 87–89.

ELLWOOD, D. C. & TEMPEST, D. W. 1972 Effects of environment on bacterial wall content and composition. *Advances in Microbial Physiology* **7,** 83–117.

EUDY, W. W. & BURROUGHS, S. E. 1973 Generation times of *Proteus mirabilis* and *Escherichia coli* in experimental infections. *Chemotherapy* **19,** 161–170.

FARWELL, J. A. & BROWN, M. R. W. 1971 Effect of inoculum history on the inhibition and destruction of the microbial cell. In *Inhibition and Destruction of the Microbial Cell*, ed. Hugo, W. B. pp. 703–752. London & New York: Academic Press.

FILIP, C., FLETCHER, G., WULFF, J. L. & EARHART, C. F. 1973 Solubilization of the cytoplasmic membrane of *Escherichia coli* by the ionic detergent sodium-lauryl sarcosinate. *Journal of Bacteriology* **115,** 717–722.

FINCH, R. 1980 Immunomodulating effects of antimicrobial agents. *Journal of Antimicrobial Chemotherapy* **6,** 691–699.

FINCH, J. E. & BROWN, M. R. W. 1975 The influence of nutrient limitation in a chemostat on the sensitivity of *Pseudomonas aeruginosa* to polymyxin and to EDTA. *Journal of Antimicrobial Chemotherapy* **1,** 379–386.

GERSON, D. F. 1980 Cell surface energy, contact angles and phase partition. 1. Lymphocytic cell lines in biphasic aqueous mixtures. *Biochimica et Biophysica Acta* **602,** 269–280.

GILBERT, P. & BROWN, M. R. W. 1978 Influence of growth rate and nutrient limitation on the gross cellular composition of *Pseudomonas aeruginosa* and its resistance to 3- and 4-chlorophenol. *Journal of Bacteriology* **133,** 1066–1072.

GILBERT, P. & BROWN, M. R. W. 1980 Cell wall mediated changes in sensitivity of *Bacillus megaterium* to chlorhexidine and 2-phenoxyethanol, associated with growth rate and nutrient limitation. *Journal of Applied Bacteriology* **48,** 223–230.

GILBERT, P. & STUART, A. 1977 Small scale chemostat for the growth of mesophilic and thermophilic microorganisms. *Laboratory Practice* **26,** 627–628.

GRAY, G. W. & WILKINSON, S. G. 1965 The action of ethylenediaminetetra-acetic acid on *Pseudomonas aeruginosa*. *Journal of Applied Bacteriology* **28,** 153–164.

GRIFFITHS, E., ROGERS, H. J. & BULLEN, J. J. 1980 Iron, plasmids and infection. *Nature, London* **284,** 508–509

HANCOCK, R. E. W. & NIKAIDO, H. 1978 Outer membranes of Gram-negative bacteria XIX. Isolation from *Pseudomonas aeruginosa* PAO1 and use in reconstitution and definition of the permeability barrier. *Journal of Bacteriology* **136,** 381–390.

HARDER, K. J., NIKAIDO, H. & MATSUHASHI, M. 1981 Mutants of *Escherichia coli* that are resistant to certain beta-lactam compounds lack the *ompF* porin. *Antimicrobial Agents and Chemotherapy* **20,** 549–552.

HASIN, M., ROTTEM, S. & RAZIN, S. 1975 The outer membrane of *Proteus mirabilis*. I. Isolation and characterization of the outer and cytoplasmic membrane fractions. *Biochimica et Biophysica Acta* **375,** 381–394.

HERBERT, D., ELSWORTH, R. & TELLING, R. C. 1956 The continuous culture of bacteria; a theoretical and experimental study. *Journal of General Microbiology* **14,** 601–622.

HUGO, W. B. & DAVIDSON, J. R. 1973 Effect of cell lipid depletion in *Staphylococcus aureus* upon its resistance to antimicrobial agents. 2. A comparison of the response of normal and lipid-depleted cells of *S. aureus* to antibacterial drugs. *Microbios* **8,** 63–72.

KENWARD, M. A. & BROWN, M. R. W. 1978 Relation between growth rate and sensitivity to cold shock of *Pseudomonas aeruginosa*. *Federation of European Microbiological Societies Microbiology Letters* **3,** 17–19.

KENWARD, M. A., BROWN, M. R. W. & FRYER, J. J. 1979 The influence of calcium or magnesium on the resistance to EDTA, polymyxin B or cold shock, and the composition of *Pseudomonas aeruginosa* in glucose or magnesium depleted batch cultures. *Journal of Applied Bacteriology* **47,** 489–503.

KLEMPERER, R. M. M. 1976–77 The development of resistance to polymyxin by *Pseudomonas aeruginosa* following sulphate depletion. *Proceedings of the Society for General Microbiology* **4,** 37.

KLEMPERER, R. M. M., GILBERT, P., MEIER, M. M., COZENS, R. M. & BROWN, M. R. W. 1979*a* Influence of suspending media upon the susceptibility of *Pseudomonas aeruginosa NCTC* 6750, and its spheroplasts to polymyxin B. *Antimicrobial Agents and Chemotherapy* **15,** 147–151.

KLEMPERER, R. M. M., ISMAIL, N. T. A. J. & BROWN, M. R. W. 1979*b* Effect of R-plasmid RP1 on the nutritional requirements of *Escherichia coli* in batch culture. *Journal of General Microbiology* **115,** 325–331.

KLEMPERER, R. M. M., ISMAIL, N. T. A. J. & BROWN, M. R. W. 1980 Effect of R-plasmid RP1 and nutrient depletion on the resistance of *Escherichia coli* to cetrimide, chlorhexidine and phenol. *Journal of Applied Bacteriology* **48,** 349–357.

KRAUSE, R. M. 1977 Cell wall antigens of Gram-positive bacteria and their biological activities. In *Microbiology*, ed. Schlessinger, D. pp. 151–157. Washington: American Society for Microbiology.

LOWRY, O. H., ROSEBROUGH, N. J., FARR, A. L. & RANDALL, R. J. 1951 Protein measurement with the folin phenol reagent. *Journal of Biological Chemistry* **193,** 265–275.

LUGTENBERG, B., MEIJERS, J., PETERS, R., VAN DER HOEK, P. & VAN ALPHEN, L. 1975 Electrophoresis resolution of the major outer membrane protein of *Escherichia coli* K-12 into four bands. *Federation of European Biochemical Societies, Letters* **58,** 254–258.

LUGTENBERG, B., PETERS, R., BERHEIMER, H. & BERENDSEN, W. 1976 Influence of cultural conditions and mutations on the composition of the outer membrane proteins of *Escherichia coli. Molecular and General Genetics* **147,** 251–262.

MAGNUSSEN, K.-L., KIHLSTROM, E., NORQVIST, A., DAVIES, J. & NORMARK, S. 1979 Effect of iron on surface charge and hydrophobicity of *Neisseria gonorrhoeae. Infection and Immunity* **26,** 402–407.

MCDONALD, P. J., WETHERALL, B. L. & PRUUL, H. 1981 Postantibiotic leukocyte enhancement: increased susceptibility of bacteria pretreated with antibiotics to activity of leukocytes. *Reviews of Infectious Diseases* **3,** 38–44.

MCGARRITY, J. T. & ARMSTRONG, J. B. 1975 The effect of salt on the phospholipid fatty acid composition in *Escherichia coli* K-12. *Biochimica et Biophysica Acta* **398,** 258–264.

MEYNELL, G. G. & SUBBIAH, T. V. 1963 The true division and death rate of *Salmonella typhimurium* in the mouse spleen determined with superinfecting phage 22. *British Journal of Experimental Pathology* **44,** 197–219.

MIÖRNER, H., MYHRE, E., BJORCK, L. & KRONVALL, G. 1980 Effect of specific binding of human albumin, fibrinogen and immunoglobulin G on surface characteristics of bacterial strains as revealed by partition experiments in polymer phase systems. *Infection and Immunity* **29,** 879–885.

MIURA, T. & MIZUSHIMA, S. 1968 Separation by density gradient centrifugation of two types of membranes from spheroplast membrane of *Escherichia coli* K-12. *Biochimica et Biophysica Acta* **150,** 159–161.

MIZUNO, T. & KAGEYAMA, M. 1978 Separation and characterization of the outer membrane of *Pseudomonas aeruginosa. Journal of Biochemistry* **84,** 179–191.

MONOD, J. 1949 The growth of bacterial cultures. *Annual Review of Microbiology* **3,** 371–394.

NICAS, T. I. & HANCOCK, R. E. W. 1980 Outer membrane protein H1 of *Pseudomonas aeruginosa*: involvement in adaptive and mutational resistance to ethylenediaminetetraacetate, polymyxin B, and gentamicin. *Journal of Bacteriology* **143,** 872–878.

NIKAIDO, H. 1979 Nonspecific transport through the outer membrane. In *Bacterial Outer Membranes*, ed. Inouye, M. Chap. 11, pp. 361–407. New York: John Wiley & Sons.

NIKAIDO, H. & NAKAE, T. 1979 The outer membrane of Gram-negative bacteria. *Advances in Microbial Physiology* **20,** 163–250.

NISHIDA, M., MINE, Y., NONOYAMA, S. & YOKOTA, Y. 1976 Effect of antibiotics on the phagocytosis and killing of *Pseudomonas aeruginosa* by rabbit polymorphonuclear leukocytes. *Chemotherapy* **22,** 203–210.

OMBAKA, E. A. 1980 The effect of environment on virulence factors and resistance of mucoid strains of *Pseudomonas aeruginosa*. Ph.D. Thesis, University of Aston in Birmingham.

OSBORN, M. J. & WU, H. C. P. 1980 Proteins of the outer membrane of Gram-negative bacteria. *Annual Review of Microbiology* **34,** 369–422.

OSBORN, M. J., GANDER, J. E., PARISI, E. & CARSON, J. 1972 Mechanism of assembly of the outer membrane of *Salmonella typhimurium*. *Journal of Biological Chemistry* **247,** 3962–3972.

PRUUL, H. & McDONALD, P. J. 1979 Enhancement of leukocyte activity against *Escherichia coli* after brief exposure to chloramphenicol. *Antimicrobial Agents and Chemotherapy* **16**, 695–700.

PRUUL, H. & REYNOLDS, B. L. 1972 Interaction of complement and polymyxin with Gram-negative bacteria. *Infection and Immunity* **6,** 709–717.

REAVELEY, D. A. & BURGE, R. E. 1972 Walls and membranes in bacteria. *Advances in Microbial Physiology* **7,** 1–81.

ROGERS, H. J., WARD, J. B. & BURDETT, I. D. J. 1978 Structure and growth of the walls of Gram-positive bacteria. In *Relations between Structure and Function in the Prokaryotic Cell*, ed. Stanier, R. Y., Rogers, H. J. & Ward, J. B. pp. 139–176. Symposium of Society for General Microbiology 28. Cambridge: University Press.

ROOT, R. K., ISTURIZ, R., MOLAVI, A., METCALF, J. A. & MALECH, H. L. 1981 Interactions between antibiotics and human neutrophils in the killing of staphylococci. *Journal of Clinical Investigation* **67,** 247–259.

ROSENBERG, M., GUTNICK, D. & ROSENBERG, E. 1980 Adherence of bacteria to hydrocarbons: a simple method for measuring cell-surface hydrophobicity. *Federation of European Microbiological Societies Microbiology Letters* **9,** 29–33.

ROTHFIELD, L. & PEARLMAN-KOTHENCZ, M. 1969 Synthesis and assembly of bacterial membrane components. A lipopolysaccharide-phospholipid-protein complex excreted by living bacteria. *Journal of Molecular Biology* **44,** 477–492.

SCHINDLER, H. & ROSENBUSCH, J. D. 1978 Matrix protein from *Escherichia coli* outer membranes forms voltage-controlled channels in lipid bilayers. *Proceedings of the National Academy of Sciences of the United States* **75,** 3751–3755.

SCHNAITMANN, C. A. 1971 Solubilization of the cytoplasmic membrane of *Escherichia coli* by Triton X-100. *Journal of Bacteriology* **108,** 545–552.

SCHÜRCH, S., GERSON, D. F. & McIVER, D. J. L. 1981 Determination of cell/medium interfacial tensions from contact angles in aqueous polymer systems. *Biochimica et Biophysica Acta* **640,** 557–571.

SLEYTR, U. B. 1978 Regular arrays of macromolecules on bacterial cell walls: structure, chemistry, assembly and function. *International Review of Cytology* **53,** 1–64.

STENDAHL, O., NORMANN, B. & EDEBO, L. 1979 Influence of O and K antigens on the surface properties of *Escherichia coli* in relation to phagocytosis. *Acta Pathologica et Microbiologica Scandinavica Section B* **87,** 85–91.

STOCK, J. B., RAUCH, B. & ROSEMAN, S. 1977 Periplasmic space in *Salmonella typhimurium* and *Escherichia coli*. *Journal of Biological Chemistry* **252,** 7850–7861.

SUGARMAN, B. 1980 Attachment of bacteria to mammalian surfaces. *Infection* **8,** 132–141.

SUTHERLAND, I. W. 1979 Microbial exopolysaccharides: control of synthesis and acylation. In *Microbial Polysaccharides and Polysaccharases*, ed. Berkeley, R. C. W., Gooday, G. W. & Ellwood, D. C. pp. 1–34. London and New York: Academic Press.

TEMPEST, D. W. 1970 The continuous cultivation of microorganisms. 1. Theory of the chemostat. In *Methods in Microbiology*, ed. Norris, J. R. & Ribbons, D. W. Vol. 2, pp. 259–276, London & New York: Academic Press.

TEUBER, M. and BADER, J. 1976 Action of polymyxin B on bacterial membranes. *Archives of Microbiology* **109,** 51–58.

TEUBER, M. and MILLER, I. R. 1977 Selective binding of polymyxin B to negatively charged lipid monolayers. *Biochimica et Biophysica Acta* **467,** 280–289.

VAN ALPHEN, W. & LUGTENBERG, B. 1977 Influence of osmolarity of the growth medium on the outer membrane protein pattern of *Escherichia coli. Journal of Bacteriology* **131,** 623–630.

VAN ALPHEN, W., VAN SELM, N. & LUGTENBERG, B. 1978 Pores in the outer membrane of *Escherichia coli* K-12: involvement of proteins b and e in the functioning of pores for nucleotides. *Molecular and General Genetics* **159,** 75–83.

VAN OSS, C. J. 1978 Phagocytosis as a surface phenomenon. *Annual Review of Microbiology* **32,** 19–39.

VAN OSS, C. J., GILLMAN, C. F. & NEUMANN, A. W. 1975 In *Phagocytic Engulfment and Cell Adhesiveness as Cellular Surface Phenomena*, Chap. 2, pp. 7–19. New York: Marcel Dekker.

VOSBECK, K., HANDSCHIN, H., MENGE, E.-B. & ZAK, O. 1979 Effects of subminimal inhibitory concentrations of antibiotics on adhesiveness of *Escherichia coli in vitro. Reviews of Infectious Diseases* **1,** 845–851.

WARREN, G. H., GRAY, J. & YURCHENCO, J. A. 1957 Effect of polymyxin on the lysis of *Neisseria catarrhalis* by lysozyme. *Journal of Bacteriology* **74,** 788–793.

WEINBERG, E. D. 1978 Iron and infection. *Microbiological Reviews* **42,** 45–66.

WEISSBACH, A. & HURWITZ, J. 1959 The formation of 2-keto-3-deoxyheptanoic acid in extracts of *Escherichia coli* B. *Journal of Biological Chemistry* **234,** 705–709.

ZAK, O. & KRADOLFER, F. 1979 Effects of subminimal inhibitory concentrations of antibiotics in experimental infections. *Reviews of Infectious Diseases* **1,** 862–879.

ZIMELIS, V. M. & JACKSON, G. G. 1973 Activity of aminoglycoside antibiotics against *Pseudomonas aeruginosa*: specificity and site of calcium and magnesium antagonism. *Journal of Infectious Diseases* **127,** 633–669.

Ionophoric Antibiotics as Experimental Tools in Microbiology

S. P. Denyer and W. B. Hugo

Department of Pharmacy, University of Nottingham, Nottingham

The ionophoric antibiotics can be divided into two main groups. One group can form complexes with ions similar to the clathrate compounds recognized by the organic chemist. The complex so formed confers a lipid solubility on the sequestered ion which is then able to traverse the lipid membrane of animal, plant and microbial cells, and the membranes of subcellular organelles such as mitochondria and chloroplasts. Among the complex-formers two subclasses can be recognized, depending on the chemical structure of the complexing molecule. In one, the complex carries a residual positive charge, in the other, due to the presence of a carboxyl group on the molecule, the final complex is neutral.

Another group acts differently, actually inserting themselves into lipid membranes and, as a result, creating channels or pores in the membrane. The molecular dimensions of the intruding molecule dictate the size of the pore, which in turn determines the size of the ion most readily accommodated and transmitted by that pore. Historically, the first ionophore to be discovered, but not so-called, was an ion-transmitting channel-forming ionophore, gramicidin A.

It should also be recorded that a number of synthetic molecules with ionophoric properties have been made. These are the cryptates and the polyethers.

The study of ionophore action contributed significantly to the substantiation and clarification of the chemiosmotic hypothesis of Mitchell (see Mitchell 1972). This has provided an answer to the problem of the mechanism by which metabolism is linked to solute transport and the generation of ATP in mitochondria, chloroplasts and bacteria. In brief, a metabolically generated proton gradient formed across the membrane was to provide the driving power for these activities (Fig. 1). Thus, an agent

ANTIBIOTICS
ISBN 0 12 604480 5

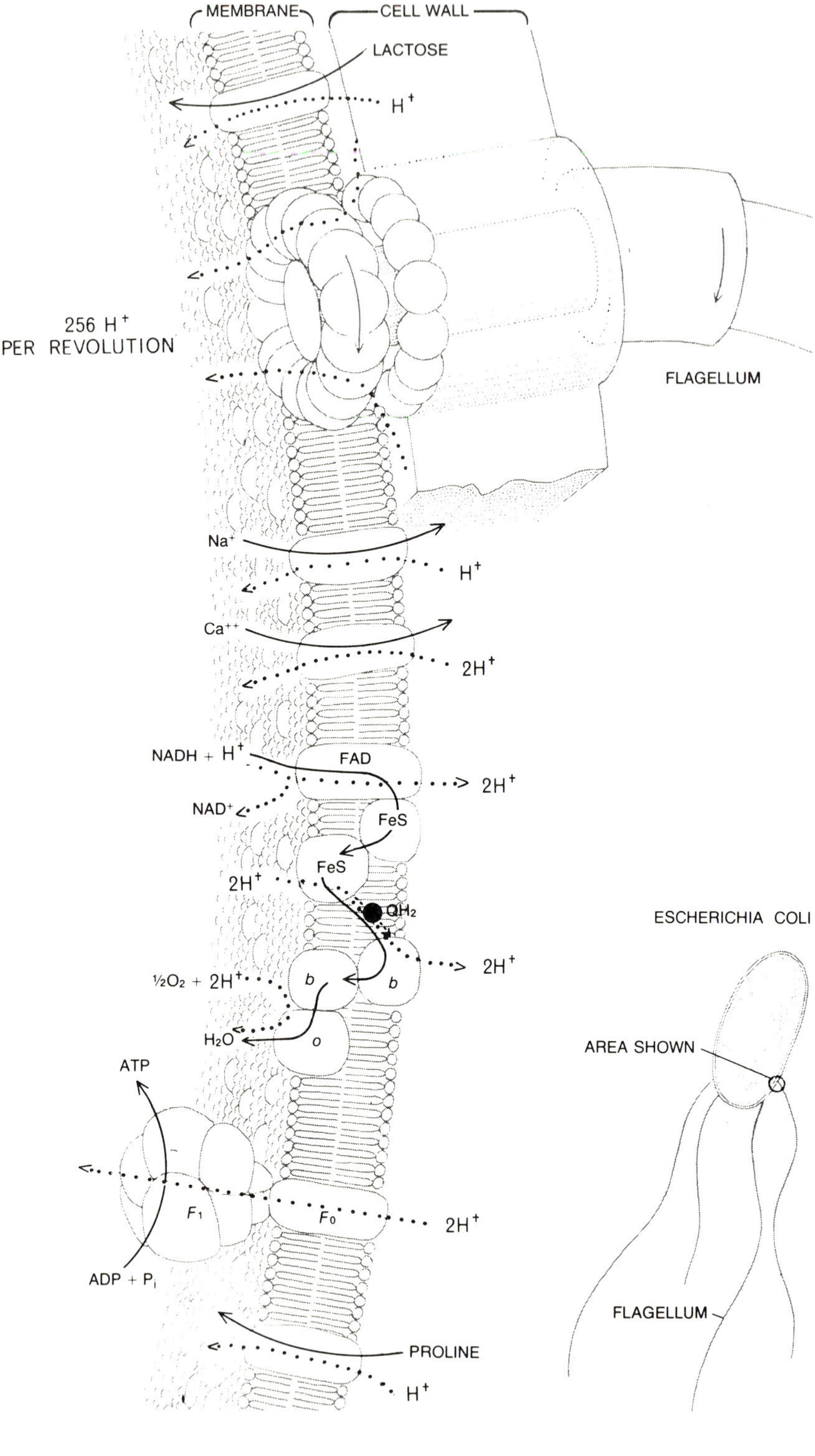

MEMBRANE
CELL WALL
LACTOSE
H^+
256 H^+
PER REVOLUTION
FLAGELLUM
Na^+
H^+
Ca^{++}
$2H^+$
NADH + H^+
FAD
$2H^+$
NAD^+
FeS
FeS
$2H^+$
QH_2
$2H^+$
$\frac{1}{2}O_2 + 2H^+$
b
b
H_2O
o
ATP
F_1
F_0
$2H^+$
ADP + P_i
PROLINE
H^+
ESCHERICHIA COLI
AREA SHOWN
FLAGELLUM

capable of destroying a proton gradient or otherwise modifying an ion gradient may well have profound biochemical consequences.

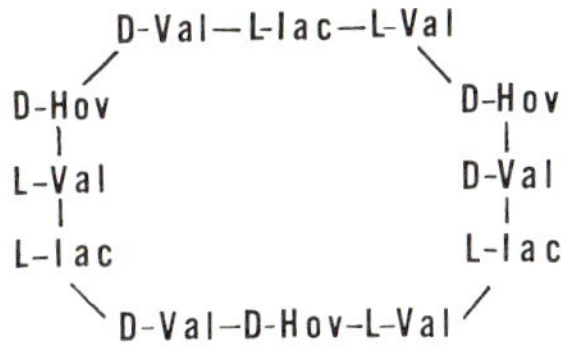

VALINOMYCIN

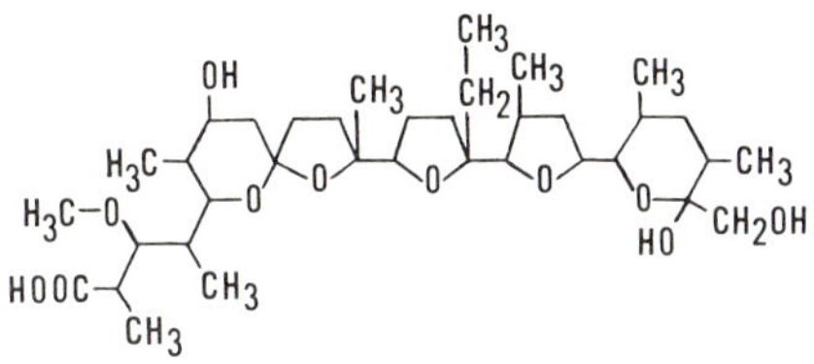

MONENSIN

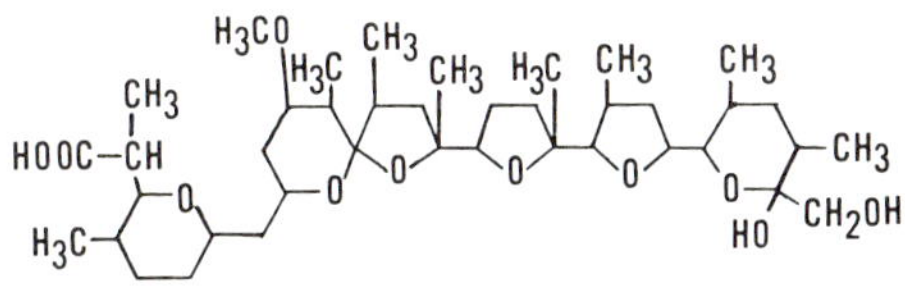

NIGERICIN

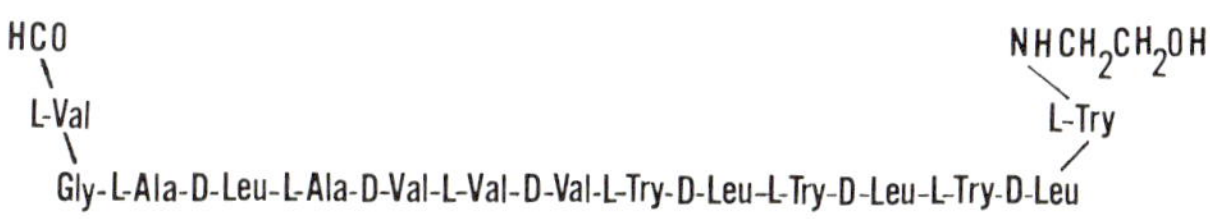

GRAMICIDIN A

FIG. 2. The structures of some ionophoric antibiotics used in membrane research. Hov = α-hydroxyisovaleric acid, Lac = lactic acid, Val = valine, Ala = alanine, Leu = leucine, Try = tryptophan, Gly = glycine.

FIG. 1. Chemiosmosis and the bacterial membrane. A proton gradient is generated by the operation of the respiratory chain. The passage of protons down this gradient can be coupled to ATP synthesis, active transport and flagellar motion. (From 'How cells make ATP' by Hinkle & McCarty. Copyright © 1978 by Scientific American, Inc. All rights reserved.)

TABLE 1

Ionophores frequently used in fundamental membrane research

Ionophore	Class	Date of discovery	Source	Ion affinity
Valinomycin	Neutral complexing agent	1955	*Streptomyces fulvissimus*	$H > Rb > K \gg NH_4 > Na > Li$
Monensin	Charged complexing agents	1967	*S. cinnamonensis*	$Na \gg K > Rb > Li > Cs$
Nigericin		1951	*Streptomyces* spp.	$K > Rb > Na > Cs > Li$
Gramicidin A	Channel-former	1939	*Bacillus brevis*	$H > Rb > NH_4 > K > Na > Li$

In this, too, a possible reason may be seen for the general toxicity of ionophores as they do not distinguish between the membranes of the host and invader, a prerequisite for a chemotherapeutic agent. However one, monensin, has found application in veterinary medicine for the treatment of coccidiosis in poultry, especially poultry reared under intensive conditions. This ionophore has also been used in beef production to induce the ruminant metabolic pathways to produce less methane which represents a loss of carbon to the general nutrition of the animal.

Individual Ionophores

There are many detailed reviews on ionophores which attempt to encompass the vast literature (e.g. Harold *et al.* 1974; Bakker 1979; Jain 1972). In this account the review will be restricted to the four representative compounds shown in Table 1 and illustrated in Fig. 2 as having probably been those most frequently used in fundamental membrane research. The antibacterial activity of this group of antibiotics is generally confined to Gram positive cells since the cell envelope of Gram negative bacteria acts as a barrier to adsorption.

Valinomycin

This compound, discovered in Germany in 1951, inhibits the growth of Gram positive bacteria at 1·0 μg/ml which is also the LD_{50} concentration towards mice (i.v. or i.p.).

Chemically it is a cyclododecadepsipeptide consisting of a trimer of the sequence D-valine, L-lactic acid, L-valine and D-α-hydroxyisovaleric acid. It has a mol. wt of 1110 daltons.

Biochemically, valinomycin was found to act as an uncoupling agent. Later studies, notably by Pressman and his school (Pressman 1963), showed that its mode of action differed from that of the 'classical' uncoupler 2,4-dinitrophenol. At physiological pH values valinomycin is able to form a lipid-soluble carrier complex with the potassium ion and transmit it across the cytoplasmic membrane of the microbial cell (Fig. 3). Depending on the external K^+ concentration the cell may be drained of its K^+ complement and protein synthesis, dependent on K^+, ceases. An efflux or influx of a charged species, whether by natural metabolism or by means of a carrier, will also modify the membrane potential ($\Delta\Psi$) which forms part of the proton motive force (Δp), the basic transducer, according to Mitchell, for many energy-requiring mechanisms in prokaryotes. The reduction of this component of Δp can account for the uncoupling action of valinomycin.

Thus, in simple summary, valinomycin can deplete the cell of essential potassium (Fig. 4*a*) and under certain conditions can destroy or seriously reduce the proton motive force.

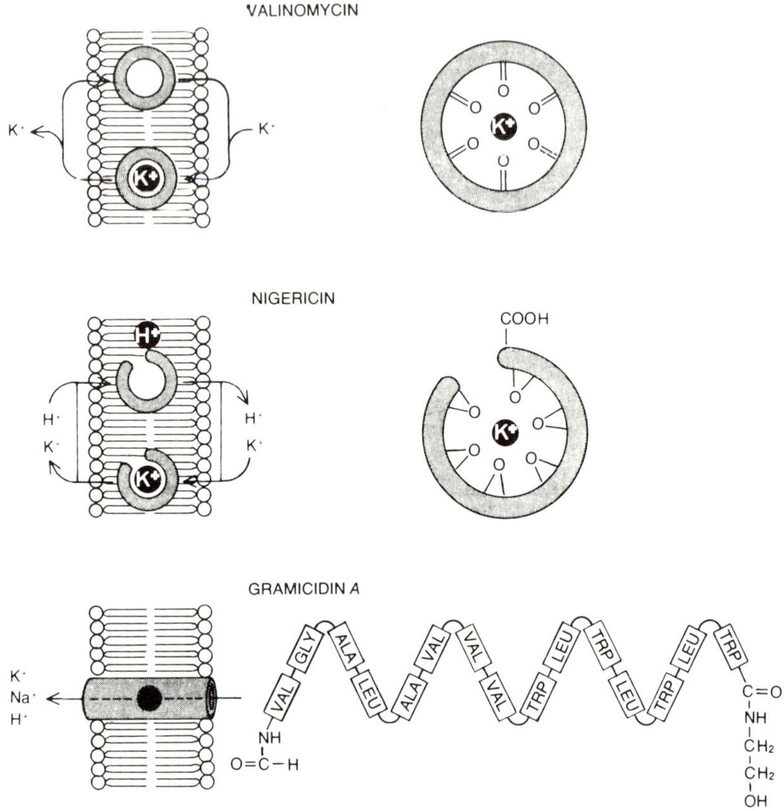

FIG. 3. Ion transport by ionophores. Valinomycin and nigericin, when complexed with potassium, act as circulating carriers within the membrane. Nigericin will only transport potassium in exchange for protons. Gramicidin A forms a pore in the membrane which is freely permeable to monovalent cations. Each pore consists of two helical molecules and has a lifetime of about half a second. (From 'How cells make ATP' by Hinkle & McCarty. Copyright © 1978 by Scientific American, Inc. All rights reserved.)

Monensin and nigericin

In contrast to valinomycin these two ionophores contain a carboxylic acid group in the molecule and therefore form a neutral complex with cations. As to their sequestering properties, monensin has a much greater affinity for the sodium ion than the potassium ion while nigericin, like valinomycin, has a high affinity for potassium ions. These ionophores can translate either

Na^+ or K^+ ions across a lipid membrane, in exchange for protons, by a circulating carrier mechanism (Fig. 3).

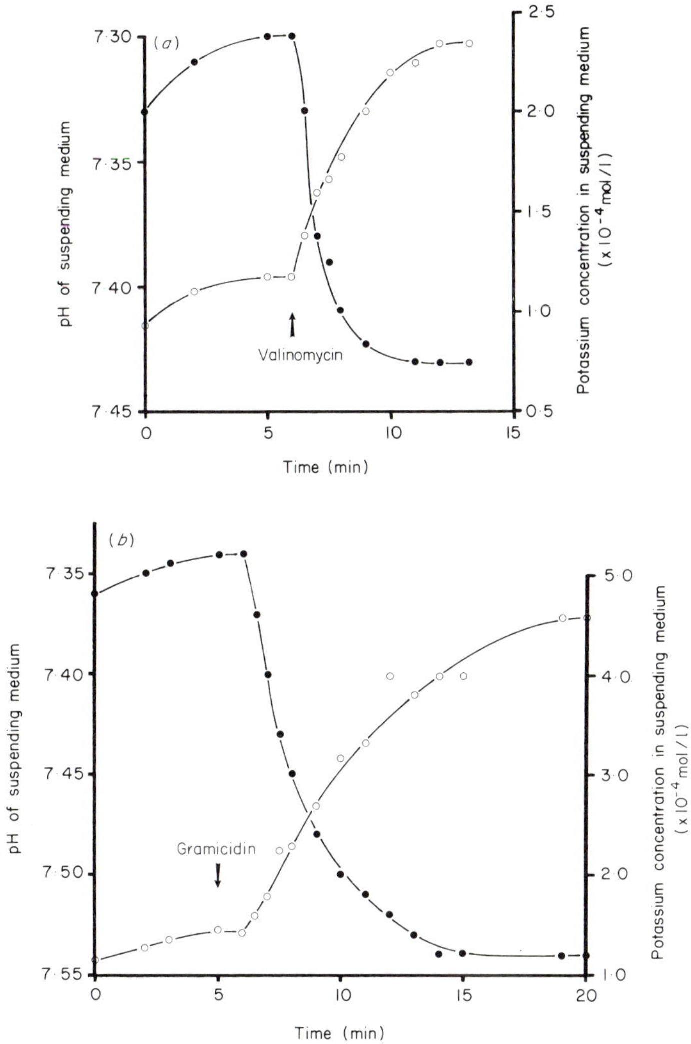

FIG. 4. Ion fluxes in the presence of ionophores. *Staphylococcus aureus* (NCTC 6571) cells were grown overnight on the surface of nutrient agar (Oxoid Ltd, Basingstoke), harvested, washed twice and finally resuspended to 4×10^9 cells/ml in 50 ml 1 mmol/l Tris–HCl buffer, pH 7·5 (25°C). The ionophores (*a*) valinomycin, and (*b*) gramicidin D, at a final concentration of 1 μg/ml, were added as a 25 μl aliquot from a stock solution in acetone. The suspension was stirred continuously with a magnetic stirrer and changes in pH (●—●) and potassium ion concentration (○—○) were followed using the appropriate ion-selective electrode. All solutions were prepared from triple distilled water.

Gramicidin A

This antibiotic has already been mentioned as an early discovery, in 1939, and it was Hladky & Haydon (1970) who first showed that it owed its biological uncoupling effect to its ability to insert itself into lipid membranes and form an ion-conducting channel. Gramicidin A forms a pore in the membrane, made up of two helical molecules, that is permeable to ions with one positive charge (Fig. 3). It is likely that all linear gramicidins act in this fashion.

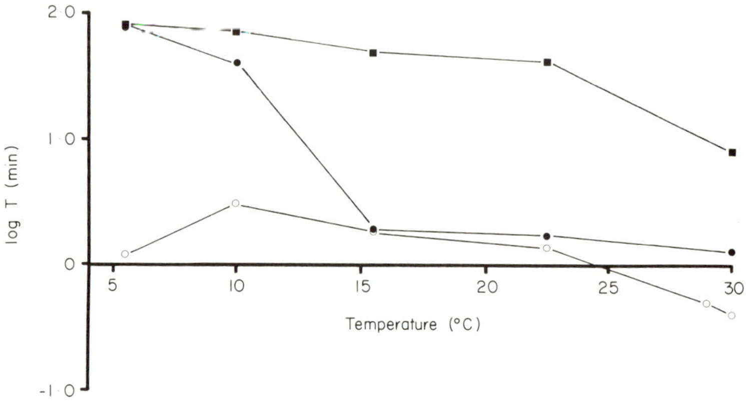

FIG. 5. The effect of temperature on ionophoric activity. *Staphylococcus aureus* cells were harvested as before (see Fig. 4), suspended in 50 ml 1 mmol/l Tris–HCl buffer, pH 7·5, and maintained at 30°C in the presence or absence of ionophore. After 10 min the suspension was removed, cooled to the required temperature and adjusted to a pH between 7·55 and 7·60 with aliquots of 0·1 mol/l HCl or Tris base. The slow flux of protons and potassium ions was monitored with ion selective electrodes. When a base line had been established and the pH returned to 7·5, 250 μl of a 2 mol/l solution of KCl in water was added. The subsequent inward passage of potassium elicited a charge-compensating efflux of protons which was recorded as a change in pH. Suspensions were stirred continuously throughout and all solutions were prepared from triple distilled water. T = time taken for the compensatory pH change to reach half its maximum value. ■—■, Control cells (ionophore absent); ○—○, gramicidin-treated cells; ●—●, valinomycin-treated cells.

The action of a pore-forming ionophore can be distinguished from that of a complex-forming carrier by observing the effect of temperature on ion conductance. At low temperatures, below its transition temperature, a membrane exists in a solid 'frozen' state. As the temperature is increased to a point above the transition temperature the membrane gradually 'melts', finally achieving a liquid or fluid state. It might be supposed that, once introduced into the membrane, a complex-forming ionophore would only conduct ions while free to move as a circulating carrier. Krasne *et al.* (1971) have shown this to be the case for an artificial membrane system, the ionophoric properties of valinomycin exhibiting a marked temperature dependence, in complete contrast to the pore-forming antibiotic gramicidin which provides an ion-transmitting channel even in the solid-state membrane.

It was considered to be of interest to apply this approach to a biological system. Figure 5 shows the results obtained from following the reflex proton flux (see Fig. 4) induced by the addition of KCl to whole cells of *Staphylococcus aureus* pretreated with either gramicidin D or valinomycin. One striking feature of this work was the almost total absence of a response to valinomycin at temperatures below 10°C, while the ionophoric properties of gramicidin remained essentially unaffected by temperature. It is most interesting that a temperature-dependent drug effect which has been noted in an entirely artificial system appears to be elicited in the intact cell. There are no conceptual reasons why this should not be the case but to the best of our knowledge this is the first time it has been demonstrated in a living system. As a cautionary note, however, it must be remembered that in a biological system the contribution made by membrane-bound carriers to ion flux may also be influenced by temperature.

Experimental Applications

In this section we have chosen to illustrate the use to which ionophores can be put with a summary of experiments employing valinomycin. Success in this field depends upon a meticulous attention to experimental detail. It will become evident that even the slightest change in ionic concentration may markedly alter the response from a given bacterial suspension.

This work is largely concerned with the practical aspects of ionophore usage and for a more extensive theoretical treatment of ionophoric antibiotics as probes of transport the reader is referred to Harold *et al.* (1974).

Manipulation of ion gradients

In brief, ionophoric antibiotics can be used to create, modify or destroy transmembrane ion gradients by a simple manipulation of experimental conditions. As a consequence the energy-generating capabilities of an organism are modified and the research microbiologist then has a biolgical system available for the study of active transport and other energy-coupled phenomena.

Thus the addition of valinomycin to potassium-replete cells results in the rapid efflux of that ion with the concomitant generation of a membrane potential ($\Delta\Psi$). This potential, similar in essence to that generated by chemiosmosis, can be detected by the uptake of protons (Fig. 4*a*) or of lipid-soluble cations (Fig. 6). Uptake can be followed by pH and ion-selective electrodes, spectrophotometry or by introducing radioactive labels. Large inoculum sizes are required, in the order of 4×10^9 cells/ml, to ensure detectable ion fluxes.

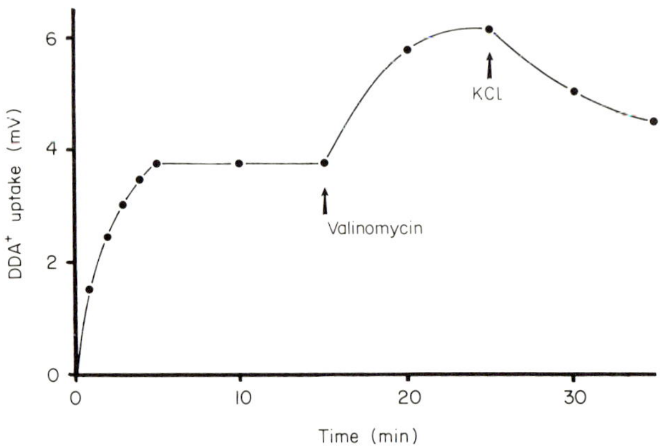

FIG. 6. The generation of a membrane potential by valinomycin. To 20 ml 0·1 mol/l glycylglycine buffer, pH 7·4 (25°C), containing 10 mmol/l glucose, 0·1 mmol/l DDA^+ and 1 μmol/l TPB^- was added sufficient *Staphylococcus aureus* cells (prepared as in Fig. 4) to give a final inoculum of 4×10^9 cells/ml. DDA^+ uptake was followed with a DDA^+ electrode (Muratsuga *et al.* 1977). Valinomycin, 20 μg, was added as a 20 μl aliquot from a stock solution in acetone. At 25 min KCl was introduced to a final concentration of 20 mmol/l. All solutions were prepared from triple distilled water. DDA^+ = dibenzyldimethylammonium, a lipid-soluble cation. TPB^- = tetraphenylboron, a lipid-soluble anion, catalyses the uptake of DDA^+.

In accordance with the principles of chemiosmosis an artificially derived membrane potential, if sufficiently large, should be able to support the active transport of essential nutrients by proton symport. The magnitude of the developed potential will depend upon counter-ion flow and the K^+ inside/K^+ outside concentration ratio. A decrease in this ratio will lead to a reduced membrane potential and an inhibition of active transport (Fig. 7). In extreme cases valinomycin can be used to collapse completely a pre-existing membrane potential, whether artificially produced (Fig. 6) or of metabolic origin, by introducing potassium into the suspending medium to a concentration approaching, or in excess of, the intracellular K^+ concentration. In *Streptococcus faecalis* for instance, Harold and co-workers (Asghar *et al.* 1973) have shown that an external concentration of 300 mmol/l was needed to inhibit accumulation of L-threonine by approximately 80%. The internal K^+ content had previously been estimated to be in the order of 400 mmol/l.

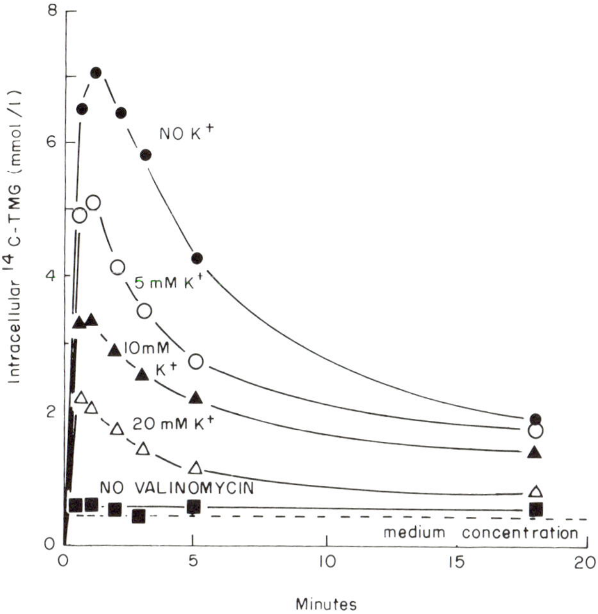

FIG. 7. Accumulation of ^{14}C–TMG on addition of valinomycin in media containing various amounts of K^+. *Streptococcus lactis* (ATCC 7962) cells were grown in the complex medium of Citti *et al.* (1965) supplemented with 1% galactose and 30 mmol/l arginine. Cells from logarithmic growth were washed and resuspended in 0·1 mol/l Tris–HCl buffer, pH 7·6. Each vessel contained: 0·2 ml of washed exponential-phase *Strep. lactis* 7962 cells at 18 mg dry weight cells/ml, 0·1–0·4 ml 50 mmol/l KCl and sufficient 0·1 mol/l Tris–HCl buffer, pH 7·6, to give a final volume of 1·0 ml; 1 μl of 1 × 10^{-2} mol/l valinomycin dissolved in 95% ethanol was added, and within 10 s, 0·1 ml of 5 mmol/l ^{14}C–TMG at 1 μCi/ml to start the reaction. Portions of 0·1 ml were removed at indicated intervals; the cells were collected on membrane filters, washed and counted (Kashket & Wilson, 1972*a*). All manipulations were carried out at 25°C. TMG = thiomethyl-β-galactoside. (Reproduced from Kashket & Wilson (1972*b*) by courtesy of Academic Press Inc. and the authors).

Determination of the membrane potential

The membrane potential generated by the distribution of a freely permeable cation across a membrane is given by the Nernst equation which, at electrochemical equilibrium, simplifies to

$$\Delta\Psi = -\frac{2{\cdot}303RT}{ZF}\log\frac{C_{IN}}{C_{OUT}}$$

where $\Delta\Psi$ = membrane potential; C_{IN} = concentration of cation inside cell; C_{OUT} = concentration of cation in suspending medium; and R, T, Z, F have their usual meanings.

For membranes rendered permeable to potassium ions by valinomycin this equation finds a direct application in the calculation of membrane potentials, the distribution of K^+ usually being determined by ion-selective electrodes, K^{42} activity or flame photometry. The method, originally applied to respiring mitochondria (Padan & Rottenberg 1973), consists of centrifugation of the cells, estimation of the intracellular water volume and pellet water content followed by determination of the K^+ distribution between the sedimented mitochondrial pellet and the supernatant fluid.

Collins & Hamilton (1976) have used the technique to study the magnitude of $\Delta\Psi$ developed in bacterial cells energized with a pulse of oxygen. In a typical experiment, *Staph. aureus* whole cells or *Escherichia coli* spheroplasts, at 0·5–1·0 mg/ml, were suspended in 25 ml lightly buffered 250 mmol/l sucrose–30 mmol/l choline chloride solution containing 0·1 mmol/l KCl, 2 μg/ml valinomycin and choline base-neutralized iodoacetic acid (1 mmol/l) to inhibit glycolysis. 2 μl of C100 catalase suspension was added and mixed by bubbling with oxygen-free nitrogen, while the pH was adjusted to approximately 7·0 with HCl or choline hydroxide. Anaerobiosis was maintained by sweeping the liquid surface with nitrogen. Oxygen to initiate metabolic energization was added as hydrogen peroxide (100 μl, 2 vol.) and changes in external K^+ concentration monitored by an ion-selective electrode technique. When the oxygen was exhausted the level of extracellular potassium increased in response to the declining membrane potential. The internal concentration of K^+ under energized conditions was calculated from these ion fluxes, due consideration being paid to the residual K^+ content after de-energization.

TABLE 2

Reported values for $\Delta\Psi$ *in energized* Staphylococcus aureus *and* Escherichia coli *cells*

Organism	Technique used for $\Delta\Psi$ determination (mV)			
	K^+/valinomycin*	DDA^+ uptake†	$TPMB^+$ uptake†	K^+ uptake†
Staph. aureus	−134 ± 10	−137	−148	−148
E. coli	−132 ± 10 (spheroplasts)	−131	—	—

* From Collins & Hamilton (1976).
† From Denyer *et al.* (1980).

$\Delta\Psi$ was estimated from the ratio of external and internal K^+ concentrations immediately preceding oxygen exhaustion. In Table 2 the results obtained by these authors are compared with values for $\Delta\Psi$ reported, in part, elsewhere (Denyer *et al.* 1980).

Manipulation of cellular internal ionic environment

The physiological importance of specific ions is implied by the sensitivity of many cells to ionophoric antibiotics; indeed under certain conditions the resultant loss of ions can be lethal to the cell. Nevertheless, if wisely employed, ionophores can offer a simple method for selectively altering the internal ionic environment of cells and their use may perhaps lead to a better understanding of the exact role played by individual ions within the bacterium. Thus, using the ionophore monactin, Harold and co-workers (Harold & Baarda 1968; Harold & Papineau 1972) have succeeded in replacing over 99% of the internal Rb^+ (K^+) of a washed suspension of *Strep. faecalis* by Na^+. Similarly, Niven & Hamilton (1974), this time using a combination of valinomycin and a proton ionophore (tetrachlorosalicylanilide) at an acid pH, have been able to reduce the internal K^+ concentration of *Staph. aureus* cells from 31 to 1·5 mmol/l. Figure 8 shows

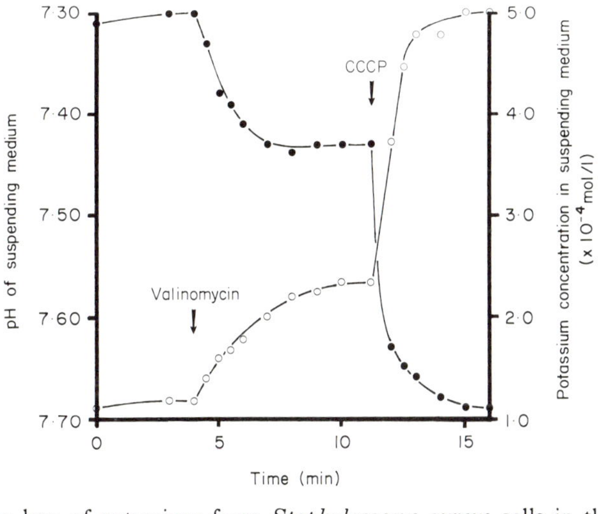

FIG. 8. The loss of potassium from *Staphylococcus aureus* cells in the presence of valinomycin and the protonophore CCCP. Experimental conditions were as in Fig. 4. Valinomycin and CCCP, both dissolved in acetone, were added as 25 µl aliquots to give final concentrations of 0·9 and 25 µmol/l respectively. The suspension was stirred continuously. pH changes (●—●) and the appearance of K^+ in the suspending medium (○—○) were followed by ion-selective electrode techniques. All solutions were prepared from triple distilled water.

the effect of suspending *Staph. aureus* NCTC 6571 cells in a medium containing 1 μg/ml (0·9 μmol/l) valinomycin and 5 μg/ml (25 μmol/l) of the protonophore carbonyl cyanide *m*-chlorophenylhydrazone (CCCP).

Summary

In the incredible research effort to find new and clinically applicable antibiotics the screening programme has thrown up a fascinating group, the ionophores, which although not finding a place in clinical medicine, have proved invaluable tools in basic biochemical studies on membrane processes. It cannot be over-emphasized that the most meticulous and rigorous attention to detail is essential for success in their application to obtain meaningful and reproducible results.

References

ASGHAR, S. S., LEVIN, E. & HAROLD, F. M. 1973 Accumulation of neutral amino acids by *Streptococcus faecalis*: energy coupling by a proton motive force. *Journal of Biological Chemistry* **248,** 5225–5233.

BAKKER, E. P. 1979 Ionophore antibiotics. In *Antibiotics Vol. V, Part I* ed. Hahn, F. E. pp. 67–97. Berlin: Springer-Verlag.

CITTI, J. E., SANDINE, W. E. & ELLIKER, P. R. 1965 β-Galactosidase of *Streptococcus lactis*. *Journal of Bacteriology* **89,** 937–942.

COLLINS, S. H. & HAMILTON, W. A. 1976 Magnitude of the proton motive force in respiring *Staphylococcus aureus* and *Escherichia coli*. *Journal of Bacteriology* **126,** 1224–1231.

DENYER, S. P., GRANT, D. J. W., GUNDIDZA, M. & HUGO, W. B. 1980 A novel technique for studying the effect of antibacterial agents on *Staphylococcus aureus*. *Journal of Pharmacy and Pharmacology* **32,** 15P.

HAROLD, F. M. & BAARDA, J. R. 1968 Effects of nigericin and nonactin on cation permeability of *Streptococcus faecalis* and metabolic capacities of potassium depleted cells. *Journal of Bacteriology* **95,** 816–823.

HAROLD, F. M. & PAPINEAU, D. 1972 Cation transport and electrogenesis by *Streptococcus faecalis*. I. The membrane potential. *Journal of Membrane Biology* **8,** 27–44.

HAROLD, F. M., ALTENDORF, K. H. & HIRATA, H. 1974 Probing membrane transport mechanisms with ionophores. *Annals of the New York Academy of Sciences* **235,** 149–160.

HINKLE, P. C. & MCCARTY, R. E. 1978 How cells make ATP. *Scientific American* **238,** 104–123.

HLADKY, S. B. & HAYDON, D. A. 1970 Discreteness of conductance change in bimolecular lipid membranes in the presence of certain antibiotics. *Nature, London* **225,** 451–453.

JAIN, M. K. 1972 Extrinsic properties of bimolecular lipid membranes. In *The Bimolecular Lipid Membrane: A System*, ed. Jain, M. K. pp. 145–252. New York: Van Nostrand Reinhold.

KASHKET, E. R. & WILSON, T. H. 1972*a* Role of metabolic energy in the transport of β-galactosides by *Streptococcus lactis*. *Journal of Bacteriology* **109,** 784–789.

KASHKET, E. R. & WILSON, T. H. 1972*b* Galactoside accumulation associated with ion movements in *Streptococcus lactis*. *Biochemical and Biophysical Research Communications* **49,** 615–620.

KRASNE, S., EISENMAN, G. & SZABO, G. 1971 Freezing and melting of lipid bilayers and the mode of action of nonactin, valinomycin and gramicidin. *Science* **174,** 412–415.

MITCHELL, P. 1972 Chemiosmotic coupling in energy transduction: a logical development of biochemical knowledge. *Journal of Bioenergetics* **3,** 5–24.

MURATSUGU, M., KAMO, N., KURIHARA, K. & KOBATAKE, Y. 1977 Selective electrode for dibenzyl dimethyl ammonium cation as indicator of the membrane potential in biological systems. *Biochimica et Biophysica Acta* **464,** 613–619.

NIVEN, D. F. & HAMILTON, W. A. 1974 Mechanisms of energy coupling to the transport of amino acids by *Staphylococcus aureus*. *European Journal of Biochemistry* **44,** 517–522.

PADAN, E. & ROTTENBERG, H. 1973 Respiratory control and the proton electrochemical gradient in mitochondria. *European Journal of Biochemistry* **40,** 431–437.

PRESSMAN, B. C. 1963 Specific inhibitors of energy transfer. In *Energy-linked Functions of Mitochondria* ed. Chance, B. pp. 181–203. New York and London: Academic Press.

Extraction and Purification of Antibiotic-destroying Enzymes

D. F. BROAD AND J. T. SMITH

Microbiology Section, Department of Pharmaceutics, The School of Pharmacy, 23–39 Brunswick Square, London, UK

Bacteria can become resistant to antibiotics as a result of possessing R-plasmids (reviewed by Falkow 1975). A variety of mechanisms exists whereby R-plasmids can mediate antibiotic resistance and with chloramphenicol and the β-lactam antibiotics (penicillins and cephalosporins) this is brought about by complete inactivation of the antibiotic. With β-lactam antibiotics this is effected by β-lactamase (penicillin/cephalosporin amidohydrolase E. C. 3.5.2.6.) enzymes which hydrolyse the β-lactam bond in the penicillin/cephalosporin nucleus. Penicillins are converted to the corresponding penicilloic acid (Fig. 1) which is devoid of antibacterial activity (Abraham & Chain 1940). The inactivation of cephalosporins by β-lactamase action is more complex; while hydrolysis of the β-lactam bond is the primary chemical reaction other chemical changes such as ring rearrangement and side-chain expulsion then follow. The sequence of these secondary reactions and the final products depend on the actual cephalosporin involved, although none of these products retains antibacterial activity (Sabbath *et al.* 1965; Newton & Hamilton-Miller 1967).

The many types of β-lactamase produced by bacteria have been extensively studied and reviewed (Hamilton-Miller & Smith 1979). This report, however, will be concerned with the study of R-plasmid-mediated β-lactamases produced in Gram negative bacteria (excluding pseudomonads) and particularly with their extraction and purification with a view to their classification.

Preparation of Crude β-Lactamase Samples by Ultrasonic Disintegration

Cells are grown for 18 h at 37°C in nutrient broth (Oxoid No. 2) and

ANTIBIOTICS
ISBN 0 12 604480 5

harvested by centrifugation at 5000 **g** for 20 min at 4°C. The supernatant fluid is discarded and the pellet resuspended in approximately 50 ml of cold 0·025 mol/l $Na_2HPO_4.NaH_2PO_4$ buffer pH 7·4 (buffer A). The resuspended cells are centrifuged as above, and this 'washing process' is repeated if required. The pellet is resuspended in a volume of cold buffer A to give the required final cell concentration (N value, where 1 N represents the cell concentration of the overnight culture). To release the enzyme, the cells are disintegrated by ultrasonic treatment using an M.S.E. 100 watt ultrasonic disintegrator (M.S.E. Ltd, UK) for 2 × 1 min at an amplitude of 6 μm peak to peak in a vessel surrounded by crushed ice and water. The disrupted sample is then centrifuged at 32,000 **g** for 60 min at 4°C to remove cell debris. The supernatant fluid, which represents the crude β-lactamase preparation, is retained and dialysed for 36 h at 4°C against two changes (200 vols) of buffer A to reduce the concentration of chloride ions. Samples are stored at −20°C.

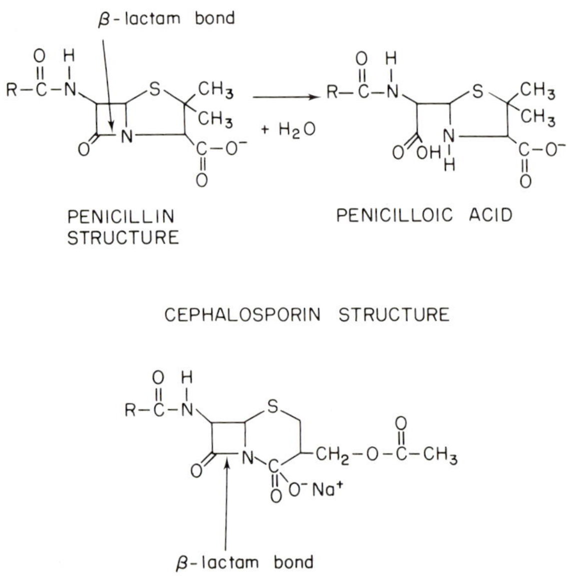

FIG. 1. Structure of penicillins and cephalosporins.

Osmotic Shock

The procedure is that of Smith & Wyatt (1974) which is based on an osmotic shock procedure for cells in the stationary phase of growth (Neu & Chou 1967).

Cells grown for 18 h at 37°C in nutrient broth (Oxoid No. 2) are centrifuged at 5000 **g** for 20 min at 4°C. The volume of the supernatant fluid is measured and the cells resuspended (using a glass rod and bench vortex mixer) in a volume of cold 0·01 mol/l Tris–HCl buffer pH 7·3, containing 0·03 mol/l NaCl equal to 1/25th of that of the supernatant (i.e. to give a 25 N suspension). If the culture contains between $0{\cdot}4 \times 10^9$ cells/ml and $1{\cdot}0 \times 10^9$ cells/ml then the 25 N culture will contain between $1{\cdot}0 \times 10^{10}$ cells/ml and $2{\cdot}5 \times 10^{10}$ cells/ml, a range that will provide an adequate sample.

At this stage the 25 N suspension is halved, one half to form the control sample and the other the test sample. Both samples are centrifuged at 5000 **g** for 20 min at 4°C and the supernatants discarded. The washed pellets are treated as follows.

Test sample

The pellet is resuspended in 0·03 mol/l Tris–HCl buffer pH 7·3, containing 20% sucrose at room temperature. EDTA solution (10 mg/ml) is added to give a final concentration of 1 mmol/l at a cell concentration of 25 N and the mixture stirred with a glass rod for 5 min at room temperature and then centrifuged at 5000 **g** for 20 min at 4°C. The supernatant fluid is discarded and the pellet rapidly resuspended (using a glass rod and bench vortex mixer) in ice-cold distilled water (to give a 25 N sample again). The cells are stirred for 5 min in a vessel surrounded by crushed ice and then centrifuged at 5000 **g** for 20 min at 4°C. The supernatant (the osmotic shock fluid) is removed carefully using a pipette and sufficient cold stock 0·5 mol/l $Na_2HPO_4.NaH_2PO_4$ buffer pH 7·4 is added to give a final molarity of 0·025 mol/l. This constitutes the 'osmotic shock supernatant' which contains any enzymes that were released by osmotic shock. The pellet (the 'osmotic shock cells') is resuspended in cold buffer A to give a 25 N sample, and then ultrasonically disintegrated for 2×1 min at an amplitude of 6 μm peak to peak.

Control sample

The washed control pellet is resuspended in cold buffer A to give a 25 N sample and then ultrasonically disintegrated as described previously.

The ultrasonic extracts from the control sample and the osmotic shock cells are then centrifuged at 32,000 **g** for 60 min at 4°C to precipitate cell debris. The supernatants, which represent the control and osmotic shock cells samples, are stored at −20°C until required.

Spheroplast Formation

The method is based on that of Lindström *et al* (1970) for *Escherichia coli* as adapted by Wyatt (1972).

Cells are grown for 18 h at 37°C in nutrient broth (Oxoid No. 2) and harvested by centrifugation at 5000 **g** for 20 min at 4°C. The volume of the supernatant is measured and the pellet resuspended in a volume of 0·01 mol/l Tris–HCl buffer pH 7·3, containing 0·03 mol/l NaCl to give 25 N cells. The suspension is then divided into two parts and centrifuged at 5000 **g** for 20 min at 4°C. The supernatants are discarded and one pellet is used as the test sample and the other as the control.

Test sample

The pellet is resuspended in 20% sucrose in 0·03 mol/l Tris–HCl buffer pH 7·3 at room temperature to give 25 N cells using a bench vortex mixer and a glass rod. Sufficient disodium EDTA solution (10 mg/ml) in distilled water is added to give a final concentration of 1 mmol/l. Immediately after this sufficient freshly prepared egg lysozyme solution (1 mg/ml) in distilled water is added to give a final concentration of 50 μg/ml. The mixture is stirred gently with a glass rod for 8 min to allow spheroplast formation, which may be monitored by measuring the extent of lysis by adding 0·1 ml of mixture to 5 ml of distilled water at intervals and measuring the optical density at 550 nm. No increase in lysis, and therefore of spheroplast formation, occurs after 8 min.

Sufficient 1·0 mol/l $CaCl_2$ is then added to give a final concentration of 0·01 mol/l to stabilize the spheroplasts. Sufficient 1·0 mol/l $MgSO_4$ is also added to give a final concentration of 5 mmol/l Mg^{2+} which may be necessary to reverse any enzyme inhibition due to EDTA. The spheroplast suspension is centrifuged at 5000 **g** for 20 min at 4°C. The supernatant fluid contains any enzymes released by spheroplast formation and the pellet constitutes the spheroplast cells which are then resuspended in 0·03 mol/l Tris–HCl buffer pH 7·3 at a cell concentration of 25 N and ultrasonically disrupted for 2 × 1 min at 6 μm peak to peak.

Control sample

The pellet is resuspended in 0·03 mol/l Tris–HCl buffer pH 7·3 at a cell concentration of 25 N and ultrasonically disrupted as for the spheroplast cells. Both the ultrasonically disrupted test (spheroplast) and control samples are then centrifuged at 32,000 **g** for 1 h at 4°C and the supernatants retained.

β-Lactamase Assay

The assay used routinely in this laboratory for estimating β-lactamase is the hydroxylamine method. Hydroxylamine reacts with a number of carboxylic acid derivatives, including penicillins and cephalosporins, to form hydroxamates which yield coloured complexes with Fe^{3+} in acidic solution. The optical density (O.D.) of these complexes (measured at 500 nm) is therefore a measure of the amount of penicillin/cephalosporin present in an assay mixture at a given time, thus allowing the rate of penicillin/cephalosporin destruction, i.e. β-lactamase activity, to be determined.

The method used is that of Dale & Smith (1971*a*) and is as follows.

The assay mixture usually contains 0·6 ml of penicillin solution (see below) and the required amount of sample to be assayed made up to 6·0 ml with buffer A. The buffer and enzyme sample are allowed to equilibrate at 30°C in a water bath and the reaction started by the addition of the penicillin solution. The reaction is allowed to proceed at 30°C and 0·8 ml samples are removed at 15–30 min time intervals. These samples are added with mixing to 2·6 ml of 'hydroxylamine reagent' (see below) and allowed to stand for 5 min (penicillins) or 3 min (cephalosporins) at room temperature. 0·8 ml of the 'ferric reagent' is then added and mixed. The O.D. of the resulting brown complex is read immediately at 500 nm on a spectrophotometer (e.g. Bausch and Lomb 'Spectronic 20') against a blank, made from a control sample containing buffer, 'hydroxylamine reagent' and 'ferric reagent'.

The rate of fall of O.D. is then plotted graphically. This rate is converted into micromoles of penicillin hydrolysed/min at 30°C in 0·025 mol/l $Na_2HPO_4.NaH_2PO_4$ buffer pH 7·4, i.e. enzyme units (Thompson 1962). In practice, milliunits (mUnits) are used and these are converted to mUnits/10^9 cells to allow comparison between different enzyme preparations.

Reagents used in the hydroxylamine assay

1. *Hydroxylamine reagent*
   (a) 5 mol/l hydroxylammonium chloride solution.
   (b) Alkaline buffer (pH 11·2):

sodium hydroxide	86·5 g
sodium acetate	10·3 g
distilled water to	500 ml

   Reagent (prepared daily):
   8 vols of 96% ethyl alcohol
   1 vol. of distilled water
   2 vols of (a) above
   2 vols of (b) above

2. *Ferric reagent*

Ferric ammonium sulphate	200 g
conc. sulphuric acid (sp. gr. 1·84)	93·4 ml
(i.e. final concentration 3·5 mol/l)	
distilled water to	1000 ml

3. *Penicillin solution*
Benzylpenicillin is made up to 18 mg/ml in buffer A and stored at −20°C. 0·6 ml of this is added to the assay mixture to give a final volume of 6 ml, i.e. a final penicillin concentration of 1·8 mg/ml which is enough to saturate the enzyme. If other penicillins and cephalosporins are used then these are made and stored as above, but at a concentration of 20 mg/ml, giving a final concentration of 2 mg/ml in the assay mixture.

Starch-gel Electrophoresis

The gels are prepared and run as described by Smithies (1955) and modified by Dale & Smith (1971b). A 10% (w/v) starch solution in gel buffer is prepared by gently heating starch/buffer mixture in a 600 ml flask over a bunsen burner. When the mixture is near to boiling it is removed from the bunsen burner and a negative pressure applied for the shortest possible time (to avoid evaporation) to remove any air bubbles present. The clear starch solution is then poured gently into a plastic tray (18 × 6 × 0·6 cm) until the starch is just above the level of the trough. The gel is allowed to set at 4°C for 30–60 min and any gel that has spilled over from the trough is removed with a scalpel blade. A transverse slit, 0·5 cm from each side of the tray, is made halfway along the length of the gel using a sharp scalpel blade. Samples, usually three per gel, are introduced by soaking a piece of Whatman No. 3 filter paper (1 × 0·6 cm) into the sample solution and carefully inserted into the transverse slit using a spatula to open the slit. The filter paper is positioned so that the 0·6 cm edge is vertical and thus fitted accurately into the cross-section of the gel. The tray containing the gel is then placed over the top of a large tray which contains the bridge buffer and two electrodes (in separate compartments) connected to a power supply. Electrical contacts between the gel and the bridge buffer and cathode consists of 8 strips of Whatman No. 3 filter paper soaked in bridge buffer. These wicks are placed in contact with each end of the gel. To prevent loss of water from the gel during electrophoresis it is covered with a sheet of thin polythene soaked in silicone oil. To avoid the formation of air bubbles the polythene is lowered very carefully from one end of the gel. A constant voltage of 200 V is applied and electrophoresis allowed to continue for a suitable period of time.

To detect β-lactamase activity the gel is sliced horizontally in two with a very fine wire. The cut surfaces are then sprayed with a penicillin/iodine solution (see below). The cut surfaces are used so that β-lactamase migration can be observed in the absence of edge effects. The β-lactamase activity is identified by the decolourization of discrete bands of the dark blue starch–iodine complex by penicilloic acid formed by the hydrolysis of penicillin by β-lactamase. The distance of the band from the origin (transverse slit) is measured and the mobilities of the individual bands are expressed as cm/h towards the cathode.

Penicillin/iodine solution

The solution used is that of Lampen (1967) and is prepared fresh daily:
0·15 mol/l penicillin solution in
0·05 mol/l $Na_2HPO_4.NaH_2PO_4$ buffer pH 7·4, containing:
0·016 mol/l iodine dissolved in 0·06 mol/l potassium iodide.

Extraction of β-Lactamases

Obviously it would be advantageous to study only pure enzymes but this is not feasible when large numbers of enzymes are being examined and compared. For this reason the R-plasmid-mediated β-lactamases have been classified using crude enzyme preparations produced by ultrasonic disintegration as described previously. These crude preparations are usually extensively dialized to remove any ions present, particularly chloride ions, which might inhibit the β-lactamases (Hedges *et al.* 1974). One problem encountered using these crude β-lactamase preparations is the presence not only of the R-plasmid-mediated β-lactamase, but also the host cell chromosomal β-lactamase. This is not usually a major problem in practice because most host cell chromosomal β-lactamases are produced in very small amounts when compared to the R-plasmid-mediated β-lactamases (Hedges *et al.* 1974). However, this is not always the case because Matthew *et al.* (1979) found that one β-lactamase, mediated by R-plasmid R997, was produced in considerably smaller amounts than the chromosomal β-lactamase. Therefore before any of its enzymic properties were studied it was necessary to separate the R-plasmid and chromosomal β-lactamases. This was achieved using Sephadex G75 chromatography followed by QAE–Sephadex ion-exchange chromatography which yielded two peaks of β-lactamase activity with the R997 β-lactamase being purified 16-fold.

These problems can possibly be circumvented either by introducing R-plasmid into a mutant *Escherichia coli* host strain which lacks a detectable level of chromosomal β-lactamase (Bobrowski *et al.* 1976), or (if the R-plasmid β-lactamase has mol. wt $< 30{,}000$) by separating it from *E. coli* chromosomal β-lactamase by osmotic shock (see below).

Another method for producing β-lactamase preparations is by techniques which disrupt the outer cell wall of Gram negative bacteria releasing enzymes that exist outside the cell cytoplasm, but causing no gross cell lysis or release of cytoplasmic enzymes (Heppel 1971). β-Lactamases, which by necessity exist outside the cell cytoplasm (the site of action of β-lactam antibiotics is the peptidoglycan layer of the outer cell wall), can therefore be released by such techniques. The two most commonly used methods of releasing such enzymes from Gram negative bacteria are osmotic shock (Fig. 2) and spheroplast formation using lysozyme (Fig. 2). Both these techniques involve pre-treatment of the cells with Tris and EDTA, a treatment which damages the outer cell wall causing the release of the acid soluble nucleotide pool (Neu *et al.* 1966) and increased sensitivity of the cells to a variety of agents (Lieve 1974). If the Tris/EDTA damaged cells are then treated with lysozyme (which degrades the cell wall peptidoglycan) spheroplasts are formed which can be stabilized in sucrose so that no significant lysis occurs (Malamy & Horecker 1961). This treatment causes the release of a considerable number of enzymes and proteins, although cytoplasmic enzymes are not believed to be released (Heppel 1971).

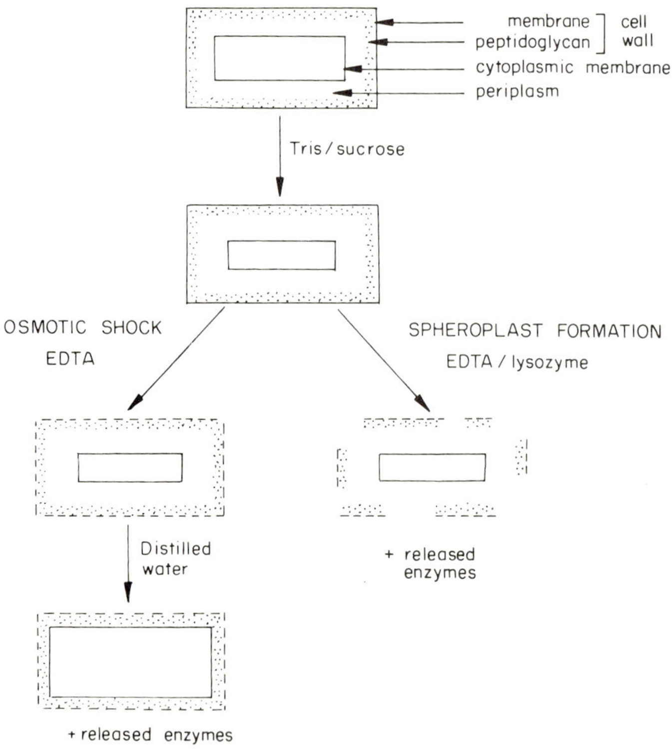

FIG. 2. Diagrammatic representation of cells during osmotic shock and spheroplast formation.

Osmotic shock also involves treating the cells with Tris and EDTA but because lysozyme is omitted no gross cell wall damage occurs and as such it is a much more gentle technique than that of spheroplast formation. In fact the cells remain viable and only 5% of the total cell protein, together with fewer enzymes and proteins, are released by osmotic shock than by spheroplast formation (Heppel 1971). After Tris/EDTA treatment the cells are then exposed to a solution containing 20% sucrose which causes the cytoplasm to plasmolyse, i.e. it contracts. The cells are then exposed to a medium of very low osmotic pressure, e.g. water for *E. coli* cells in the stationary phase of growth (Neu & Heppel 1965) and dilute $MgCl_2$ solution for *E. coli* cells in the exponential phase of growth (Nossal & Heppel 1966). This causes a rapid influx of water into the cytoplasm causing the cytoplasm to expand and forcing enzymes that exist outside the cytoplasmic membrane through the Tris/EDTA damaged cell wall.

TABLE 1

Release of β-lactamase by osmotic shock treatment

β-Lactamase	Genetic location of β-lactamase genes*	Mol. wt	Release (%)
R6K	R	20,500	96·2
RP1	R	19,500	94·2
RGN238	R	23,300	83·8
R46	R	44,600	11·2
R55	R	41,200	52·0
R22Ka	R	31,800	0
K. aerogenes 418	C	20,080	74·4†
E. coli D3	C	31,800	0

* R represents R-plasmid, C chromosomal, β-lactamases.

† This probably represents the maximum release of enzymes from *K. aerogenes* since Neu & Chou (1967) showed that enzymes totally released by osmotic shock of *E. coli* were at best only 50% released in *K. pneumoniae* and 70–80% released in *Enterobacter aerogenes*.

Both osmotic shock and spheroplast formation yield enzyme preparations with increased specific activities and greater purity than those obtained using ultrasonically disrupted cell extracts (Broad & Smith 1981). Because osmotic shock is a less drastic technique than spheroplast formation it would be preferable to use osmotic shock in the preparation of β-lactamase samples; however, not all β-lactamases are released by this technique. Smith & Wyatt (1974) found that there was a permeability barrier to the release of β-lactamases by osmotic shock, with those enzymes of mol. wt 20,000 being totally released, whereas those of mol. wt 30,000 were not released, irrespective of the genetic location of the gene(s) for β-lactamase formation (Table 1). This is, however, a useful purification step because most R-plasmid-mediated β-lactamases found in Gram negative bacteria have mol. wt approx. 20,000 whereas those of chromosomally mediated β-lactamases are 30,000 (Smith & Sykes 1979), thus allowing the preparation of R-plasmid-mediated β-lactamase extracts with no contaminating chromosomally-mediated β-lactamase. Nevertheless, some R-plasmid-mediated β-lactamases are known which have mol. wt > 40,000 (Dale & Smith 1974) and these are not completely released by osmotic shock treatment (Table 1). With these larger plasmid-mediated β-lactamases a small proportion is consistently released by osmotic shock treatment. The fraction released has been explained in terms of molecular shape and sub-unit structure of these enzymes (Broad & Smith 1979; 1981). These β-lactamases and other β-lactamases of smaller molecular weight can all, however, be released by spheroplast formation (Smith & Wyatt 1974).

Classification of R-Plasmid-mediated β-Lactamases

Having obtained β-lactamase preparations (which can be stored for considerable lengths of time at −20°C) it is then necessary to consider which criteria are to be used in classifying them. Because these enzyme preparations are impure in practice it is necessary to use a variety of techniques to obtain an overall pattern of classification. The first stage in classification is to determine a "substrate profile", i.e. the hydrolytic activity of the β-lactamases against a range of β-lactam antibiotics is measured and compared, usually against benzylpenicillin which is given an arbitrary value of 100.

From Table 2 it can be seen that two major groups of R-plasmid-mediated β-lactamases are obtained; one, the TEM-type, hydrolyses penicillins and cephalosporins but not the isoxazoyl penicillins such as oxacillin; the other group, the OXA-type, hydrolysing oxacillin. These two major groups of β-lactamases can then be further subdivided on the basis of substrate profile and sensitivity to inhibitors such as chloride ions and *para*-chloromercuribenzoate (*p*CMB) The use of *p*CMB as a β-lactamase inhibitor has led to the discovery of an unusual type of β-lactamase (Matthew *et al.* 1979), the SHV-1 group, as exemplified by the p453 β-lactamase. The ability of this enzyme to hydrolyse cephaloridine is completely abolished by incubating the enzyme preparation for 10 min at 30°C in the presence of 0·5 mmol/l *p*CMB, whereas its activity against benzylpenicillin is unaffected by this treatment.

TABLE 2

Classification of R-plasmid-mediated β-lactamases

β-Lactamase type	R-Plasmid	Relative rate of hydrolysis*				Inhibited by		Mol. wt	Mobility† (cm/h) towards cathode	Isoelectric point pI
		Oxa	Amp	Ceph	Meth	*p*CMB‡	chloride ions§			
TEM-1	R6K	5	106	76	0	R	R	20,500	−1·7	5·4
TEM-2	RP1	5	107	74	0	R	R	19,500	−1·4	5·6
OXA-1	RGN238	197	382	30	332	5	8	23,300	−0·08	7·4
OXA-2	R46	646	179	36	23	R	15	44,600	+0·51	7·45 7·7
OXA-3	R55	376	173	44·7	32·8	R	49	41,200	−0·13	7·1
SHV-1	p453	0	212	56	< 2	R/S	R	17,000	−0·03	7·6
HMS-1	R997	< 2	253	183	< 2	S	R	21,000	−2·8	5·2

Results from Sykes & Smith (1979), Matthew *et al.* (1979) and this paper.

* Benzylpenicillin = 100. Oxa represents oxacillin, Amp ampicillin, Ceph cephaloridine, Meth methicillin.

† During starch gel electrophoresis at pH 8·5.

‡ R, resistant (100% of control activity); S, sensitive (0% of control activity) when incubated for 10 min at 30°C in the presence of 0·5 mmol/l *p*CMB.

§ R, resistant to 100 mmol/l NaCl (100% control activity). The values for the OXA-1, -2 and -3 type β-lactamase are the NaCl concentrations (mmol/l) which give 50% inhibition of the control enzyme activity.

The ability of the SHV-1 β-lactamase to hydrolyse benzyl penicillin is resistant to this treatment whereas its ability to hydrolyse cephaloridine is not.

There are, however, problems in comparing enzymic properties because the conditions used vary from laboratory to laboratory, which led Dale & Smith (1971*b*) to conclude that physical properties such as molecular weight and electrophoretic mobility as well as enzymic properties must be taken into account. Although Dale & Smith (1972) were able to differentiate between two apparently similar β-lactamases, the RGN238 and R46 β-lactamases (OXA-1 and OXA-2 types, respectively) on the basis of molecular weight this criterion can normally only be used to provide confirmatory evidence of β-lactamase identity because many β-lactamases which have different enzymic properties have similar molecular weights (Table 2). Furthermore, molecular weight estimates of β-lactamases vary significantly with the technique used (Dale & Smith 1976; Broad & Smith 1981). Therefore molecular weight estimates must be obtained using the same technique, normally Sephadex gel exclusion chromatography (which can be used with crude enzyme preparations), although molecular weight estimates obtained by the same technique for the same enzyme can vary from laboratory to laboratory. For instance, Neu (1970), who studied an R-plasmid-mediated β-lactamase in *Pseudomonas aeruginosa* which was later termed RP1 (Sykes & Richmond 1970), obtained molecular weight estimates of 24,000 and 29,000 for this β-lactamase by gel exclusion chromatography, although when its molecular weight was estimated by the gel exclusion chromatography method described by Dale & Smith (1971*a*) it was found to be 19,500 (Broad & Smith unpublished). This latter value would appear to be correct because the RP1-mediated β-lactamase is very similar to other TEM-type β-lactamases (see below) which all have mol. wt of approx. 20,000 (Table 2).

Perhaps a better technique for identifying β-lactamases is electrophoresis. Both starch gel electrophoresis (Dale & Smith 1974) and analytical isoelectric focusing in polyacrylamide gels (Matthew & Hedges 1976) have been used for this purpose. Both techniques are extremely sensitive and can be used with crude enzyme preparations. For instance, using analytical isoelectric focusing, Matthew *et al.* (1975) were able to separate two TEM-type β-lactamases, the R6K- and RP1-mediated enzymes, which had previously been thought to be identical because they exhibited (1) no significant difference in their enzymic properties (Hedges *et al.* 1974), (2) serological cross-reactivity (Sykes & Richmond 1970) and (3) DNA specifying the production of these β-lactamases was found to be homologous by heteroduplex analysis (Heffron *et al.* 1975). It is in fact probable that there are only minor differences in the amino acid composition of these two enzymes.

The RP1 and R6K β-lactamases can also be separated readily by starch gel electrophoresis (Fig. 3), having mobilities of −1·4 and −1·7 cm/h

FIG. 3. Starch gel electrophoresis of RP1- and R6K-mediated β-lactamases. (*a*) 30 μl of a 200 N crude preparation of *Escherichia coli* K12 J62 (R6K). (*b*) 22 μl of a 200 N crude preparation of *Escherichia coli* K12 J62 (R6K) mixed with 8 μl of a 200 N crude preparation of *E. coli* K12 J62 (RP1). (*c*) 30 μl of a 200 N crude preparation of *Escherichia coli* K12 J62 (RP1) diluted 1:3 in cold buffer A. Electrophoresis was performed at a constant voltage of 200 V. The gel buffer was 0·03 mol/l boric acid–NaOH buffer pH 8·5 and the bridge buffer was 0·3 mol/l boric acid–NaOH buffer pH 8·5.

towards the cathode, respectively (Table 2). (The mobilities in the SHV-1 and HMS-1 β-lactamases, −0·03 and −2·8 cm/h towards the cathode, respectively, previously undetermined are included in Table 2.) Thus, although isoelectric focusing has largely superseded starch gel electrophoresis because of the very small amounts of enzymes required (during isoelectric focusing proteins are focused and thus concentrated during this process) and also absolute values (i.e. pI values) are obtained, starch gel electrophoresis remains a valid technique for identifying β-lactamases. In addition, care must be exercised when interpreting pI values obtained by analytical isoelectric focusing because the mobility of some β-lactamases is affected by the position of application of the samples onto the gels (Barthelmy *et al.* 1978). Isoelectric focusing also suffers from the drawback that multiple bands of β-lactamase activity are seen using this technique, e.g. two bands of R46 β-lactamase activity (Table 2), whereas only one band is seen after starch gel electrophoresis.

Further Purification of β-Lactamases

For some studies of β-lactamases, e.g. amino acid sequencing, X-ray crystallography and quaternary structure determinations, the enzymes must be further purified, usually to homogeneity. Several R-plasmid-mediated β-lactamases have been purified to apparent homogeneity (reviewed by Dale 1979), normally using a variety of combinations of gel exclusion chromatography and ion-exchange chromatography, although affinity chromatography using ampicillin and cephalosporin C coupled to Indubiose 4A has been used to purify the R6K (RTEM) β-lactamase (Le Goffic *et al.* 1973, 1975).

It is, however, not apposite to describe each and every purification procedure here, although the method used in this laboratory originally for the purification of the R46- (R1818-)mediated β-lactamase (Dale & Smith 1971*a*) and later for the R55-mediated β-lactamase (Dale & Smith 1976) will be described as an indication of the techniques available and also because the R46 and R55 β-lactamases so purified were shown to consist of sub-units and, as such, are the only β-lactamases known to do so (Dale & Smith 1976). A typical purification is shown in Table 3 and it can be seen that the R46-mediated β-lactamase was purified 312-fold and had a specific activity of 143 units/mg protein. This enzyme preparation was pure as judged by polyacrylamide gel electrophoresis.

Dale & Smith (1976) subjected a pure R46-mediated β-lactamase preparation and also an R55-mediated β-lactamase preparation obtained by the same procedure to polyacrylamide gel electrophoresis in the presence of SDS. This yielded a single band of protein in each case with

TABLE 3

Purification of R46 (R1818) β-lactamase

Step	Volume (ml)	Total protein (mg)	Total enzyme activity (units)	Specific activity (units/mg protein)	Purification
Crude enzyme	360	13,460	6190	0·46	1
50% saturation ammonium sulphate precipitate	46	2 320	4070	1·76	4
First DEAE–cellulose column	80	72·5	1649	22·7	49
Second DEAE–cellulose column	50	19·9	760	38·2	83
Sephadex G100	28	6·0	410	68·3	148
60% saturation ammonium sulphate precipitate	3·5	4·0	577	143·2	312

From Dale & Smith (1971*a*).

that in the R46 sample having mol. wt 28,400, the one for R55 being 29,000. Their molecular weights obtained by gel exclusion chromatography were 44,600 and 41,200, respectively, which led these authors to conclude that these two enzymes are dimeric, each consisting of identical sub-units, although the sub-units of each individual enzyme appeared to be different. This was confirmed by constructing a bacterial strain containing both R-plasmids and subjecting a crude enzyme preparation to starch gel electrophoresis. They found not only two β-lactamase bands, one with a mobility corresponding to the R46 β-lactamase and the other with a mobility corresponding to the R55 β-lactamase, but also a band with an intermediate mobility which presumably corresponds to a hybrid β-lactamase consisting of a sub-unit from both enzymes.

The authors are grateful to Miss Kim Holdsworth for expert technical assistance, and Mr C. Upton for photography.

References

ABRAHAM, E. P. & CHAIN, E. 1940 An enzyme from bacteria able to destroy penicillin. *Nature, London* **146,** 837.

BARTHELMY, M., GUIONIE, M. & LABIA, R. 1978 β-lactamases: determination of their isoelectric points. *Antimicrobial Agents and Chemotherapy* **13,** 695–698.

BOBROWSKI, B. B., MATTHEW, M. BARTH, P. T., DATTA, N., GRINTER, N. J., JACOB, A. E., KONTAMICHALOU, P., DALE, J. W. & SMITH, J. T. 1976 Plasmid-determined β-lactamase indistinguishable from the chromosomal β-lactamase of *Escherichia coli. Journal of Bacteriology* **125,** 149–157.

BROAD, D. F. & SMITH, J. T. 1979 Release of enzymes from bacteria. *Journal of Pharmacy and Pharmacology* **31,** 30P.

BROAD, D. F. & SMITH, J. T. 1981 *Escherichia coli* 5′-nucleotidase: purification, properties and its release by osmotic shock. *Journal of General Microbiology* **123,** 241–247.

DALE, J. W. 1979 In *Beta-lactamases* eds Hamilton-Miller, J. M. T. and Smith, J. T. Chap. 4, pp. 73–98. London & New York: Academic Press.

DALE, J. W. & SMITH, J. T., 1971*a* The purification and properties of the β-lactamase specified by the resistance factor R-1818 in *Escherichia coli* and *Proteus mirabilis. Biochemical Journal* **123,** 493–500.

DALE, J. W. & SMITH, J. T. 1971*b* Some relationships between R-factor and chromosomal β-lactamase in Gram-negative bacteria. *Biochemical Journal* **123,** 507–512.

DALE, J. W. & SMITH, J. T. 1972 A direct comparison of two unusual R-factor mediated β-lactamases. *Biochemical Journal* **128,** 173–174.

DALE, J. W. & SMITH, J. T. 1974 R-factor-mediated β-lactamases that hydrolyze oxacillin: evidence for two distinct groups. *Journal of Bacteriology* **119,** 351–356.

DALE, J. W. & SMITH, J. T. 1976 The dimeric nature of an R-factor mediated β-lactamase. *Biochemical and Biophysical Research Communications* **68,** 1000–1005.

FALKOW, S. 1975 *Infectious Multiple Drug Resistance.* London: Pion.

HAMILTON-MILLER, J. M. T. & SMITH, J. T. 1979 *Beta-lactamases*. London & New York: Academic Press.

HEDGES, R. W., DATTA, N., KONTAMICHALOU, P. & SMITH, J. T. 1974 Molecular specificities of R-factor-determined β-lactamases: correlation with plasmid compatibility. *Journal of Bacteriology* **117,** 56–62.

HEFFRON, F., SUBLETT, R., HEDGES, R. W., JACOB, A. & FALKOW, S. 1975 Origin of the TEM beta-lactamase gene found on plasmids. *Journal of Bacteriology* **122,** 250–256.

HEPPEL, L. A. 1971 In *Structure and Function of Biological Membranes* ed. Rothfield, L. I. Ch. 5, pp. 223–247. New York & London: Academic Press.

LAMPEN, J. O. 1967 Cell bound penicillinase of *Bacillus licheniformis*: properties and purification. *Journal of General Microbiology* **48,** 249–259.

LE GOFFIC, F., LAKIW, R. & ANDRILLON, J. 1973 Affinity chromatography of β-lactamases. *Biochimica et Biophysica Acta* **315,** 439–442

LE GOFFIC, F., ANDRILLON-SPIEGEL, J. & LETARTE, R. 1975 Purification des β-lactamases par chromatographie d'affinité. *Biochimie* **57,** 29–34.

LIEVE, L. 1974 The barrier function of the Gram-negative envelope. *Annals of the New York Academy of Sciences* **235,** 109–127.

LINDSTRÖM, E. B., BOMAN, H. G. & STEELE, B. B. 1970 Resistance of *Escherichia coli* to penicillins. VI. Purification and characterization of the chromosomally mediated penicillinase present in *ampA*-containing strains. *Journal of Bacteriology* **101,** 218–231.

MALAMY, M. & HORECKER, B. L. 1961 The localization of alkaline phosphatase in *E. coli* K12. *Biochemical and Biophysical Research Communications* **5,** 104–108.

MATTHEW, M. & HEDGES, R. W. 1976 Analytical isoelectric focusing of R factor-determined β-lactamases: correlation with plasmid compatibility. *Journal of Bacteriology* **125,** 713–718.

MATTHEW, M., HARRIS, A. M., MARSHALL, M. J. & ROSS, G. W. 1975 The use of analytical isoelectric focusing for detection and identification of β-lactamases. *Journal of General Microbiology* **88,** 169–178.

MATTHEW, M., HEDGES, R. W. & SMITH, J. T. 1979 Types of β-lactamase determined by plasmids in Gram-negative bacteria. *Journal of Bacteriology* **138,** 657–662.

NEU, H. C. 1970 *Antimicrobial Agents and Chemotherapy, Annual,* ed. Hobby, G. pp. 534–538. American Chemical Society.

NEU, H. C. & CHOU, J. 1967 Release of surface enzymes in Enterobacteriaceae by osmotic shock. *Journal of Bacteriology* **94,** 1934–1945.

NEU, H. C. & HEPPEL, L. A. 1965 The release of enzymes from *Escherichia coli* by osmotic shock and during the formation of spheroplasts. *Journal of Biological Chemistry* **240,** 3685–3692.

NEU, H. C., ASHMAN, D. F. & PRICE, T. D. 1966 The release of the acid-soluble nucleotide pool of *E. coli* by EDTA-Tris. *Biochemical and Biophysical Research Communications* **25,** 615–621.

NEWTON, G. G. F. & HAMILTON-MILLER, J. M. T. 1967 Cephaloridine: chemical and biochemical aspects. *Postgraduate Medical Journal* **43,** 10–17.

NOSSAL, N. G. & HEPPEL, L. A. 1966 The release of enzymes by osmotic shock from *Escherichia coli* in exponential phase. *Journal of Biological Chemistry* **241,** 3055–3062.

SABBATH, L. D., JAGO, M. & ABRAHAM, E. P. 1965 Cephalosporinase and penicillinase activities of a β-lactamase from *Pseudomonas pyocyanea*. *Biochemical Journal* **96,** 739–752.

SMITH, J. T. & WYATT, J. M. 1974 Relation of R-factor and chromosomal β-lactamase with the periplastic space. *Journal of Bacteriology* **117,** 931–939.

SMITHIES, O. 1955 Zone electrophoresis in starch gels: group variations in serum proteins in normal human adults. *Biochemical Journal* **6,** 629–641.

SYKES, R. B. & RICHMOND, M. H. 1970 Intergeneric transfer of a β-lactamase gene between *P. aeruginosa* and *E. coli*. *Nature, London* **226,** 952–954.

SYKES, R. B. & SMITH, J. T. 1979 Biochemical aspects of β-lactamases from Gram negative organisms. In *Beta-Lactamases* ed. Hamilton-Miller, J. M. T. and Smith, J. T. pp. 369–402. London & New York: Academic Press

THOMPSON, R. H. S. 1962 Classification and nomenclature of enzymes and coenzymes. *Nature, London* **193,** 1227–1231.

WYATT, J. M. 1972 *Episomal and chromosomal bacterial enzymes: their retention and release*. Ph.D. thesis. University of London.

The Detection of Bacterial β-Lactamases and their Identification by Analytical Isoelectric Focusing

S. J. PLESTED, I. N. SIMPSON AND MARTINE JAMES

Chemotherapy Department, Microbiology Division, Glaxo Group Research Limited, Greenford, Middlesex, UK

β-Lactam antibiotics are susceptible to enzymic attack by β-lactamases, acylases and esterases (Fig. 1). Clinically, the most important of these enzymes are the β-lactamases which are believed to be produced by all bacteria (Matthew & Harris 1976). β-Lactamases produced by Gram positive organisms are generally extracellular and can be induced with predominantly penicillinase activity (Citri & Pollock 1966). Hence detection of such β-lactamases is relatively simple in the presence of an inducing agent and with benzylpenicillin or ampicillin as substrate. In contrast, Gram negative β-lactamases are generally intracellular and may be inducible or constitutive (Sykes & Matthew 1976). To facilitate detection of Gram negative β-lactamases it is often necessary to release any enzyme by cell disruption. Ultrasonic treatment is generally the most efficient technique for release of β-lactamase activity (Simpson & James, unpublished results). The main exceptions to this are the enzymes produced by *Bacteroides fragilis*, *Neisseria gonorrhoeae*, *Haemophilus influenzae* and strains producing particularly inducible or constitutively high levels of β-lactamase (Sykes & Percival 1978).

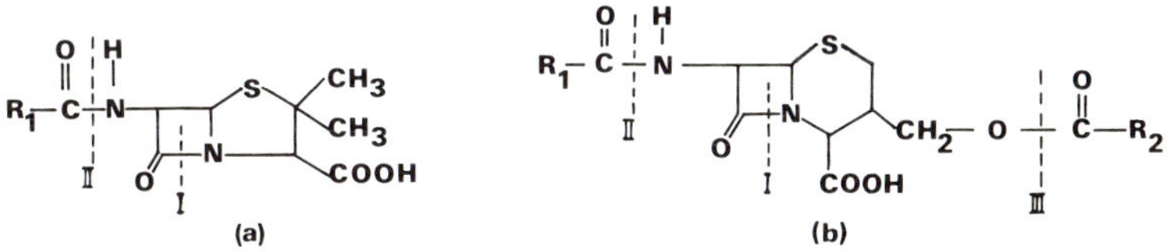

FIG. 1. Sites of action of degrading enzymes on (*a*) penicillins and (*b*) cephalosporins. I, β-lactamases; II, acylases; III, esterases.

ANTIBIOTICS
ISBN 0 12 604480 5

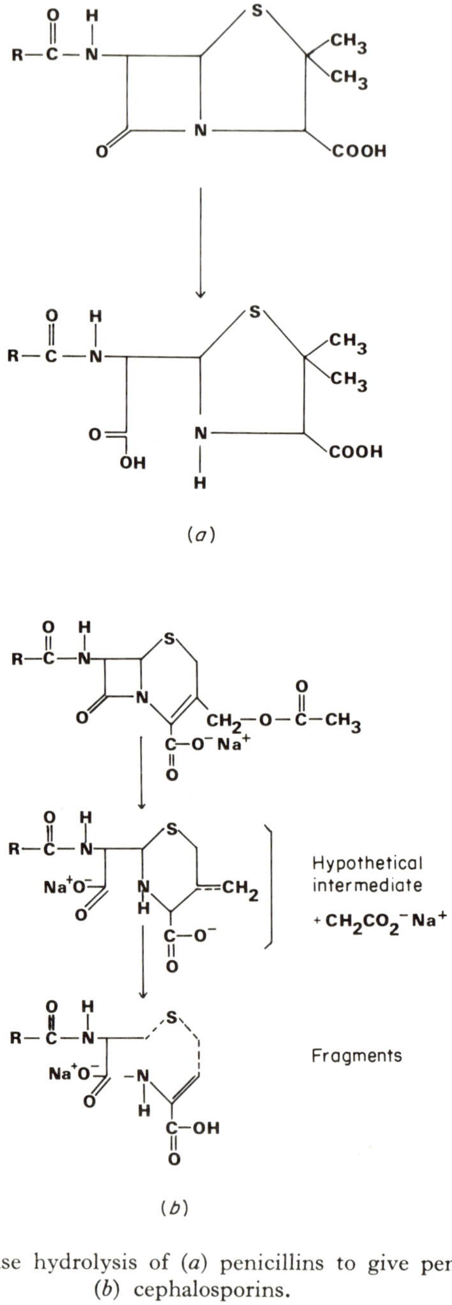

FIG. 2. β-Lactamase hydrolysis of (*a*) penicillins to give penicilloic acids, (*b*) cephalosporins.

β-Lactamases hydrolyse the cyclic amide bond of susceptible penicillins and cephalosporins which results in loss of antibacterial activity. In the case of a penicillin this reaction results in the formation of a stable penicilloic acid (Fig. 2*a*). The situation is more complex with cephalosporins. The first product of β-lactamase hydrolysis is hypothetically a cephalosporoic acid; however this is usually unstable and undergoes rapid decomposition (Fig. 2*b*) (Hamilton-Miller *et al.* 1970).

Acylases (Hamilton-Miller 1966) are also produced by a range of Gram negative micro-organisms. These enzymes remove the acyl side chain, which usually results in loss of antibacterial activity. In many cases significant amounts of β-lactamase and acylase are produced in the same strain (Cole & Sutherland 1965), and hence it can be important to distinguish between these two types of enzymes. Microbial esterases cleave the ester bond at position 3 in certain cephalosporins. However, these enzymes are relatively rare and unlikely to affect methods for detection of β-lactamase.

β-Lactamases are an extremely diverse group of enzymes and several methods for detection are available. The choice of detection system varies according to enzyme type, the material being assayed and the speed with which an answer is required.

Detection of β-Lactamases

β-Lactamases can be detected using both microbiological and biochemical systems.

Microbiological detection

Hydrolysed β-lactam antibiotics lose antibacterial activity. Hence β-lactamase-producing organisms can be detected by their ability to support the growth of a β-lactam-sensitive control organism on media containing otherwise inhibitory concentrations of β-lactam antibiotic. Two main methods are available.

Clover leaf (McGhie *et al.* 1977)

An agar plate is spread with the Oxford staphylococcus (NCTC 6571) and an ampicillin disc (30 μg) placed in the centre. A heavy inoculum of each test strain is streaked radially from the disc and the plate incubated at 37°C overnight. Deep indentations of growth of the staphylococcus in an otherwise circular zone of inhibition indicate β-lactamase production by the test strain (Fig. 3).

Detection time: 18 h.

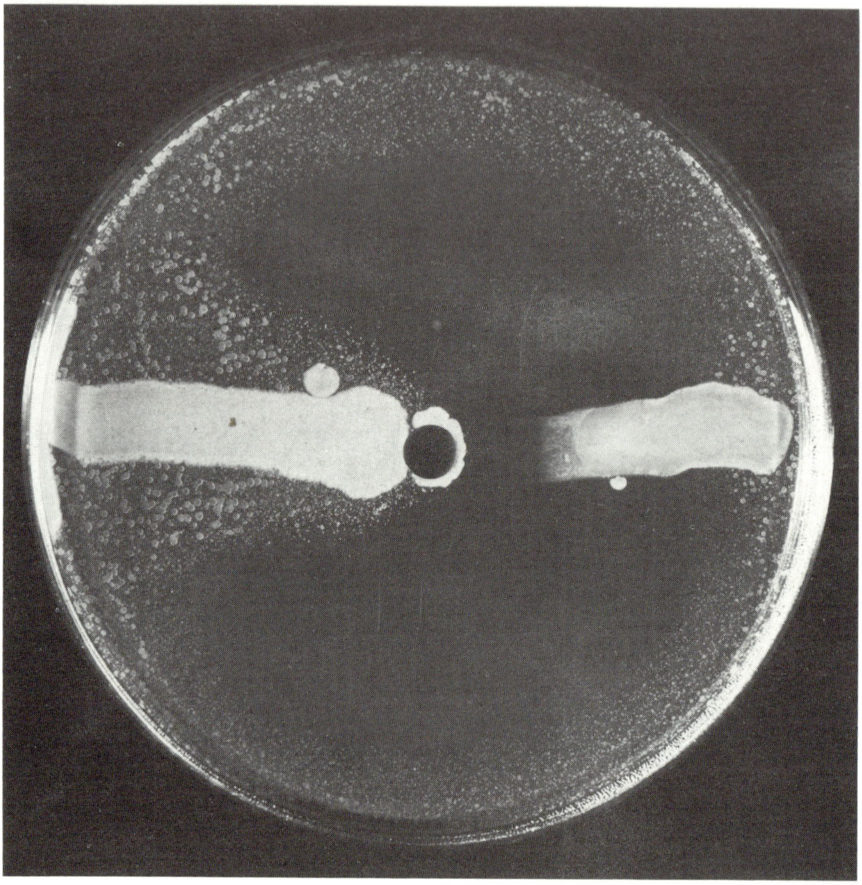

FIG. 3. Clover leaf method for β-lactamase detection. Test strains inoculated radially round the 30 μg ampicillin disc. Indentations of growth of the seeded staphylococcus along these streaks indicate β-lactamase producing organisms.

Double disc (Masuda 1976)

Agar plates are seeded with a culture of the Oxford staphylococcus (NCTC 6571) and antibiotic discs (30 μg ampicillin or cephaloridine) placed in the centre. Filter paper discs dipped into 6h broth cultures of test organism are placed radially around the antibiotic disc. After overnight incubation at 37°C growth of the staphylococcus around the outer satellite discs indicates β-lactamase production by the test strains (Fig. 4).

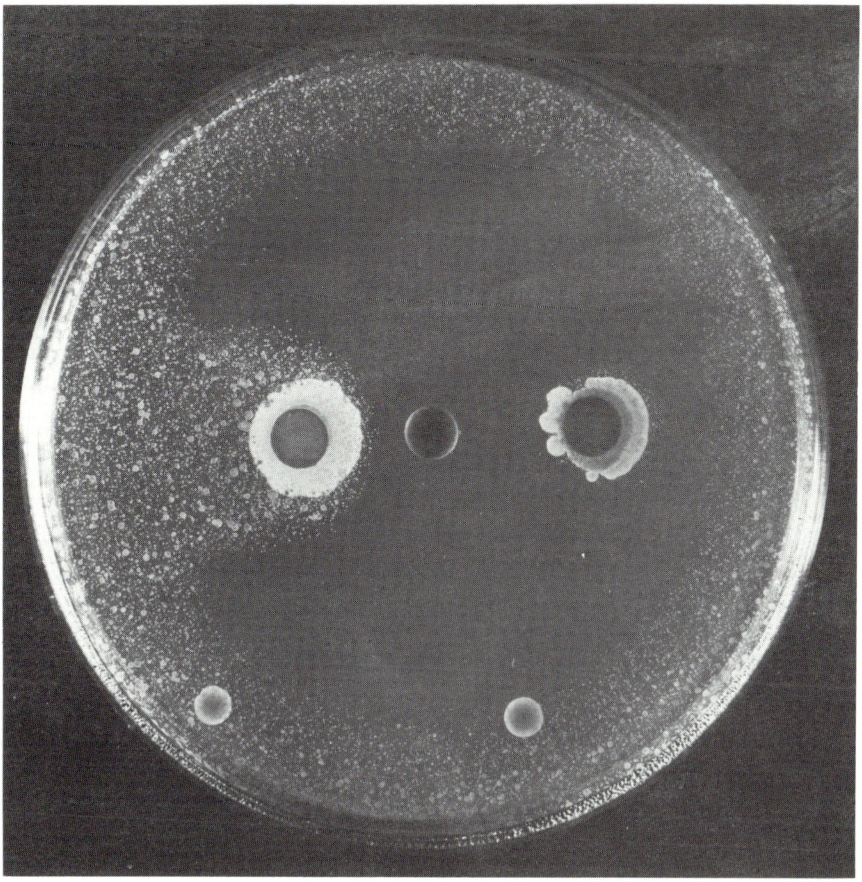

FIG. 4. Double disc method for β-lactamase detection. The central disc contained 30 μg ampicillin, the outer ones were dipped in cultures of test strains. Growth of the seeded staphylococcus around the outer discs indicates β-lactamase producing organisms.

Biochemical detection

Routine biochemical techniques can be subdivided into the following three groups: (a) Chromogenic β-lactams. Hydrolysis of certain β-lactam compounds leads to a distinct colour change in the visible region. (b) Acidimetric. β-Lactamase hydrolysis of β-lactam antibiotic leads to the formation of at least one extra carboxyl group which can be detected using pH indicators. (c) Iodometric. The products of β-lactamase hydrolysis act as reducing agents and can be used to remove iodine from a blue starch/iodine complex, resulting in loss of colour.

Each of the above biochemical detection techniques can be employed in a variety of methods. In each case β-lactamase-'producing' and 'non-producing' control organisms should be screened in conjunction with the test strains.

Techniques with chromogenic β-lactams

Reagents. The most widely used compound in this category is nitrocefin (O'Callaghan *et al.* 1972).

In aqueous solution, this cephalosporin has an absorption peak at 386 nm (yellow), which disappears on hydrolysis by β-lactamase. There is a simultaneous appearance of a new peak at 482 nm (red). The compound is dissolved initially in dimethyl sulphoxide and then diluted in 0·05 mol/l phosphate buffer, pH 7·0.

Another cephalosporin, PADAC (Calbiochem-Behring Corp.), behaves in a similar manner to nitrocefin, changing from a deep violet to pale yellow upon hydrolysis by β-lactamase.

Method. Nitrocefin (50 mg/l) solution is applied direct to plate or broth culture and the light yellow to deep red colour change observed. This is by far the most sensitive and simplest method for this reagent but all the methods applicable to acidimetric reagents can also be used.

Acidimetric techniques

Reagents. Several possibilities are available. For penicillin–phenol red test reagent (Rosen *et al.* 1972), 600 mg of benzylpenicillin is added to 16·6 ml distilled water and 2 ml 0·5% w/v phenol red solution. The pH is adjusted to 8·5 using 1·0 mol/l sodium hydroxide. Hydrolysis of the benzylpenicillin is detected by a violet to yellow colour change. Alternative indicators include bromocresol purple giving a purple to yellow colour change (Slack *et al.* 1977), Andrade's indicator, yellow to pink (Knox & Smith 1961) and *N*-phenyl-1-naphthylamine-azo-O-carboxybenzene which forms a purple precipitate that stains β-lactamase-producing bacterial colonies (Adams *et al.* 1970).

Filter paper strips (Slack *et al.* 1977). Whatman's No. 1 filter papers (9 cm diam.) are immersed in the reagent and immediately dried in a desiccator. Once dry the paper is cut into strips of *ca.* 0·6 × 1·2 cm and stored at 4°C over silica gel. The strips remain active for several months. Tests are performed by placing a drop of distilled water on a clean microscope slide and covering it with a test strip, ensuring the paper is moistened but not saturated. A bacteriological loop is used to remove a few colonies from a fresh culture of the test strain and then streaked across one end of the strip. β-Lactamases are detected by the appropriate colour change.

Detection time: 5–10 min.

Test tube or microtitre tray (Escamilla 1976; Skinner & Wise 1977). Colonies of an overnight agar culture of the test organism are suspended in a small amount of normal saline. A few drops of the reagent are then added to the test suspension either in a test tube or in a microtitre tray.

Detection time: 1 min.

Capillary tube (Rosen *et al.* 1972). A capillary tube is dipped into the reagent and the liquid allowed to flow by capillary action 1–2 cm into the tube. The tip of the capillary is then scraped across several colonies of the test strain, growing on a solid medium. Care should be taken to ensure that the resulting plug of bacteria is in direct contact with the reagent, so that no air is trapped between the two. The tubes are incubated at room temperature in a vertical position by securing the empty end in plasticine.

Detection time: up to 1 h.

Membrane filter (Knox & Smith 1961). Cellulose acetate membranes (Oxoid Ltd, 8 cm, 0·2 μm pore size) are placed on nutrient agar plates. Ten to twelve drops, each 50–100 μl, of overnight cultures are put on the membranes. The inoculated membranes are incubated overnight at 37°C, removed with forceps and placed on 2 or 3 layers of Whatman No. 1 filter paper previously moistened with the test reagent.

Detection time: 24 h.

Iodometric techniques

The composition of the test reagents varies according to the methods employed.

Filter strips (Jorgensen *et al.* 1977). A solution of 0·2% w/v soluble starch and 1% w/v benzylpenicillin plus Lugol's iodine (2 g potassium iodide and 1 g iodine dissolved in 100 ml of distilled water) are the reagents required.

Filter paper strips are immersed in the starch–penicillin solution, dried and stored at −20°C for up to a year. For use, strips are placed in a Petri dish and moistened with the Lugol's iodine. Approximately 10 colonies of overnight growth of the test organism on solid agar are applied to the centre of the strip with a bacteriological loop. β-Lactamase production is detected by decolourization of the purple reagent.

Detection time: 1 min.

Tubes (Catlin 1975). The starch indicator is a 1% solution of soluble starch, prepared fresh each day. The iodine reagent is 2·03 g iodine and 53·2 g potassium iodide dissolved in 100 ml distilled water. A solution of 6 g/l benzylpenicillin or ampicillin in 0·05 mol/l phosphate buffer pH 7·0 is also required.

The penicillin solution is dispensed into small tubes or into a microtitre tray. Test bacteria are removed from fresh agar cultures and suspended in the penicillin solution at a concentration of 10^9 cells/ml. Following incubation for at least 1 h at room temperature, two small drops of starch indicator and one drop iodine reagent are added giving a blue colour. Rapid decolourization indicates β-lactamase. Two additional controls of penicillin solution without bacteria should be included, one receiving drops of starch indicator and iodine at the start of the hour's incubation and the other at the end.

Detection time: up to 10 min.

Agar plates (Foley & Perret 1962). Fresh 1% w/v soluble starch solution, 0·04 mol/l iodine solution and benzylpenicillin solution (6 mg/l) are required.

Plates with single sparse colonies of the test organisms are covered with strips of Whatman No. 1 filter paper excluding air bubbles. The strips, previously impregnated with starch solution and dried, are immersed in the penicillin solution and drained prior to placing on the plates. After 30 min at room temperature the iodine solution is pipetted on to the paper. β-Lactamase-producing isolates form white spots on the blue paper.

Detection time: up to 10 min.

Another modification involves growing the test organisms on plates containing 2% starch (Sykes & Matthew 1979). After overnight incubation at 37°C the plates are flooded with the penicillin solution and left for 15 min at room temperature. The penicillin solution is then removed and replaced by the iodine reagent. β-Lactamase-producing colonies have colourless halos against a blue background.

A summary of the various detection systems is provided in Table 1.

Identification of β-Lactamases using Analytical Isoelectric Focusing

Analytical isoelectric focusing (IEF) is a technique whereby proteins align themselves as sharp bands according to their isoelectric points (pIs) in an electrophoretically produced pH gradient. A high degree of resolution is obtained because focusing is effected by forces that act against diffusion and the proteins are concentrated during their separation. For identification of β-lactamases, focusing is conducted upon thin layers of polyacrylamide gel and the focused enzymes are located using nitrocefin. The β-lactamases appear as a pattern of bands (usually a group comprising a main band and several satellite bands). Purification of crude β-lactamase extracts is unnecessary and the technique is sufficiently sensitive to detect β-lactamase activity in mutants previously reported to lack the enzyme (Matthew *et al.* 1975). The technique is also capable of distinguishing between enzymes indistinguishable by other biochemical and immunological means.

TABLE 1

Summary of applicability of detection systems

Criterion	Detection system: Microbiological	Chromogenic β-lactam	Acidimetric	Iodometric
Specificity	Acylases and β-lactamases	β-lactamases only	Acylases and β-lactamases	β-lactamases only
Sensitivity to β-lactamases	All types	All types	Preferentially for penicillinases and broad spectrum β-lactamases*	
Misleading results	Biologically active products of hydrolysis	Reacts with serum and some sulphur-containing molecules	Reacts with acidic groups of general metabolic products	Reacts with other reducing groups
Applicable methods				
Filter paper	Not applicable	√	√	√
Tube/microtitre		√	√	√
Membrane filter		√	√	√
Agar plate		√	×	√

* Sensitivity to cephalosporinases instead of penicillinases may be increased by using a cephalosporin substrate.

Preparation of crude β-lactamase extracts

A loop of cells is taken from a fresh plate culture and used to inoculate a 250 ml Ehrlenmeyer flask containing 100 ml of nutrient broth. After overnight incubation at 37°C on an orbital shaker, the bacterial cells are harvested by centrifugation at 5000 **g** for 45 min at 4°C. For extracellular β-lactamases, the supernatant fluid constitutes the crude β-lactamase extract. For preparation of intracellular enzymes the cell pellet is resuspended in 10 ml of 0·02 mol/l neutral phosphate buffer, and the cells disrupted by ultrasonic treatment (100 W Ultrasonic Disintegrator, MSE) for 3 min in an ice-water bath. Cell debris is removed by centrifugation at 17,000 **g** for 60 min at 4°C. Crude enzymes are stored at −20°C (Simpson *et al.* 1980).

Assessment of β-lactamase activity of crude enzyme preparation

Samples of 0·1 ml of crude β-lactamase extract are added to 0·3 ml nitrocefin at a concentration of 50 μg/ml in a microtitre tray. The time required for the colour change is taken as an indication of the β-lactamase activity of the crude enzyme preparation. All β-lactamase preparations that fail to give a positive response within 2 min are concentrated by freeze-drying.

Concentration of β-lactamase preparations with low activity

Samples of 10 ml of crude β-lactamase extract are placed in sealed lengths of 8/32 in (*ca.* 0·64 cm) Visking Tubing (The Scientific Instrument Centre, London) and dialysed overnight at 4°C against distilled water to remove excess salts. Each dialysed β-lactamase preparation is distributed equally between three 12 ml conical-based centrifuge tubes and frozen rapidly in an acetone–dry ice freezing mixture. The frozen extracts are placed overnight in a freeze-drier. Freeze-dried preparations are stored at 4°C and reactivated by the addition of 0·1 to 0·5 ml of 0·02 mol/l neutral phosphate buffer.

Analytical isoelectric focusing

The following method is taken from Matthew *et al.* (1975).

Apparatus

This is home-made to the design of Williamson and co-workers (Awdeh *et al.* 1968; Salaman & Williamson 1971). Alternatively, multi-purpose electrophoretic kits are available from LKB Instruments (South Croydon, Surrey, UK) or Bio-Rad Laboratories Ltd (Bromley, Kent, UK).

Isoelectric focusing is performed on sheets of polyacrylamide gel (21·5 × 16·5 × 0·15 cm) supported on glass plates. The composition of the gel mixture is given in Table 2. The gel sets within 1 h in daylight. A graph paper life-size layout is used when loading the plate so that pH values can be noted on this same piece of paper and it can be compared easily with photographs, provided the plate is photographed beside a ruler. Samples, up to 100 μl, are loaded on the gel surface 2 cm from the anode and 25 μl myoglobin (20 mg/ml) is loaded 1 cm from each side edge as a visible guide to focusing. The gel is inverted onto the carbon electrodes for running. Focusing is carried out at a constant power of 1·0 W (max voltage setting: 500 V) for 18 h at 4°C. As soon as the current is switched off the pH gradient is read at 0·5 cm intervals from cathode to anode using a flat-end electrode.

TABLE 2

Composition of gel for isoelectric focusing

Material	Volume used (ml)	Final concentration
5% Tetramethyl-ethylenediamine (TEMED) in distilled water	0·2	0·25 mg/l
40% Ampholine w/v (various pH ranges available)	2·0	2% w/v
Acrylamide (100 g) plus methylene bis acrylamide (2·7 g) in water (300 ml)	9	Acrylamide 70 g/l, bis acrylamide 2 g/l
Distilled water	25	
	The mixture is degassed at this point	
Riboflavin (2 mg/100 ml water)	4	2×10^{-3} g/l

Staining the gels for β-lactamase activity.

Detection of β-lactamases is most easily achieved using nitrocefin (O'Callaghan *et al.* 1972). A sheet of Whatman No. 54 paper is dipped in a solution of this chromogenic cephalosporin (500 mg/l) and laid over the gel surface. The focused β-lactamases appear as red bands against a yellow background.

Staining gels for protein

Gels are immersed for 1 h in Coomassie brilliant blue G (0·1%, w/v dissolved in ethanol/acetic acid/water, 35:10:55, v/v). They are destained in ethanol/acetic acid/water (30:5:65, v/v).

Photography

A precise record of the results can be obtained only if the plates are photographed, because bands associated with β-lactamase activity cannot be fixed. When a focused gel is treated with β-lactam substrate the β-lactamase bands appear gradually and by the time the weakest bands are visible, the strongest bands have diffused. Serial photographs using a green filter and Agfa Ortho film are taken to obtain a complete record. Figure 5 shows common marker enzymes: see Broad & Smith (this volume, pp. 93–110).

Discussion

Detection of β-lactamases

Microbiological detection tests are relatively time consuming, whilst the majority of biochemical tests can be conducted in less than ten minutes. Of the biochemical tests, the iodometric and chromogenic β-lactam detection techniques are specific for β-lactamases, whereas acidimetric and microbiological techniques do not distinguish between β-lactamase and acylase activity (Table 1). Chromogenic and microbiological techniques are sensitive for all types of β-lactamase activity, but iodometric and acidimetric techniques are less sensitive for enzymes with predominantly cephalosporinase activity. The cephalosporinase sensitivity of the iodometric and acidimetric techniques can be improved by the use of a cephalosporin substrate but this may result in reduced overall sensitivity due to the non-specific hydrolysis of cephalosporins (Fig. 2*b*). Each of the detection techniques may yield misleading results owing to antibacterial activity of hydrolysis products (microbiological tests) or interference by other chemical groups (biochemical tests). It is likely that the factors affecting nitrocefin detection methods are less of a problem in these cases (O'Callaghan *et al.* 1972).

Although each of the three biochemical tests can be implemented theoretically in at least four ways, i.e. filter strips, tubes, membrane filter and direct upon agar plates, it is our experience that some combinations are significantly better than others. The filter paper strip method is most successful using a bromocresol purple pH indicator. Mast Laboratories Ltd (Bootle, Merseyside, UK) market this combination as 'Intralactam' (Wheldon & Slack 1979; Shannon & Phillips 1980). Phenol red reagent is the best indicator for capillary tube and microtitre methods, whereas nitrocefin is the most effective reagent for direct application to agar plates. This is the simplest and most rapid of the detection methods. The membrane filter test and the nitrocefin plate test are the only methods which reliably detect small numbers of β-lactamase-'producing' or -'non-producing' organisms in mixed cultures.

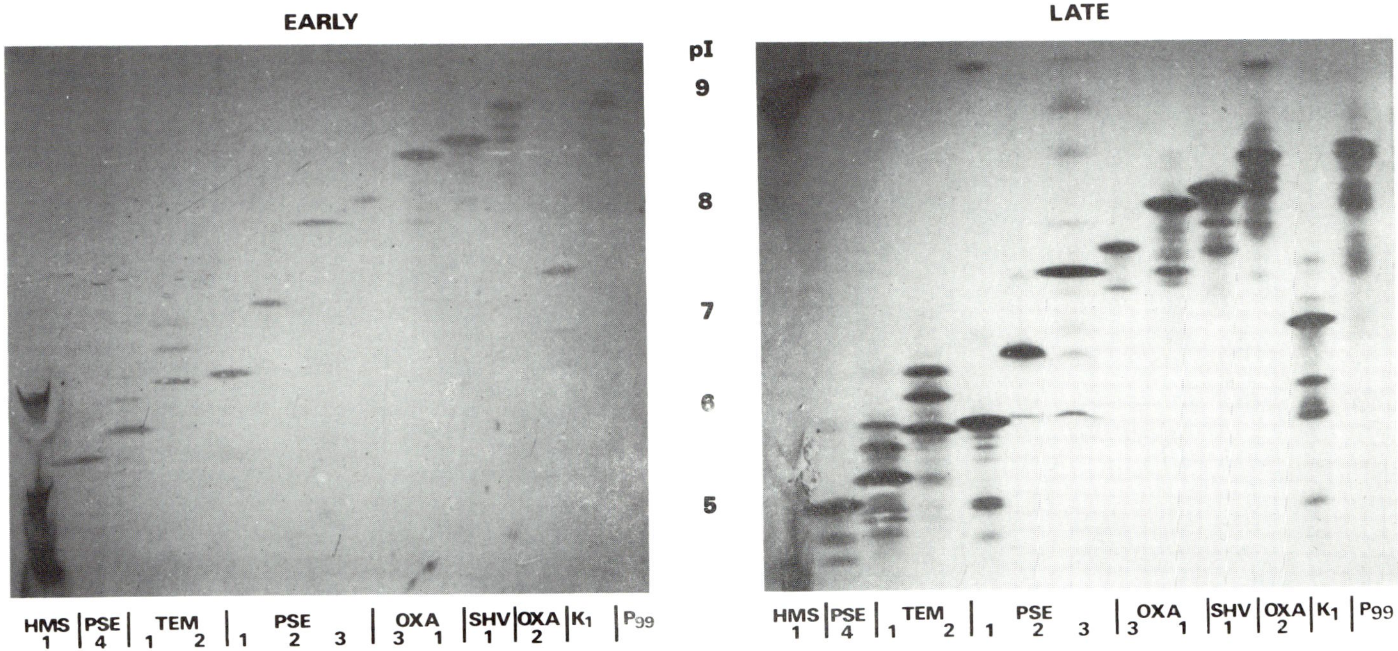

FIG. 5. Isoelectric focusing patterns of common R-plasmid- and chromosomally mediated β-lactamases.

Analytical isoelectric focusing

Many biochemical criteria have been used to characterize and hence classify β-lactamases (Hamilton-Miller 1967; Jack & Richmond 1970; O'Callaghan & Morris 1972; Richmond & Sykes 1973; Sykes & Matthew 1976). Clinically the most important criterion is the substrate profile, i.e. relative activity against various penicillins and cephalosporins as substrates. Until the advent of isoelectric focusing, determination of the substrate profile of an enzyme had always necessitated relatively laborious techniques (this volume, pp. 127–139). Isoelectric focusing permits rapid comparison of test enzymes with a range of known and well-characterized enzymes. Should identity be found, the necessity for substrate profile studies is removed since the test enzyme will exhibit the same biochemical properties as the marker enzyme. This application is essentially limited to R-plasmid-mediated rather than chromosomally mediated β-lactamases, because distinct R-plasmid β-lactamases are few in number and readily recognized (Matthew *et al.* 1979), whereas chromosomally mediated β-lactamases are species specific and hence extremely diverse and numerous (Matthew & Harris 1976). Isoelectric focusing can also be used to determine the number of different β-lactamases produced by a strain and to study transfer of plasmids mediating β-lactamases.

Summary

β-Lactam antibiotics are susceptible to enzymic attack by β-lactamases, acylases and esterases. Clinically the most important of these are the β-lactamases which are produced by all bacteria.

Several techniques are available for detection of β-lactamases. Microbiological techniques are very sensitive but slow and not specific for β-lactamases. Biochemical techniques are much more rapid and each may be implemented in several ways, e.g. filter paper strips, tubes, membrane filters and agar plates. Methods involving chromogenic β-lactams, e.g. nitrocefin and PADAC are specific for β-lactamases and generally the simplest to use.

Isoelectric focusing is a technique for rapid identification of β-lactamases. The technique can also be used to determine the number of β-lactamases produced by a strain and to study transfer of R-plasmids mediating β-lactamases.

References

Adams, A. P., Barry, A. L. & Benner, E. J. 1970 A simple, rapid test to differentiate penicillin-susceptible from penicillin resistant *Staphylococcus aureus. Journal of Infectious Diseases* **122,** 544–546.

AWDEH, Z. L., WILLIAMSON, A. R. & ASKONAS, P. A. 1968 Isoelectric focusing in polyacrylamide gel and its application to immunoglobulins. *Nature, London* **219,** 66–67.

CATLIN, W. 1975 Iodometric detection of *Haemophilus influenzae* beta-lactamase: rapid presumptive test for ampicillin resistance. *Antimicrobial Agents and Chemotherapy* **7,** 265–270.

CITRI, N. & POLLOCK, M. R. 1966 The biochemistry and function of β-lactamase (penicillinase). *Advances in Enzymology* **28,** 237–323.

COLE, M. & SUTHERLAND, R. 1965 The role of penicillin acylase in the resistance of Gram-negative bacteria to penicillin. *Journal of General Microbiology* **42,** 345–356.

ESCAMILLA, J. 1976 Susceptibility of *Haemophilus influenzae* to ampicillin as determined by use of a modified, one minute β-lactamase test. *Antimicrobial Agents and Chemotherapy* **9,** 196–198.

FOLEY, J. M. & PERRETT, C. J. 1962 Screening bacterial colonies for penicillinase production. *Nature, London* **195,** 287–288.

HAMILTON-MILLER, J. M. T. 1966 Penicillin acylase. *Bacteriological Reviews* **30,** 761–771.

HAMILTON-MILLER, J. M. T. 1967 Hydrolysis of cephalosporins by β-lactamases from Gram-negative bacteria. *Nature, London* **214,** 1333–1334.

HAMILTON-MILLER, J. M. T., NEWTON, G. G. F. & ABRAHAM, E. P. 1970 Products of aminolysis and enzymic hydrolysis of the cephalosporins. *Biochemical Journal* **116,** 371–384.

JACK, G. W. & RICHMOND, M. H. 1970 A comparative study of eight distinct β-lactamases synthesised by Gram-negative bacteria. *Journal of General Microbiology* **61,** 43–61.

JORGENSEN, J. H., LEE, J. C. & ALEXANDER, G. A. 1977 Rapid penicillinase paper strip test for detection of β-lactamase producing *Haemophilus influenzae* and *Neiserria gonorrhoeae*. *Antimicrobial Agents and Chemotherapy* **11,** 1083–1088.

KNOX, R. & Smith, J. T. 1961 Use of cellulose acetate membranes for detecting penicillinase producing organisms. *Nature, London* **191,** 926–927.

MASUDA, G. 1976 Studies on bactericidal activities of β-lactam antibiotics on agar plates: the correlation with the antibacterial activities determined by the conventional methods. *Journal of Antibiotics* **29,** 1237–1240.

MATTHEW, M. & HARRIS, A. M. 1976 Identification of β-lactamases by analytical isoelectric focusing: Correlation with bacterial taxonomy. *Journal of General Microbiology* **94,** 55–67.

MATTHEW, M., HARRIS, A. M., MARSHALL, M. J. & ROSS, G. W. 1975 The use of analytical isoelectric focusing for detection and identification of β-lactamase. *Journal of General Microbiology* **88,** 169–178.

MATTHEW, M., HEDGES, R. W. & SMITH, J. T. 1979 Types of β-lactamase determined by plasmids in Gram-negative bacteria. *Journal of Bacteriology* **138,** 657–662.

MCGHIE, D., CLARKE, P. D., JOHNSON, T. & HUTCHINSON, J. G. P. 1977 Detection of beta-lactamase activity of *Haemophilus influenzae*. *Journal of Clinical Pathology* **30,** 585–586.

O'CALLAGHAN, C. H. & MORRIS, A. 1972 Inhibition of β-lactamases by β-lactam antibiotics. *Antimicrobial Agents and Chemotherapy* **2,** 442–448.

O'CALLAGHAN, C. H., MORRIS, A., KIRBY, S. M. & SHINGLER, A. H. 1972 Novel method for detection of β-lactamases by using a chromogenic cephalosporin substrate. *Antimicrobial Agents and Chemotherapy* **1,** 283–288.

RICHMOND, M. H. & SYKES, R. B. 1973 The β-lactamases of Gram-negative bacteria and their possible physiological role. *Advances in Microbial Physiology* **9,** 31–88.

ROSEN, I. G., JACOBSON, J. & RUDDERMAN, R. 1972 Rapid capillary tube method for detecting penicillin resistance in *Staphylococcus aureus. Applied Microbiology* **23,** 649–650.

SALAMAN, M. R. & WILLIAMSON, A. R. 1971 Isoelectric focusing of proteins in the native and denatured states. *Biochemical Journal* **122,** 93–99.

SHANNON, K. & PHILLIPS, I. 1980 β-lactamase detection by three simple methods: Intralactam, nitrocefin and acidimetric. *Journal of Antimicrobial Chemotherapy* **6,** 617–621.

SIMPSON, I. N., HARPER, P. B. & O'CALLAGHAN, C. H. 1980 Principal β-lactamases responsible for resistance to β-lactam antibiotics in urinary tract infections. *Antimicrobial Agents and Chemotherapy* **17,** 929–936.

SKINNER, A. & WISE, R. 1977 A comparison of three rapid methods for the detection of β-lactamase activity in *Haemophilus influenzae. Journal of Clinical Pathology* **30,** 1030–1032.

SLACK, M. P. E., WHELDON, D. B. & TURK, D. C. 1977 A rapid test for β-lactamase production by *Haemophilus influenzae. Lancet* **2,** 906

SYKES, R. B. & MATTHEW, M. 1976 The β-lactamases of Gram-negative bacteria and their role in resistance to β-lactam antibiotics. *Journal of Antimicrobial Chemotherapy* **2,** 115–151.

SYKES, R. B. & MATTHEW, M. 1979 Detection, assay and immunology of β-lactamases. In *Beta-Lactamases*, ed. Hamilton-Miller, J. M. T. & Smith, J. T. pp. 17–49. London & New York: Academic Press.

SYKES, R. B. & PERCIVAL, A. 1978 Studies on gonococcal β-lactamases. In *Immunobiology of* N. gonorrhoeae, ed. Brooks, G. F., Gotschlich, E. C., Holmes, K. K., Sawyer, W. D. & Young, F. E. p. 68. Washington: American Society of Microbiology.

WHELDON, D. B. & SLACK, M. P. E. 1979 An evaluation of Intralactam, a preparation for the detection of β-lactamase production by *Haemophilus influenzae. Journal of Clinical Pathology* **32,** 738–740.

Quantitative Methods for Assessing Stability of β-Lactam Antibiotics to Cell-free β-Lactamase Extracts

JUDITH HOLT, I. N. SIMPSON AND P. B. HARPER

Chemotherapy Department, Microbiology Division, Glaxo Group Research Ltd, Greenford, Middlesex, UK

Introduction

Production of β-lactamases is a major factor responsible for bacterial resistance to β-lactam antibiotics. Quantitative techniques are necessary for characterizing β-lactamases and assessing the stability of β-lactam antibiotics to these enzymes. Both applications are important in the screening of new β-lactam antibiotics and in the choice of antimicrobial agents for infections involving β-lactamase-producing organisms.

Penicillins are hydrolysed by β-lactamases to give their corresponding penicilloic acids in stoichiometric proportions; the product has two acidic groups whereas the parent compound has only one such group (as shown in Fig. 1*a*). Whereas penicilloic acids are chemically stable, the products of hydrolysis of cephalosporins are generally unstable owing to the presence of the substituent at position 3 of the cephalosporin nucleus, as depicted in Fig. 1*b*.

The techniques currently available for determination of β-lactamase activities fall into two categories: (a) microbiological (bioassay); (b) biochemical—spectrophotometric, acidimetric, iodometric and hydroxylamine techniques, and high pressure liquid chromatography (HPLC).

The method of choice is dependent upon the range of substrates and β-lactamases involved and the desired rapidity and sensitivity of the assay.

Microbiological Methods

Bioassay

β-Lactamase hydrolysis of penicillin and cephalosporin antibiotics

ANTIBIOTICS
ISBN 0 12 604480 5

results in loss of antibacterial activity. Residual compound can be determined using microbiological plate assay.

Method (Ross & O'Callaghan 1975)
Choice of assay organism. This will vary according to the concentration and intrinsic activity of the antibiotic involved. Gram positive organisms are generally more reliable than Gram negatives.
Reagents. 1 mmol/l substrate prepared in 0·02 mol/l phosphate buffer pH 7·0. Iodine reagent (17·8 mg iodine dissolved in 100 ml of 0·06% w/v potassium iodide solution).
Procedure. Substrate and β-lactamase are incubated together for 30 min. Samples are removed at 5 min intervals and diluted 100-fold with iodine reagent to stop the reaction. Replicate aliquots of 0·1 ml of test samples and standard substrate solutions are applied to 8 × 8 assay plates using randomized or Latin square designs (Lees & Tootill, 1955*a*, *b*, *c*). The plates are incubated at 37°C overnight. Zones of inhibition are measured and residual substrate determined following calibration against the substrate standards.

Biochemical Methods

Spectrophotometric

Hydrolysis of the cyclic amide bond in the β-lactam ring of penicillins and cephalosporins (Figs 1*a*, *b*) results in a detectable shift in the u.v. absorption spectrum (Fig. 2). The wavelength at which maximum decrease in absorption occurs is termed λmax and is determined by comparing spectra of intact and fully hydrolysed substrate. The rate of substrate hydrolysis is determined by measuring the rate of fall in optical density (O.D.) at λmax.

Method (O'Callaghan *et al.* 1969)
Equipment. Double beam recording spectrophotometer with thermostatically controlled cell carrier.
Reagents. Cephalosporin and penicillin substrates are prepared at 10^{-3} and 10^{-2} mol/l respectively in 0·02 mol/l phosphate buffer, pH 7·0. Enzyme concentration is adjusted to hydrolyse completely the substrate in 10–20 min.

Procedure. Two cuvettes, one containing 0·3 ml substrate and 2·6 ml buffer (test) and the other containing 2·9 ml buffer (blank) are equilibrated at 37°C. 0·1 ml of enzyme solution is then added to both cuvettes and the rate of decrease in O.D. at λmax monitored over the initial linear part of the reaction to obtain a value for change in O.D./min.

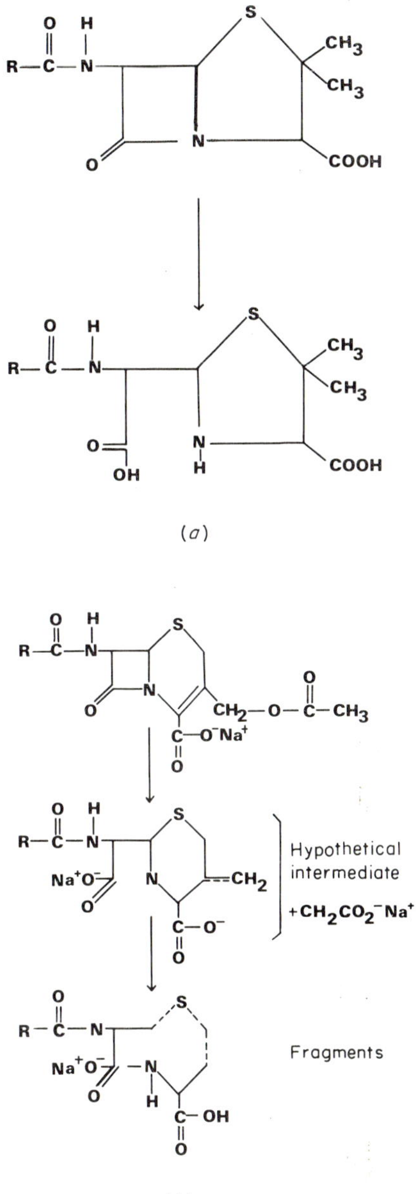

FIG. 1. β-Lactamase hydrolysis of (*a*) penicillins to give penicilloic acids, (*b*) cephalosporins.

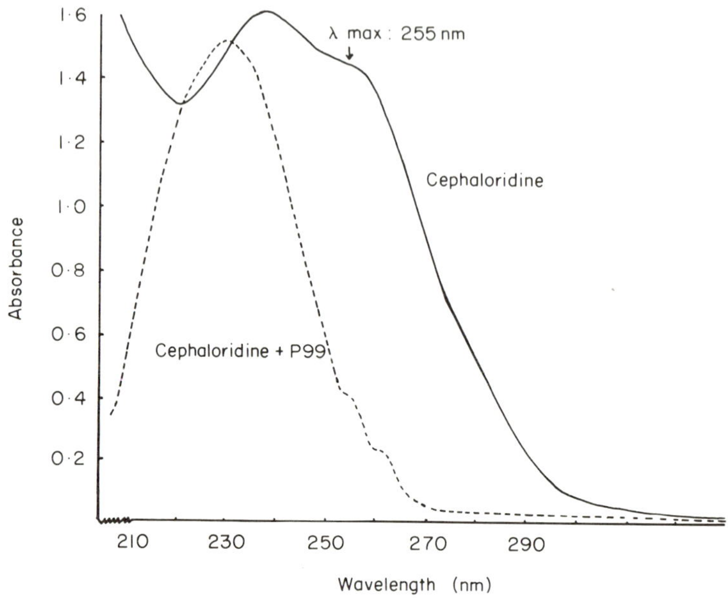

FIG. 2. Ultraviolet spectrum of intact and fully hydrolysed cephaloridine.

Calculation. $$R = \frac{\Delta \text{O.D.} \times N \times \text{enzyme dilution}}{\text{O.D.}_{\cdot 1} \times \text{time}}$$

where R = μmoles of substrate hydrolysed/min/ml enzyme, ΔO.D. = change in optical density, N = μmoles of substrate in cuvette (0·3 for cephalosporins, 3·0 for penicillins), $\text{O.D.}_{\cdot 1}$ = optical density of intact substrate.

In the original method (O'Callaghan *et al.* 1969), the divisor used was the difference in O.D. between intact and fully hydrolysed substrate, termed 'total destruction'. However, with the evolution of β-lactams particularly stable to β-lactamases, e.g. ceftazidime (O'Callaghan *et al.* 1980) and moxalactam (Yoshida *et al.* 1980), the change in O.D. associated with 'total destruction' cannot easily be determined using routine β-lactamase preparations. In addition the products of hydrolysis may themselves absorb u.v. light, giving misleading results. Hence the best compromise is to assume that total hydrolysis gives total loss of u.v. absorption.

Special case: chromogenic compounds

Certain β-lactam compounds also have significant absorption spectra in the visible region, which can be utilized instead of their u.v. spectra.

Nitrocefin (O'Callaghan *et al.* 1972) is a cephalosporin which changes from yellow (intact compound) to red (fully hydrolysed). Hence for this compound the rate of hydrolysis can be determined by decrease in O.D. at 386 nm (yellow) or increase in O.D. at 482 nm (red). Similarly another cephalosporin (Schlindler & Huber 1980) PADAC forms a violet solution (λmax 573 nm) which changes to yellow (λmax 463 nm) following hydrolysis.

Acidimetric

β-Lactamase hydrolysis of penicillins and cephalosporins results in an increase in the number of acidic groups. Hence the reaction rate can be determined by monitoring change in pH. Several methods are available.

pH Stat titration (Hou & Poole 1972; Konecny & Schneider 1978)
Equipment. pH meter, automatic titrator, titration assembly, titrigraph, autoburette, water-jacketed reaction cell.
Reagent. Potassium hydroxide solution (0·04 mol/l), 5·0 mmol/l substrate prepared in pH 7·0 phosphate buffer.
Procedure. 20 ml of substrate solution are equilibrated to operating temperature by stirring in a water-jacketed reaction vessel. A slow stream of nitrogen gas is passed over the surface of the substrate solution and the pH adjusted to the set point by automatic titration. Enzyme solution (less than 0·5 ml, and capable of hydrolysing 2–10 μmoles of substrate/min) is added to initiate the reaction. The rate of substrate hydrolysis is directly proportional to the rate of alkali addition required to maintain a constant pH.
Calculation. The initial rate (about 50% of the entire course of the reaction) is usually followed. The rate V (in μmoles/min) is calculated from the following equation:

$$V = \frac{M \times v \times X}{\text{time (min)}}$$

where M = molarity of titrant, v = volume of titrant, X = mole–molar conversion factor (2 for penicillin, 4 for cephalosporins).

Indicator method

The concentration of acid formed during the β-lactamase reaction correlates directly with the decrease in absorption at a particular wavelength of the alkaline form of a pH indicator. This can be followed spectrophotometrically choosing an indicator whose pK coincides with the reaction

pH, e.g. phenol red (pK = 7·8) at pH 7·6, bromothymol blue (pK = 7·0) at pH 7·0.
Method. (Rubin & Smith 1973)
Equipment. Double beam recording spectrophotometer with thermostatically controlled cell carrier.
Reagents. A solution of substrate (0·2 mmol/l) and phenol red (0·0013% w/v) prepared in 0·4 mmol/l phosphate buffer pH 7·6.
Procedure. 0·01 ml enzyme solution is added to a cuvette containing 1·2 ml of reagent mixture and the change in absorption at 558 nm followed. The assay is initially standardized for each substrate by measuring the total change in O.D. following the addition of excess HCl to the phenol red reagent. The assay is then repeated substituting β-lactamase for HCl.

An alternative indicator technique using bromothymol blue (λmax 620 nm) has also been described by Imsande (1965).

Iodometric

The acidic products of β-lactamase hydrolysis reduce iodine whereas the intact substrates generally do not (Grove & Randall 1955). The reduction reaction has been used to determine rates of β-lactamase hydrolysis using two methods.

Micro-iodometric (Sykes & Nordstrom 1972)

In this method the rates of hydrolysis of compounds can be determined by measuring the rate of decolourization of a starch–iodine complex by hydrolysed substrate.
Equipment. Double beam recording spectrophotometer with thermostatically controlled cell carrier.
Reagents. 0·2 mmol/l substrates prepared daily in phosphate buffer (0·05 mol/l) pH 7·0 and kept on ice. Starch–iodine solution, prepared by adding 0·15 ml of iodine reagent (0·68 ml/l in 3·2 mol/l potassium iodide) to 100 ml of 0·2% w/v hydrolysed starch solution. The final iodine concentration is 120 μmol/l.
Procedure. Two 1-cm cuvettes, one containing 2·9 ml phosphate buffer (blank) and the other 1 ml starch–iodine solution, 1 ml substrate solution and 0·9 ml phosphate buffer (test), are equilibrated. A 100 μl aliquot of enzyme is added to each cuvette. The decrease in absorption at 620 nm is followed giving a measure of the rate of hydrolysis.

Decolourization of the starch–iodine complex is a slow process and does not give an accurate measure of the rate of hydrolysis until a steady state is obtained between formation of penicilloic acid and its oxidation by iodine. This takes about 15–20 min.

In the presence of excess enzyme the starch–iodine is completely decolourized before a steady state is reached.

Calculation. $O.D._{620}$ decreases from 1·2 to 0 when a penicillin is completely destroyed by a β-lactamase.

$$\therefore N = \frac{\Delta O.D._{620} \times 0{\cdot}03 \times 10}{1{\cdot}2 \times \text{time}}$$

where N = μmol of substrate destroyed/min/ml of enzyme, $\Delta O.D._{620}$ = change in optical density.

Macro-iodometric (Perret 1954; Matthew *et al.* 1979)

The amount of iodine reduced by hydrolysed substrate in a given time can be determined by back-titration with sodium thiosulphate, using a starch indicator.

Equipment. Shaking water bath.

Reagents. Substrate prepared at 5 mmol/l in 0·05 mol/l phosphate buffer pH 7·0. Iodine reagent (0·0166 mol/l iodine, 0·06 mol/l potassium iodide in 2·0 mol/l acetate buffer pH 4·0). 0·0166 mol/l sodium thiosulphate. 2% w/v starch solution.

Procedure. Test and control flasks containing 5 ml substrate are equilibrated at 37°C in a shaking water bath before adding 1 ml of enzyme to each of the test flasks. Following a reaction period of 30 min, 10 ml of iodine reagent are added to all the flasks to stop the enzymic reaction. At this stage 1 ml aliquots of crude enzyme are also added to the control flasks. A further incubation period (10 min for penicillins and 20 min for cephalosporins) is then required for completion of the reaction between the hydrolysis products and iodine. The flasks are then removed from the water bath and titrated with sodium thiosulphate using a starch indicator. If the titration is $< 4{\cdot}5$ ml or $> 8{\cdot}0$ ml the assay needs to be repeated either using an appropriately diluted enzyme or a different incubation period.

Calculations. Under the conditions cited, 1 ml of 0·0166 mol/l iodine reduced is equivalent to 2 μmol of penicillin substrate or 4 μmol of cephalosporin substrate. Corrections need to be made for spontaneous decay of β-lactam substrate and uptake of iodine by the enzyme. If t is the incubation time (min), and control—test = X ml of iodine consumed, then $2X/t$ = μmol of penicillin substrate destroyed per min and $4X/t$ = μmol of cephalosporin substrate destroyed per min.

Hydroxylamine

Hydroxylamine reacts with a number of carboxylic acid derivatives to form hydroxamic acids which yield coloured complexes with Fe^{3+} in acidic

solutions. Only molecular species having an intact β-lactam ring will react with hydroxylamine and hence the residual substrate is assayed.
Reaction. Shown in Fig. 3.
Method for penicillins (Dale & Smith 1971)
Equipment. Double beam spectrophotometer.
Reagents. Substrate (2 mg/ml) in 25 mmol/l sodium phosphate buffer. Hydroxylamine hydrochloride (prepared by adding 173·8 g hydroxylamine hydrochloride to 500 ml of water). Sodium acetate buffer pH 11·2 (173 g of sodium hydroxide and 20·6 g of anhydrous sodium acetate in 1 litre of water). Ferric reagent (prepared by adding 200 g of ferric ammonium sulphate and 93·4 ml of concentrated H_2SO_4 to distilled water to give 1 litre of solution).

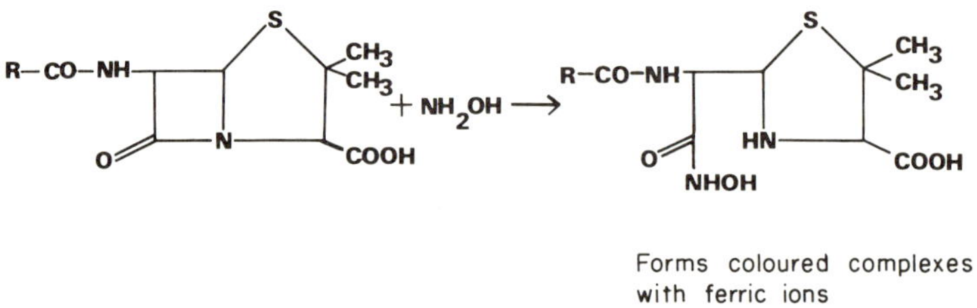

FIG. 3. Reaction of penicillins with hydroxylamine.

Procedure. At suitable time intervals following addition of enzyme to substrate solution, 2 ml aliquots of the reaction mixture are pipetted into 6·5 ml of a fresh mixture of hydroxylamine hydrochloride : sodium acetate buffer : water : ethanol (2 : 2 : 1 : 8 by vol.), and allowed to stand for 7 min. 2 ml of ferric reagent are then added, mixed thoroughly and the absorbance at 500 nm read immediately against a blank in which 2 ml of buffer has been treated in an identical manner.
Calculation. Residual substrate is determined from a reference calibration curve.

Cephalosporins are generally more stable than penicillins and hence the reaction with hydroxylamine is usually slower, resulting in reduced sensitivity and reproducibility. The following method, using a nickel (II) catalyst, has been devised for cephalosporins.

Method for cephalosporins (Mays *et al.* 1975)
Equipment. Double beam spectrophotometer.
Reagents. Substrate 1 mg/ml in 1% w/v sodium bicarbonate solution. Hydroxylamine–nickel reagent (6·95 g hydroxylamine hydrochloride and 2·39 g $NiCl_2.6H_2O$ are dissolved in 50 ml of water, and the pH

adjusted with concentrated sodium hydroxide). Iron reagent (15% w/v ferric ammonium sulphate hydrate dissolved in sulphuric acid).

Procedure. 2 ml aliquots of substrate solution are added to 0·9 ml of 1% w/v sodium bicarbonate solution. 2 ml hydroxylamine–nickel reagent is added to each sample along with 0·1 ml enzyme and allowed to react at room temperature for exactly 20 min. 5·0 ml of iron reagent are then added to each sample, mixed and allowed to stand for 5 min. The absorbance at 470 nm is then determined against a blank containing enzyme + buffer which has been treated in an identical manner.

Calculation. A standard curve of absorbance against concentration of the reference substrate is prepared from which the sample concentration can be calculated.

HPLC

Residual intact substrate and products of hydrolysis are separated chromatographically on the basis of their differing partition-coefficients and molecular weights.

Method. (A. M. Pastorino, Glaxo, Verona: pers. comm.)

Equipment. HPLC system comprising column with reverse phase support, u.v. detector, thermostatically controlled reaction vessel.

Reagents. Methanol/acetic acid mixture (100 : 1), substrates at 1·28 mmol/l, in 0·02 mol/l phosphate buffer pH 7·0, enzyme solution (activity adjusted to hydrolyse *ca.* 30% of the substrate in 10 min). Eluent, 0·03 mol/l NaH_2PO_4 (pH 4·5)/CH_3OH (variable composition depending on substrate).

Procedure. Aliquots of 3 ml of substrate are equilibrated at 37°C. 0·1 ml of enzyme and 0·1 ml of buffer are added to test and control samples respectively. After a reaction period of 10 min, 4 ml of methanol/acetic acid mixture are added to each sample to stop the reaction. Samples are stored at 0°C prior to HPLC, which is conducted at an eluent flow rate of 1–1.5 ml/min.

Calculation. Quantitation of hydrolysis products and intact substrate is by measurement of their u.v. peak heights or areas. Sample concentration is determined by calibration against a standard curve of internal or external standard solutions. External standards, i.e. dilutions of intact test substrate, are treated identically to test samples without addition of enzyme and applied to the HPLC column on separate occasions. Internal standards are dilution ranges of a compound with similar properties to the test substrate, which are added to the "stopped" reaction mixtures prior to HPLC, i.e. run on the same occasion.

TABLE 1

Summary of versatility, limitations and requirements of current techniques for assay of β-lactamase activity

Technique	Principal substrate	Amount of compound required (mg)	Compound assayed	Assay time	Accuracy	Continuous monitoring	Expensive equipment	Complications
Microbiological	Penicillins and cephalosporins	5	Residual substrate	Several hours	Good	×	×	Acylases. Products with antibacterial activity
Spectro-photometric	Better for cephalosporins	1 cephs 10 pens	Residual substrate	10 min	Good	√	√	Products may absorb u.v.
Acidimetric								
pH-stat	Better for penicillins	50	Hydrolysis products	30 min		√	√	Acylases. Substrates with buffering capacity
indicator	Better for penicillins	20	Hydrolysis products	15 min		√	√	
Iodometric								
macro-	Better for penicillins	50	Hydrolysis products	60 min	Poor	×	×	
micro-	Better for penicillins	1	Hydrolysis products	20 min	Poor	×	√	Amylases
Hydroxylamine	Penicillins and cephalosporins	10	Residual substrate	10–30 min	Poor	×	√	Unstable chromagens. Precipitation
HPLC	Penicillins and cephalosporins	10	Residual substrate and hydrolysis products	15 min	Good	×	√	Unsuitable for crude enzymes. Penicillins may require to be derived

Discussion

Despite the range of techniques currently available for assay of β-lactamase activity, none has proven ideal for all situations. A summary of the versatility and limitations of the techniques described in this chapter is given in Table 1.

The fact that β-lactamase hydrolysis of penicillins generally results in stable penicilloic acid products, permits the use of techniques (acidimetric, iodometric) which measure product formation. Such methods are less reliable for cephalosporins because of the chemically unstable nature of the hydrolysis products. Hence assay of cephalosporins is restricted to techniques which measure residual substrate.

The conjugated system associated with the β-lactam ring of cephalosporins gives rise to an easily detectable u.v. spectrum (typically 1–1·5 absorbance units for λmax at 10^{-4} mol/l) by direct spectrophotometry in the region 250–270 nm. Penicillins absorb less u.v. irradiation at their λmaxs than cephalosporins (typically 0·8–1·2 absorbance units at 10^{-3} mol/l). In addition, their λmaxs fall in the region 230–240 nm where many organic molecules absorb and may cause interference. These spectral differences make direct u.v. detection techniques, i.e. spectrophotometric and HPLC, more suitable for cephalosporins than penicillins.

Microbiological techniques are very sensitive for antibiotics with high intrinsic activity and can be used to compare rates of hydrolysis of penicillins and cephalosporins. However, they do not distinguish between β-lactamase and acylase activity in crude enzyme preparations (Cole & Sutherland 1965; Holt & Stewart 1964) or between residual substrate and hydrolysis products which may retain some antibacterial activity. In addition, the assays are extremely slow (>6 h) and it is difficult to assay compounds with low antibacterial activity and samples displaying a wide range of activities.

Only the u.v. spectrophotometric and acidimetric techniques permit continuous monitoring of β-lactamase reactions which is necessary for accurate determination of K_m and V_{max} values. The u.v. spectrophotometric technique is highly suitable for rapid determination of the activity of β-lactamase preparations and assessment of the stability of a compound to a range of β-lactamases. The major disadvantage is the necessity to use penicillins at 10^{-3} mol/l, i.e. ten times more concentrated than cephalosporins, due to their inferior u.v. absorption. This concentration difference prevents reliable comparison of the rates of hydrolysis of penicillins and cephalosporins.

Acidimetric techniques are effectively restricted to penicillins. These techniques also suffer from the disadvantages that they do not differentiate between β-lactamases and acylases. Although rapid, indicator techniques are unsuitable for compounds which have buffering capacity, e.g. ampicillin and cephalexin.

The macro-iodometric method is relatively slow, requires large amounts of compound and gives poor reproducibility. However, the equipment involved is inexpensive, simple to use and the reproducibility can be improved by increased replication. The method permits reasonable assessment of the relative rates of hydrolysis of penicillins and cephalosporins and has been used extensively for β-lactamase substrate profile studies (Matthew *et al.* 1979). The micro-iodometric technique is not suitable for cephalosporins, primarily because the decolourization reaction is much slower than with penicillins. Reproducibility is poor for penicillins and may be further impaired by non-specific decolourization of the starch–iodine complex by other proteins in crude enzyme extracts.

The hydroxylamine technique measures intact substrate and can be used for both penicillins and cephalosporins, although slightly different reagents are necessary. The technique is relatively insensitive. Inaccuracies are enhanced by the formation of unstable chromogens and precipitation problems. The main advantage of this technique is its application in the presence of high protein concentrations.

HPLC is the only technique whereby both products and residual substrate can be co-monitored. The technique is relatively fast, accurate, and can be used at concentrations in excess of those possible using spectrophotometric or microbiological assay. A further major advantage is that fully automated operation is possible. Major disadvantages are the need to use pre-columns or purified enzymes and to make derivatives of some hydrolysed penicillins to enhance their u.v. absorption.

References

Cole, M. & Sutherland, R. 1965 The role of penicillin acylase in the resistance of Gram-negative bacteria to penicillins. *Journal of General Microbiology* **42,** 345–356.

Dale, J. W. & Smith, J. T. 1971 The purification and properties of the β-lactamase specified by the resistance factor R-1818 in *Escherichia coli* and *Proteus mirabilis. Biochemical Journal* **123,** 493–500.

Grove, D. C. & Randall, W. A. 1955 Chemical method for penicillin. In *Assay Methods of Antibiotics*, ed. Welch, H. & Martí-ibáñez, F. p. 16. Chicago: Medical Encyclopedia Inc.

Holt, R. J. & Stewart, G. T. 1964 Production of amidase and β-lactamase by bacteria. *Journal of General Microbiology* **36,** 203–213.

Hou, J. P. & Poole, J. W. 1972 Measurement of β-lactamase activity and rate of inactivation of penicillins by a pH-stat alkalimetric titration method. *Journal of Pharmaceutical Sciences* **61,** 1594–1598.

IMSANDE, J. 1965 New assay for penicillinase and some results on penicillinase induction. *Journal of Bacteriology* **89**, 1322–1327.

KONECNY, J. & SCHNEIDER, A. 1978 Alkalimetric microassay of cephalosporins. *The Journal of Antibiotics* **31**, 776–782.

LEES, K. A. & TOOTILL, J. P. R. 1955*a* Microbiological assay on large plates. I. General considerations, with particular reference to routine assay. *Analyst* **80**, 95–110.

LEES, K. A. & TOOTILL, J. P. R. 1955*b* Microbiological assay on large plates. II. Precise assay. *Analyst* **80**, 110–117.

LEES, K. A. & TOOTILL, J. P. R. 1955*c* Microbiological assay on large plates. III. High throughput, low precision assays. *Analyst* **80**, 531–535.

MATTHEW, M., HEDGES, R. W. & SMITH, J. T. 1979 Types of β-lactamase determined by plasmids in Gram-negative bacteria. *Journal of Bacteriology* **138**, 657–662.

MAYS, D. L., BANGERT, F. K., CANTRELL, W. C. & EVANS, W. G. 1975 Hydroxylamine determination of cephalosporins. *Analytical Chemistry* **47**, 2229–2234.

O'CALLAGHAN, C. H., MUGGLETON, P. W. & ROSS, G. W. 1969 Effects of β-lactamase from Gram-negative organisms on cephalosporins and penicillins. In *Antimicrobial Agents and Chemotherapy* 1968 ed. Hobby, G. L. pp. 57–63. Bethesda, Maryland: American Society for Microbiology.

O'CALLAGHAN, C. H., MORRIS, A., KIRBY, S. M. & SHINGLER, A. H. 1972 Novel method for detection of β-lactamases by using a chromogenic cephalosporin substrate. *Antimicrobial Agents and Chemotherapy* **1**, 283–288.

O'CALLAGHAN, C. H., ACRED, P., HARPER, P. B., RYAN, D. M., KIRBY, S. M. & HARDING, S. M. 1980 GR 20263, a new broad-spectrum cephalosporin with anti-pseudomonal activity. *Antimicrobial Agents and Chemotherapy* **17**, 876–883.

PERRET, C. J. 1954 Iodometric assay of penicillinase. *Nature, London* **174**, 1012–1013.

ROSS, G. W. & O'CALLAGHAN, C. H. 1975 β-lactamase assays. *Methods in Enzymology* **43**, 69–85.

RUBIN, F. A. & SMITH, D. H. 1973 Characterisation of R factor β-lactamases by the acidimetric method. *Antimicrobial Agents and Chemotherapy* **3**, 68–73.

SCHLINDLER, P. & HUBER, G. 1980 Use of PADAC, a novel chromogenic β-lactamase substrate, for the detection of β-lactamase-producing organisms and the assay of β-lactamase inhibitors/inactivators. In *Enzyme Inhibitors* ed. Brodbeck, U. pp. 169–176. Berlin: Verlag Chemie.

SYKES, R. B. & MATTHEW, M. 1979 Detection, assay and immunology of β-lactamases. In *Beta-Lactamases*, ed. Hamilton-Miller, J. M. T. & Smith, J. T. pp. 17–49. London & New York: Academic Press.

SYKES, R. B. & NORDSTROM, K. 1972 Micro-iodometric determination of β-lactamase activity. *Antimicrobial Agents and Chemotherapy* **1**, 94–99.

YOSHIDA, T., MATSUURA, S., MAYAMA, M., KAMEDA, Y. & KUWAHARA, S. 1980 Moxalactam (6059-S), a novel 1-oxa-β-lactam with an expanded antibacterial spectrum: laboratory evaluation. *Antimicrobial Agents and Chemotherapy* **17**, 302–312.

The Biochemical Evaluation of β-Lactamase Inhibitors

C. READING AND T. FARMER

Beecham Pharmaceuticals, Research Division, Chemotherapeutic Research Centre, Brockham Park, Betchworth, Surrey, UK

The β-lactamase enzymes occur widely in bacteria of clinical importance. These enzymes hydrolyse the cyclic amide bond in the β-lactam ring of penicillin, cephalosporins and related compounds to produce an antibacterially inactive degradation product (Fig. 1). The production of β-lactamase by bacteria therefore plays a prime role in their resistance to the β-lactam antibiotics. During the past twenty years considerable effort has been devoted to the preparation of penicillins and cephalosporins which are stable to β-lactamase and hence retain their antibacterial activity. An alternative approach to the β-lactamase problem has been the search for inhibitors of these enzymes which, when combined with a β-lactamase labile antibiotic, protect it from degradation and allow the penicillin or cephalosporin to exert its antibacterial effect.

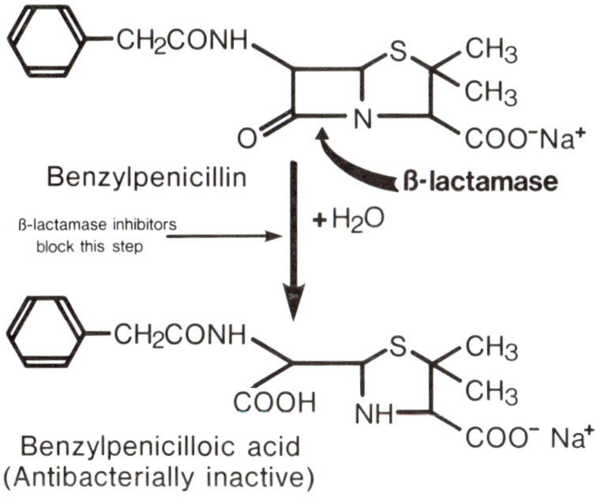

FIG. 1. The action of β-lactamase on penicillin.

ANTIBIOTICS
ISBN 0 12 604480 5

TABLE 1

β-Lactamase classification

β-Lactamase type	Example	Relative rate of amoxycillin hydrolysis (Pen G = 100)	Inhibition by low concs. of clavulanic acid
Cephalosporinase*	*Enterobacter cloacae* P99	5	−
	Pseudomonas aeruginosa A	10	−
	Escherichia coli JT410	2	−
	Bacteroides fragilis	> 100	+
Penicillinase*	*Proteus mirabilis* C889	142	+
Broad-spectrum β-lactamase*	*Klebsiella pneumoniae* E70	127	+
	Branhamella catarrhalis 1908	120	+
Plasmid-mediated β-lactamase	TEM-I and II	86	+
	SHV-1	126	+
	OXA type, e.g. OXA-2	162	+
	PSE type, e.g. PSE-4 (Dalgleish)	92	+
Gram positive penicillinase	*Staphylococcus aureus* Russell	168	+

* Chromosomal.

The discovery of the naturally occurring β-lactamase inhibitor, clavulanic acid (Reading & Cole, 1977) has revitalized interest in this approach to overcoming bacterial resistance. Apart from derivatives of clavulanic acid, further inhibitors have now been reported such as 6-β-bromopenicillanic acid (Pratt & Loosemore 1978), penicillanic acid sulphone (English *et al.* 1978) and the olivanic acids, which, like clavulanic acid, are naturally occurring β-lactam compounds (Butterworth *et al.* 1979) with potent inhibitory activity (Hood *et al.* 1979). For a recent review of β-lactamase inhibition the reader is referred to Cole (1981). The biochemical evaluation of compounds with β-lactamase inhibitory activity centres on their ability to protect a labile β-lactam from enzymic degradation. In the present paper we describe the methods we have used to provide a preliminary evaluation of these properties.

The Enzymes

Enzyme type

The β-lactamases are a diverse group of enzymes and various classification systems have been introduced. The classification of Richmond & Sykes (1973) and of Sykes & Matthew (1976) form the basis of a recent review of this subject (Sykes & Smith 1979) to which the reader is referred for further information. An outline of this scheme is shown in Table 1.

In order to obtain information on the spectrum of inhibitory activity, various enzyme types can be included at the preliminary screening stage. The enzymes we have used routinely are listed in Table 2. When selecting enzymes, the β-lactam substrate with which the inhibitor is to be combined should also be considered. When a specific β-lactam antibiotic is to be combined with an inhibitor, the enzyme types which hydrolyse that particular substrate should be included. Secondary evaluation of an inhibitor would include a wider range of enzymes from Gram negative bacteria including further plasmid-mediated types such as SHV-1 which occurs widely in resistant *Klebsiella* and also the OXA-types. Further chromosomal enzymes such as those from *Bacteroides* and *Proteus* spp. could also be examined.

Enzyme preparation

For routine testing we have used simple cell extracts of the various bacterial strains prepared as shown in Scheme 1. Although the use of purified enzyme preparations is generally considered to be desirable we have found little advantage in undertaking such procedures. Crude preparations from bacterial strains which produce predominantly one type of β-lactamase enzyme, such as those listed in Table 2, provide a satisfactory source of enzyme for inhibition studies. Obviously when bacteria produce significant amounts of more than one enzyme this must be taken into consideration. For instance, some bacterial strains producing TEM β-lactamase also produce significant amounts of a chromosomally mediated cephalosporinase. By using a substrate such as ticarcillin, which is highly stable to cephalosporinases, the rate of hydrolysis and its inhibition will reflect only the TEM activity of the preparation. Misleading results can be obtained with mixed enzymes if substrates such as benzylpenicillin or cephaloridine are employed which are hydrolysed by both enzymes. In such instances inhibitory activity should be assessed against the separated enzymes as well as against the enzyme mixture.

TABLE 2

β-Lactamases used in the primary screen

Source of β-lactamase	Type	Classification of Sykes & Smith (1979) (when applicable)
Enterobacter cloacae P99	Chromosomally mediated cephalosporinase	I (constitutive)
Pseudomonas aeruginosa A	Chromosomally mediated cephalosporinase	I (inducible)
Proteus mirabilis C889	Chromosomally mediated penicillinase	II
Klebsiella pneumoniae E70	Chromosomally mediated broad-spectrum β-lactamase	IV
Escherichia coli JT4	Plasmid-mediated broad-spectrum β-lactamase (TEM)	TEM
Pseudomonas aeruginosa Dalgleish	Plasmid-mediated penicillinase (PSE-4)	—
Staphylococcus aureus Russell	Gram positive penicillinase	—

SCHEME 1. Preparation of bacterial β-lactamases* (Reading & Cole 1977)

Enriched tryptone media

↓ culture grown 7 h, 37°C, shaken (induced after 2·5 h if necessary)†

Cell culture

↓ centrifuge

Cells

↓ resuspend in 1/50th volume and sonicate for 5 min

Sonicated cells

↓ centrifuge and discard debris

Supernatant enzyme preparation

* Except for *Bacteroides fragilis*.
† For example, 1 μg/ml methicillin for *Staphylococcus aureus* Russell and 500 μg/ml 6-APA for *Pseudomonas aeruginosa* A.

Determination of Inhibitory Activity

The concentration of inhibitor which reduces either the rate of substrate hydrolysis by 50% or alternatively reduces loss of substrate by 50% after a given enzymation period is termed the I_{50} value of the inhibitor. I_{50} values are not kinetic constants and depend entirely on the test conditions under which they were determined. For this reason, I_{50} values should be accompanied by a full description of the assay methodology employed. Further information on the nature of the inhibition may be obtained by obtaining I_{50} values with and without pre-incubation of the enzyme with the inhibitor. Assays with pre-incubation are carried out by reacting enzyme with inhibitor for a set time period and then adding the substrate to measure the residual enzyme activity. When pre-incubation is not used the enzyme is added to premixed inhibitor and substrate.

In the presence of substrate (no pre-incubation) it would be satisfactory to measure inhibition of initial velocities when examining simple competitive reversible inhibitors. For inhibitors whose mode of action is time dependent and which react with the enzyme to form relatively stable covalent complexes, the time course of substrate hydrolysis in the presence

SCHEME 2. The hydroxylamine assay

Reaction tube

- ← 1·8 ml 0·05 mol/l NaH_2PO_4/Na_2HPO_4 pH 7·3 buffer
- ← 0·1 ml inhibitor
- ← 0·1 ml β-lactamase (to give 50–70% hydrolysis of substrate for uninhibited enzyme reactions)
- ← 0·5 ml 5 mg/ml benzylpenicillin (final concentration in reaction 1 mg/ml)
- ← 6 ml Hydroxylamine reagent (1 vol. of hydroxylamine hydrochloride (347·6 g/l H_2O), +1 vol. of alkaline buffer (173 g NaOH + 20·6 g anhydrous sodium acetate/litre of H_2O) + 4 vols ethanol)
- ← 2 ml Ferric reagent (200 g ferric ammonium sulphate + 93·4 ml conc. H_2SO_4 per litre H_2O)

Steps:

- Pre-warm to 37°C → (after inhibitor)
- Pre-incubate for 15 min (inhibition reaction) → (after β-lactamase)
- Incubate for 30 min (substrate hydrolysis reaction) → (after benzylpenicillin)
- Reagent reaction 10 min → (after hydroxylamine reagent)

Read absorbance at 490 nm

The method described above is for the pre-incubation assay (the time may be varied). When no pre-incubation is required, the inhibitor and substrate are mixed first then enzyme added.

of the inhibitor is non-linear. Measurement of initial velocities may not therefore reveal the full extent of the ability of this type of compound to inhibit enzyme activity. In order to obtain a better assessment of the inhibitory ability of such compounds the determination of the inhibitor concentration required to reduce substrate loss by 50% after a set time provides a more meaningful I_{50} value. In our I_{50} determinations we have used a minimum time of 5 min for the enzyme reaction stage before measuring the residual substrate.

Assay Methods

Any assay system which reliably measures penicillin or cephalosporin concentration or their ring opened degradation products (e.g. penicilloic acids in the case of penicillins), may be used to measure β-lactamase activity and the effect of inhibitors on this activity. Such assay systems are numerous and have recently been reviewed (Sykes & Matthew 1979). We have used three main types of assay in our laboratories when evaluating β-lactamase inhibitors and these are described below.

Hydroxylamine assay

This method for the assay of penicillin (Boxer & Everett (1949) can be used to measure β-lactamase activity. The method is based on the reaction of hydroxylamine with the β-lactam ring to yield hydroxamates which when further reacted with ferric salts produce a coloured product. This method assays only intact penicillins and not the enzymic hydrolysis products. The application of the procedure to the determination of I_{50} values of β-lactamase inhibitors is described in Scheme 2, where benzylpenicillin is used as the substrate. The method is easy to use and requires no sophisticated equipment, a simple colorimeter being quite adequate to measure the reaction samples. It is useful for crude β-lactamase preparations containing high protein concentrations which can interfere in some assay systems. An automated version of this assay for I_{50} determination has been described by Reading & Hepburn (1979).

Direct spectrophotometric assay

Enzyme activity and hence its inhibition may be measured by following the decrease in the u.v. maximum of a cephalosporin which occurs on hydrolysis by β-lactamase (O'Callaghan *et al.* 1968). Penicillins have no specific u.v. maxima but changes in end absorbance occur on hydrolysis of the β-lactam ring (Samuni 1975). An example of this type of assay using benzylpenicillin as the substrate is shown in Scheme 3.

SCHEME 3. The direct spectrophotometric assay

10 mm Silica cuvette

← 2·2 ml 0·05 mol/l NaH_2PO_4/Na_2HPO_4 pH 7·3 buffer

← 0·1 ml Inhibitor

Pre-warm to 37°C →

← 0·1 ml β-lactamase (diluted to give an easily measurable rate in uninhibited enzyme reactions)

Pre-incubate for 5 min (inhibition reaction) →

← 0·1 ml benzylpenicillin 6·25 mg/ml (final concentration in reaction 250 μg/ml)

(Substrate hydrolysis reaction) →

↓

Measure fall in absorbance at 240 nm

As with the hydroxylamine assay, the method described refers to the pre-incubation (+) assay. In the case of a no pre-incubation (−) assay, inhibitor and substrate are mixed first then β-lactamase added. Using cephaloridine as substrate, reactions can be followed at the absorbance maximum of 255 nm for dilute solutions (40 μg/ml) or off peak at 290 nm for higher concentrations (250 μg/ml).

By comparing the u.v. spectra of intact and hydrolysed β-lactam, the method may be adapted for use with a variety of penicillins and cephalosporins. A wavelength is chosen which gives a readily measurable change in absorbtion after complete hydrolysis of the antibiotic. The direct spectrophotometric methods are rapid, require few reagents and with modern equipment are extremely sensitive which allows the assays to be carried out at very low substrate concentrations. When studying the kinetic aspects of β-lactamase inhibition these methods have proved particularly useful. Crude enzyme preparations which contain high protein concentrations and have low β-lactamase activity can cause problems in these u.v. assays due to their high background absorbance.

Automated chromogenic substrate (nitrocefin) assays

A further direct assay of β-lactamase activity employs the chromogenic cephalosporin, nitrocefin (O'Callaghan *et al.* 1972). On hydrolysis by β-lactamase this substrate yields a red degradation product which is readily measurable spectrophotometrically. The assay has the advantage of an absorbance change in the visible region and so the background u.v. absorbance of crude enzyme preparations presents no problem. We have adapted this simple assay for the routine determination of I_{50} values using a Pye Unicam AC-30 discrete analyser. This automated method is described in Scheme 4. A solution of the inhibitor to be tested is serially half diluted to give ten concentrations which are placed in the sample cups and then loaded into the equipment. In the pre-incubation assay, the racks containing sample cups plus reaction tubes reach the sampler/dilution station where an aliquot of inhibitor sample is mixed with the enzyme solution in a reaction tube. After a 5 min pre-incubation, the substrate (nitrocefin) is added by a further syringe station and 5 min later the reaction is diluted and transferred to the spectrophotometer. The absorbance of the sample at 482 nm is measured and the result recorded either on a chart recorder or as a print-out. Results may also be recorded using a data-logger and processed later using a small computer. Each set of inhibitor dilutions is separated by two sample cups containing buffer to provide a washing stage. Standard compounds are run with each set of assays. Clavulanic acid and cloxacillin standards are used routinely in our system and between them provide reference inhibitory activity for all the enzymes under test. A base line for an uninhibited control reaction is provided by running a rack of buffer samples and 100% inhibition is measured by running samples of a high concentration of clavulanate or cloxacillin depending on the type of enzyme under test.

SCHEME 4. Automated assay for I_{50} determination using nitrocefin

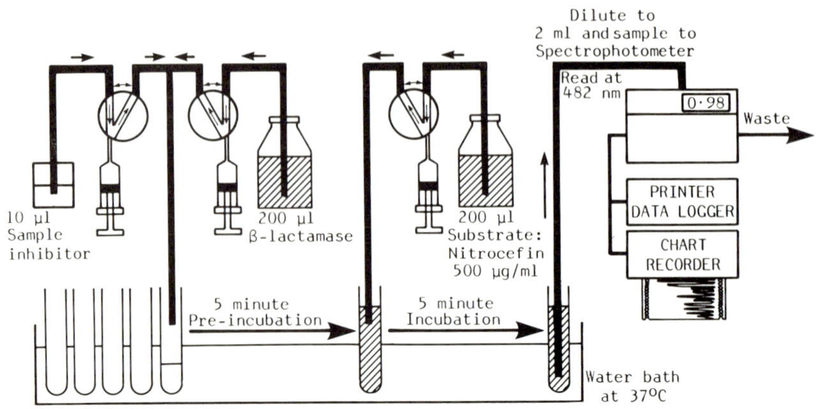

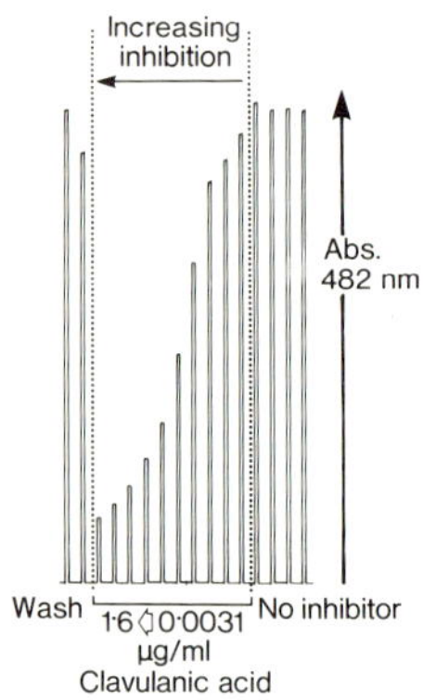

FIG. 2. Results from the automated assay for the determination of I_{50} values. A chart recorder trace shows the decrease in nitrocefin hydrolysis with increasing inhibitor concentration.

The compounds to be tested as inhibitors are all assayed against one β-lactamase type. The enzyme type is then changed and the sample racks are reloaded with fresh reaction tubes and then reprocessed. This is repeated for each of the enzymes under test. When an inhibitor is suspected of having poor stability in aqueous solution freshly prepared sample dilutions are used for each enzyme assay. Enzyme concentrations in the assay are adjusted to give an O.D. of 0·6–0·8 after a 5 min reaction with the nitrocefin substrate at 37°C in the absence of inhibitor. For the determination of I_{50}

values, both with and without a pre-incubation stage, the system is set up initially for the pre-incubation assays and all the samples are tested against all the enzymes in this mode. The system is then run using the 'without pre-incubation mode', usually with freshly prepared samples on a separate day depending on the number of compounds to be assayed. Assays without pre-incubation are obtained by replacing the enzyme solution in the sample/dilution station with the substrate as the diluent. Substrate and sample are then mixed and enzyme is added by the next syringe station. After a 5 min enzymation period the reaction is diluted and absorbance measured and recorded as described previously.

A typical recorder trace from the automated nitrocefin assay is shown in Fig. 2. This illustrates the decreasing level of absorbance due to decreased enzyme activity as the inhibitor concentration rises.

Results and Calculation of I_{50} values

I_{50} values can be obtained from each of the previously described assay systems. Percentage inhibition for each concentration can be calculated using the general equation

$$\% \text{ Inhibition} = \frac{V_0 - V_i}{V_0} \times 100,$$

where V_0 = the amount of, or rate of, substrate hydrolysis in the uninhibited reaction and V_i = the amount of, or rate of, substrate hydrolysis in the inhibited reaction.

In the automated nitrocefin assay, depending on enzyme type, an excess of clavulanate or cloxacillin is used in order to obtain a measure of absorbance at 100% inhibition. This is necessary because of slight background colour drift which can occur if the procedure is operated over a period of several hours. In this situation percentage inhibition is given by

$$\frac{\text{(absorbance of uninhibited control)} - \text{(absorbance of inhibited test sample)}}{\text{(absorbance of uninhibited control)} - \text{(absorbance at 100\% inhibition)}} \times 100.$$

A graph is then constructed by plotting percentage inhibition versus inhibitor concentration as illustrated in Fig. 3. The I_{50} value can then be read from the graph. I_{50} values which were obtained using the automated system with various inhibitors and with a number of β-lactamase enzyme types are given in Table 3.

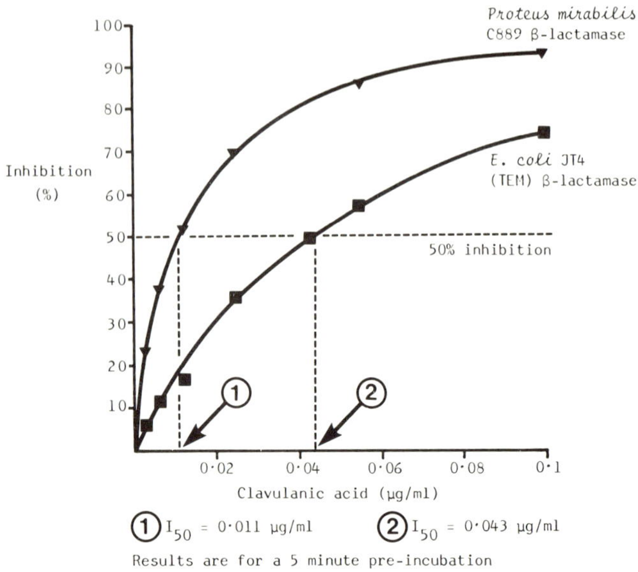

FIG. 3. Inhibition curves for clavulanic acid. The results were obtained using the automated nitrocefin assay in the with pre-incubation mode.

Interpretation of Results

The determination of I_{50} values in both the with and without pre-incubation modes can provide preliminary information about the type of inhibition which has occurred. Reactions of inhibitors such as clavulanic acid with β-lactamase have proved to be complex (Fisher *et al.* 1978; Reading & Farmer 1981). It is our experience, from studies with a large number of β-lactamase inhibitors of varying types, that the interpretations listed in Table 4 can be made. It must be stressed, however, that such interpretations must be confirmed by more detailed studies.

The Effect of Substrate on Inhibitory Activity

The β-lactamase stability of a β-lactam antibiotic formulated with a β-lactamase inhibitor depends on the kinetic properties of both components. The degree of substrate protection that an inhibitor achieves against a particular β-lactamase is highly dependent on the V_{max} and K_m values of the antibiotic with which it is combined. The kinetic properties of the substrate

TABLE 3

Inhibition of selected β-lactamases by different types of inhibitor as determined using the automated nitrocefin assay

Source of β-lactamase	I_{50} values (μg/ml) for inhibitors							
	Clavulanic acid		Cloxacillin		Olivanic acid, MM 4550		Penicillin, BRL 1437	
	(+)*	(−)	(+)	(−)	(+)	(−)	(+)	(−)
Enterobacter cloacae P99	110	4000	0·043	0·038	0·002	0·28	6·5	7·0
Staphylococcus aureus Russell	0·033	75	> 50	> 50	0·003	20	> 50	> 50
Escherichia coli JT4 (TEM)	0·06	1·2	> 50	> 50	0·0008	0·004	0·21	0·26
Proteus mirabilis C889	0·015	2·3	19	> 50	0·0003	0·002	0·15	5
Klebsiella pneumoniae E70	0·007	0·63	> 50	50	0·0002	0·0043	0·45	0·78

* (+), with pre-incubation; (−), without pre-incubation.

TABLE 4

Interpretation of results

Result*†	Possible interpretation
I_{50} values are similar with and without pre-incubation	Competitive and reversible
	Transiently stable enzyme-inhibitor complex with short half-life
+ = −	
	Progressive inhibition with inhibitor turnover, where rate of inhibition reaction is slow
I_{50} value with pre-incubation is significantly lower than without pre-incubation	Progressive inhibition where rate of inhibition reaction is fast
+ < −	
I_{50} value with pre-incubation is higher than without pre-incubation	Competitive substrate
+ > −	

* +, with 5 min pre-incubation; −, no pre-incubation.
† If with pre-incubation (+) and without pre-incubation (−) assays are carried out a comparison of the I_{50} values can provide preliminary information about the type of inhibition which has occurred. These indications, however, must be confirmed by more detailed studies.

will markedly affect the performance of the inhibitor and such effects have been illustrated for staphylococcal β-lactamase and clavulanic acid (Reading & Hepburn 1979). These substrate effects are most obvious in the assays without pre-incubation where substrate and inhibitor are competing for the active site of the β-lactamase enzyme. With time-dependent β-lactamase inactivators, assays with pre-incubation essentially measure the amount of enzyme inactivated during the pre-incubation stage. The addition of excess assay substrate after the pre-incubation stage markedly reduces further reaction by competition and essentially measures residual enzyme activity. In assays without a pre-incubation stage the substrate is present throughout. Under these conditions inhibition of the enzyme by 50% will require a higher concentration of a time-dependent, active site-directed inhibitor. In this competitive situation the relative affinities of both the substrate and the inhibitor are important factors in determining the degree of inhibition that is obtained. With simple competitive reversible inhibitors, the I_{50}

values obtained with and without a pre-incubation stage will be the same.

The biochemical assessment of a β-lactamase inhibitor must therefore also include a consideration of the type of β-lactam antibiotic with which the inhibitor would be most effectively combined. A number of factors would of course influence such a choice, not least the intrinsic antibacterial activity of the antibiotic.

Substrate Protection Experiments

The determination of I_{50} values, using the unusual cephalosporin nitrocefin, provides a satisfactory method for the routine assessment of the activity of large numbers of β-lactamase inhibitors. At the further evaluation stage the kinetics of inhibition may be considered and also the ability of the inhibitor to protect the specific β-lactam antibiotic with which it is to be combined to provide a potential chemotherapeutic agent. Substrate protection experiments can also provide information on the nature of the inhibition. We have carried out such studies using two main methods to follow the time course of antibiotic loss due to β-lactamase in the absence of inhibitor.

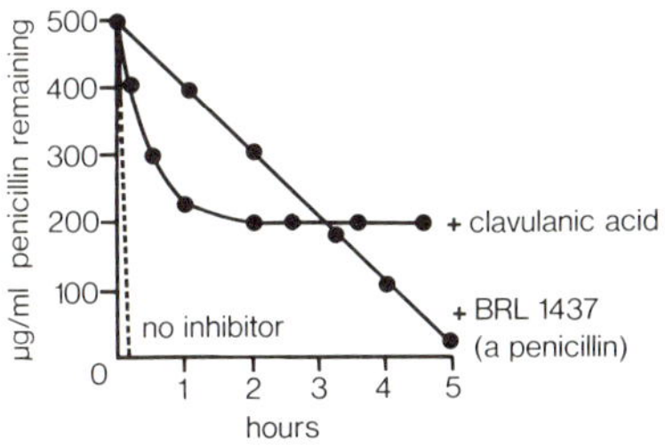

FIG. 4. The protection of benzylpenicillin from degradation by TEM-1 β-lactamase. Hydrolysis of the penicillin (500 µg/ml) was followed by measuring fall in absorbance at 240 nm on a recording spectrophotometer at 37°C and pH 7·3. Reactions were carried out in the absence of inhibitor and in the presence of 20 µg/ml of clavulanic acid or the penicillin inhibitor BRL 1437.

The direct spectrophotometric assay of penicillins described earlier provides a useful method for following the time course of antibiotic destruction by β-lactamase and the effect of an inhibitor on this reaction. Such an experiment is illustrated in Fig. 4 where the effect of two inhibitors, clavulanic acid and BRL 1437 (2-isopropoxy-1-napthyl penicillin, Cole *et al.* 1972) are compared. In this experiment, TEM-1 β-lactamase has been used at a concentration sufficient to hydrolyse 500 µg/ml of benzylpenicillin within 5 min. The differences between the β-lactamase inactivator, clavulanate, and the competitive penicillin inhibitor BRL 1437 are clearly demonstrated. While BRL 1437 efficiently slows the rate of penicillin destruction, clavulanic acid removes enzyme activity in a time-dependent fashion until the penicillin becomes completely stable. The reaction containing BRL 1437 continues slowly until all the penicillin has disappeared.

High performance liquid chromatography (HPLC) provides a further technique which can be used to measure the stability of an antibiotic to β-lactamase in the presence of an enzyme inhibitor. We have found this technique particularly useful for reactions with very low substrate concentrations, e.g. 4 μg/ml amoxycillin, and where interference from protein in crude enzyme preparations has occurred. This technique, as applied to the stability of a moderate concentration of amoxycillin (50 μg/ml) in the presence of clavulanic acid, is illustrated in Fig. 5. Reaction samples (25 μl) were injected at various times onto a Waters C_{18} μ-bondapak, reverse phase column eluted at 2·5 ml/min with 0·05 mol/l sodium acetate buffer pH 5·0, containing 4% v/v methanol. The eluent was monitored at 227 nm. Reactions of amoxycillin alone (retention time, 4 min) and amoxycillin with various concentrations of clavulanic acid were all in 0·05 mol/l phosphate buffer pH 7·3 at 37°C. The TEM-1 β-lactamase preparation was added at a concentration sufficient to completely hydrolyse 50 μg amoxycillin/ml within 5 min. The enzyme was added to pre-mixed substrate and inhibitor, i.e. without pre-incubation. Both the disappearance of the penicillin peak and the appearance of the amoxycillin penicilloic acid peak (retention time, 2·5 min) may be used to measure β-lactamase activity in this system.

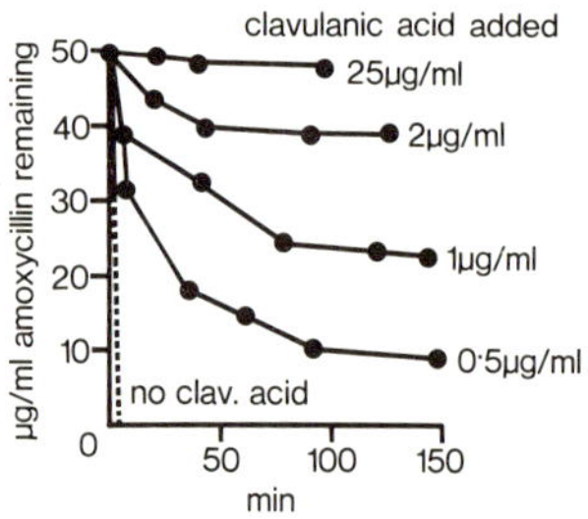

FIG. 5. Protection of amoxycillin from degradation by TEM-1 β-lactamase. The results were obtained using HPLC to follow loss of amoxycillin.

With TEM-1 β-lactamase and amoxycillin as the substrate (Fig. 5), increasing concentrations of inhibitor give reductions in amoxycillin hydrolysis until at a ratio of amoxycillin to clavulanate of 2 : 1, the substrate has been completely protected. It can be seen that at the lower clavulanate concentrations enzyme activity is completely removed and amoxycillin becomes stable. However, some amoxycillin loss occurs during the inactivation period. The concentration of inhibitor required to ensure no substrate loss in this competitive situation is, in part, a measure of the affinity of the inhibitor relative to that of the β-lactam substrate. For active site-directed inhibitors which progressively inactivate the enzyme, their affinity can be seen to play an important role in their overall performance. Assessment of such compounds must therefore take into account both affinity and the rate at which enzyme activity is removed as a stable covalent complex. The substrate protection data can be seen to illustrate both these aspects.

Conclusions

The methods described above are designed to give preliminary information on the activity of β-lactamase inhibitors. These studies are essentially comparative using known compounds such as cloxacillin, clavulanic acid and the naphthyl penicillin, BRL 1437, as reference standards. Data are obtained on the spectrum of inhibitory activity and this is also quantified in terms of an I_{50} value. The ability of the inhibitor to protect a specific β-lactam antibiotic has also been discussed and this may be expressed again using I_{50} values or may be defined by following the time course of antibiotic destruction by β-lactamase in the presence and absence of the inhibitor. The methods also provide an indication of the mode of action of inhibitors, differentiating between simple competitive inhibitors and compounds which progressively remove enzyme activity by reaction with the β-lactamase to form stable inactive covalent complexes.

Further studies dealing with the kinetics and mode of action of inhibitors of β-lactamases are beyond the scope of this present paper. Such studies, however, provide useful information in terms of structure–activity relationships and an understanding of the enzyme chemistry involved can contribute to the design of new agents in a chemical synthetic programme. However active an inhibitor of β-lactamase may be against cell-free enzyme preparations, it must also have the ability to protect a β-lactam antibiotic from degradation by growing bacterial cells which produce β-lactamase. It does not necessarily follow that an inhibitor will have this synergistic activity *in vivo*. In Gram negative bacteria, β-lactamase is located in the periplasmic space, a region between the inner and outer membranes of the bacterial cell wall and successful synergy depends on the ability of the inhibitor to neutralize this intracellular enzyme. The permeability of β-lactamase inhibitors is a further and important property which should also be considered at the further evaluation stage.

References

BOXER, G. E. & EVERETT, P. M. 1949 Colorimetric determinations of benzylpenicillin. Colorimetric determination of total penicillins. *Analytical Chemistry* **21,** 670–673.

BUTTERWORTH, D., COLE, M., HANSCOMB, G. & ROLINSON, G. N. 1979 Olivanic acids, a family of β-lactam antibiotics with β-lactamase inhibitory properties produced by *Streptomyces* species. I. Detection, properties and fermentation studies. *Journal of Antibiotics* **32,** 287–297.

COLE, M. 1981 Inhibitors of bacterial β-lactamases. *Drugs of the Future,* **6,** 697–727.

COLE, M., ELSON, S. & FULLBROOK, P. D. 1972 Inhibition of the β-lactamases of *Escherichia coli* and *Klebsiella aerogenes* by semi-synthetic penicillins. *Biochemical Journal* **127,** 295–308.

ENGLISH, A. R., RETSEMA, J. A., GIRARD, A. E., LYNCH, J. E. & BARTH, W. E. 1978 CP-45,899 a beta-lactamase inhibitor that extends the antibacterial spectrum of beta-lactams: initial bacteriological characterisation. *Antimicrobial Agents and Chemotherapy* **14,** 414–419.

FISHER, J., CHARNAS, R. L. & KNOWLES, J. R. 1978 Kinetic studies on the inactivation of *Escherichia coli* R TEM β-lactamase by clavulanic acid. *Biochemistry* **17,** 2180–2184.

HOOD, J. D., BOX, S. J. & VERRALL, M. S. 1979 Olivanic acids, a family of β-lactam antibiotics with β-lactamase inhibitory properties produced by *Streptomyces* species. II. Isolation and characterisation of the olivanic acids MM 4550, MM 13902 and MM 17880 from *Streptomyces olivaceus. Journal of Antibiotics* **32,** 295–304.

O'CALLAGHAN, C. H., MUGGLETON, P. W. & ROSS, G. W. 1968 Effects of β-lactamase from Gram-negative organisms on cephalosporins and penicillins. *Antimicrobial Agents and Chemotherapy* ed. G. Hobby, pp. 57–63. Washington, D.C.: American Society for Microbiology

O'CALLAGHAN, C. H., MORRIS, A., KIRBY, S. & SHINGLER, A. H. 1972 Novel method for detection of β-lactamases by using a chromogenic cephalosporin substrate. *Antimicrobial Agents and Chemotherapy* **1,** 283–288.

PRATT, R. F. and LOOSEMORE, M. J. 1978 6β-Bromopenicillanic acid, a potent β-lactamase inhibitor. *Proceedings of the National Academy of Sciences, USA* **75,** 4145–4194.

READING, C. & COLE, M. 1977 Clavulanic acid: a β-lactamase inhibiting beta lactam from *Streptomyces clavuligerus. Antimicrobial Agents and Chemotherapy* **11,** 852–857.

READING, C. & HEPBURN, P. 1979 The inhibition of staphylococcal β-lactamase by clavulanic acid. *Biochemical Journal* **179,** 67–76.

READING, C. & FARMER, T. 1981 The inhibition of β-lactamases from Gram-negative bacteria by clavulanic acid. *Biochemical Journal* **199,** 779–787.

RICHMOND, M. H. & SYKES, R. B. 1973 The β-lactamases of Gram-negative bacteria and their possible physiological role. In *Advances in Microbial Physiology* ed. Rose, A. H. & Tempest, D. W. Vol. 9, pp. 31–88. London and New York: Academic Press.

SAMUNI, A. 1975 A direct spectrophotometric assay and determination of Michaelis constants for the β-lactamase reaction. *Analytical Biochemistry* **63,** 17–26.

Sykes, R. B. & Matthew, M. 1976 The β-lactamases of the Gram-negative bacteria and their role in resistance to β-lactam antibiotics. *Journal of Antimicrobial Chemotherapy* **2**, 115–117.

Sykes, R. B. & Matthew, M. 1979 Detection, assay and immunology of β-lactamases. In *Beta-Lactamases* ed. Hamilton-Miller, J. M. T. & Smith, J. T. pp. 17–49. London and New York: Academic Press.

Sykes, R. B. & Smith, J. T. 1979 Biochemical aspects of β-lactamases from Gram-negative organisms. In *Beta-Lactamases* ed. Hamilton-Miller, J. M. T. & Smith, J. T. pp. 369–401. London and New York: Academic Press.

Detection of Bacterial Penicillin-binding Proteins and their Role in the Interpretation of the Mode of Action of β-Lactam Antibiotics

M. G. Boulton and D. C. Orr

Microbiology Division, Glaxo Group Research Limited, Greenford, Middlesex, UK

The different morphological effects observed in cultures of *Escherichia coli* K12 grown in the presence of β-lactam antibiotics are dependent on both the particular antibiotic used and its concentration (Spratt 1975, 1977*a*, *b*). This suggests that β-lactam inhibition of bacterial growth is a complex mechanism involving the inactivation of more than one enzyme. Understanding of this mechanism is difficult even with the advances in knowledge of the penicillin-sensitive enzymic reactions of the final stages of peptidoglycan biosynthesis (Izaki *et al.* 1968). The progress in the identification of 'killing' targets for β-lactam antibiotics in *E. coli* and other Gram negative bacteria has been largely due to the development of a system whereby individual penicillin-sensitive enzymes (PSEs) can be detected and studied. The method is based on the covalent binding of penicillin to the PSEs. Penicillin is thought to be a structural analogue of part of the peptide substrate of PSEs. The antibiotic is thus bound by the enzyme to form a stable penicilloyl–enzyme complex (Tipper & Strominger 1965) which is analogous to the transient substrate enzyme complex formed during the normal final stages of peptidoglycan biosynthesis. The PSEs can therefore be detected as those proteins that covalently bind penicillin and other β-lactam antibiotics. The detection is facilitated by the use of radioactively labelled penicillin to bind to the proteins and then, after fractionation on sodium dodecyl sulphate–polyacrylamide gels, visualization by scintillation autoradiography (Spratt & Pardee 1975). The PSEs that are detected in this manner are called penicillin-binding proteins (PBPs), and all known examples of PSEs can be detected as PBPs.

ANTIBIOTICS
ISBN 0 12 604480 5

Properties of Penicillin-binding Proteins

The majority of the work in elucidating the roles of these PBPs has been carried out on *E. coli* K12 and the work described here will be largely confined to this organism.

The inner membrane of *E. coli* K12 contains at least seven distinct PBPs with molecular weights between 40,000 and 91,000 (Spratt & Pardee 1975; Spratt *et al.* 1977). These proteins (numbered 1a, 1bs, 2, 3, 4 and 5/6 in order of decreasing molecular weight) covalently bind β-lactam antibiotics with varying affinities.

Some of these PBPs perform 'essential' functions in bacterial elongation (PBPs 1a/1bs) (Tamaki *et al.* 1977), shape (PBP 2) (Spratt & Pardee 1975) and division (PBP 3) (Spratt 1977*b*; Suzuki *et al.* 1978). Other PBPs (PBPs 4 and 5/6) appear to be 'non-essential' (Iwaya & Strominger 1977; Matsuhashi *et al.* 1977; Spratt 1977*a*). The properties of the PBPs of *E. coli* K12 are summarized in Fig. 1.

The 'essential' nature of certain PBPs has been confirmed by the isolation of temperature-conditional point mutants with lesions in the structural genes for the different PBPs (Matsuhashi *et al.* 1977; Tamaki *et al.* 1977; Spratt 1977*a*, *b*; Suzuki *et al.* 1978). These 'essential' PBPs, inhibition of any one of which leads to cell death (albeit through varying physiological mechanisms (Tomasz 1979)), are only minor components of the total PBPs which themselves are only a minor proportion of the total inner membrane protein.

The enzymic activities of both the 'essential' and 'non-essential' PBPs in peptidoglycan biosynthesis have yet to be elucidated fully. *In vitro* studies, however, have shown that both PBPs 1a and 1bs possess peptidoglycan transglycosylase and penicillin-sensitive transpeptidase activities (Ishino *et al.* 1980; Spratt 1980; Suzuki *et al.* 1980), and that the 'non-essential' proteins (PBPs 4 and 5/6) are responsible for D-alanine carboxypeptidase 1B-C and D-alanine carboxypeptidase 1A activities, respectively (Iwaya & Strominger 1977; Spratt & Strominger 1976; Matsuhashi *et al.* 1979).

Theoretical considerations

Since radioactive derivatives of β-lactam antibiotics of sufficient specific activity (other than benzylpenicillin) are not easily obtainable, the binding of different penicillin and cephalosporin derivatives to the PBPs of various bacterial strains is determined by competition with (^{14}C)-benzylpenicillin. The PBP assays are carried out as described later and the concentration of β-lactam antibiotic required to reduce the binding of (^{14}C)-benzyl-penicillin to each discrete PBP by 50% (I_{50}) is determined from the fluorogram.

PBP	Molecular Weight	Molecules per cell	Gene and map position (min)		Cellular function
1a	91, 000		ponA	73·5	PBPs 1a/1bs are 'essential' proteins involved in the biosynthesis of peptidoglycan associated with cell elongation. Combined inhibition causes spheroplasting and lysis.
1bs	86, 500 84, 000 81, 500	230	ponB	3·3	
2	66, 000	20	rodA	14·4	'Essential' protein involved in shape maintainance. Inhibition leads to 'round-form' production and eventually cell death.
3	60, 000	50	fts	1·8	'Essential' protein involved in cell division. Inhibition leads to filamentation and eventually cell death.
4	49, 000	110	dacB	68	'Non-essential'. Responsible for D-alanine carboxypeptidase 1B-C activity.
5	42, 000	1 800	dacA	13·7	'Non-essential'. Responsible for D-alanine carboxypeptidase 1A activity.
6	40, 000	570	?	?	'Non-essential' (?). Not involved in β-lactam action.

FIG. 1. Properties of the penicillin-binding proteins of *Escherichia coli* K12. Data taken from Spratt (1977*a*), Suzuki *et al.* (1978) and Matsuhashi *et al.* (1979).

One of the interacting factors attributed to the resistance shown by Gram negative bacteria to β-lactam antibiotics is the presence of periplasmically located β-lactamase enzyme (Curtis *et al.* 1972; Richmond & Sykes 1973). In whole cells this β-lactamase can either be constitutively expressed, or induced by the presence of suitable concentrations of β-lactam antibiotics. Liberation of this enzyme usually occurs during membrane preparation, but a significant amount may remain associated with the envelope and interfere with the determination of PBP affinity either by hydrolysis of the 'test' compound, or of the (^{14}C)-benzylpenicillin. Therefore for extrapolation of data obtained from the PBP assay it is necessary to use β-lactamase negative or non-inducible mutants (Curtis *et al.* 1979*c*). The extremely low level of expression of the chromosomal type Ib β-lactamase found in all *E. coli* K12 strains (Boman *et al.* 1974; Richmond & Sykes 1973) has little effect upon resistance (Nguyen-Distèche *et al.* 1974) and the PBP assay.

The penicillin-binding protein assay, performed using isolated envelopes of *E. coli*, is a 'cell-free' system (Curtis *et al.* 1979*a*) the permeability barrier operating in the intact bacterium being disrupted during envelope preparation. The I_{50} binding concentration of a penicillin or cephalosporin for its primary 'lethal' target (PBPs 1a/1bs or PBP 2 or PBP 3) can usually be correlated with the minimum concentration of the antibiotic required to kill the organism. This is assuming the compound is not excluded from the intact bacteria by the outer membrane permeability barrier (Richmond & Curtis 1974; Zimmermann & Rosselet 1977).

A comparison of the I_{50} binding concentration of a given β-lactam antibiotic for its primary 'essential' PBP target with the minimum inhibitory concentration (MIC) of the compound against intact bacteria, is an estimate of the ability of the compound to penetrate the outer membrane of the bacteria. The MIC of a given β-lactam antibiotic against *E. coli* is the concentration of the compound outside the cell which is required to produce a concentration inside, at the 'essential' PBP target, which is just sufficient to prevent its physiological function. The difference in PBP I_{50} binding concentration and MIC reflects the envelope permeability barrier, which is rendered non-functional in the PBP assay.

In order to gain further insight into the effectiveness of this barrier in excluding β-lactam antibiotics we have studied the PBP affinities and MICs of a strain of *E. coli* K12 (UB 1005, hereafter called *E. coli* DCO) in which the permeability barrier is intact and functional, and its 'permeability' mutant (*E. coli* DC2) in which lesions in the outer membrane allow easier access into the bacterial cell (Curtis *et al.* 1979*a*). Both of these strains were isolated by Richmond *et al.* (1976).

Bacterial strains

Escherichia coli DCO (methionine$^-$ nalidixic acid^r) and its permeability mutant *E. coli* DC2 were obtained from Professor M. H. Richmond, Bacteriology Department, University of Bristol. Both strains are grown at 37°C in Penassay broth (Difco Antibiotic Medium No. 3) with shaking.

Determination of minimum inhibitory concentration

MICs are determined by serial dilution of antibiotics in Penassay broth, and inoculation of the tubes with exponentially growing bacteria to a density of 10^5 organisms/ml. The tubes are incubated at 37°C overnight, and MICs recorded as the lowest concentration to impair growth significantly.

Detection of Penicillin-binding Proteins

The experimental work described will be confined to the PBPs of *E. coli* DCO. The method outlined, however, can be applied to other Gram negative bacteria, and, with slight modification, to Gram positive bacteria.

Membranes of *E. coli* DCO are mixed with a serial dilution of the antibiotic such that the different PBPs are bound to a greater or lesser extent depending on the compound on test. Any PBPs remaining free after the first step are bound by addition of a saturating concentration of (^{14}C)-benzylpenicillin. After addition of the anionic detergent sarkosyl, which both denatures the PBPs (thus preventing release of bound antibiotic molecules) and specifically solubilizes the inner membrane leaving the outer membrane and peptidoglycan fraction insoluble (Filip *et al.* 1973), the PBPs are separated according to their molecular weights using sodium dodecyl sulphate–polyacrylamide gel electrophoresis (SDS–PAGE). The radioactively labelled proteins are detected by fluorography as dark bands on X-ray emulsions. The sarkosyl treatment is not required for Gram positive bacteria since they do not have an outer membrane, the PBPs being denatured by SDS present in the buffer system.

Preparation of bacterial membranes

The method used for the preparation of bacterial membranes is essentially that described by Spratt (1977*a*).

Three litres of Penassay broth distributed in 500 ml amounts in sterile one litre conical flasks, are pre-warmed to 37°C. Each flask is inoculated with 15 ml of an overnight culture of *E. coli* DCO grown at 37°C with shaking in Penassay broth, and then shaken vigorously at 37°C until the culture is in late exponential phase (O.D.$_{675\ nm}$ 1·1–1·3) which is usually after 3½–4 h.

The cells are harvested (10,000 **g**/5 min/4°C), resuspended in 160 ml ice-cold 10 mmol/l sodium phosphate buffer pH 7·0, containing 140 mmol/l 2-mercaptoethanol and broken by ultrasonication for 3 min with constant cooling in an ice-bath. Unbroken bacteria are removed by centrifugation (8000 **g**/10 min/4°C), resuspended using an homogenizer in 100 ml 10 mmol/l phosphate buffer and sonicated and centrifuged as before. The cell envelopes contained in the combined supernatants are pelleted by ultracentrifugation (100,000 **g**/30 min/4°C) and washed by resuspension in 150 ml fresh 10 mmol/l phosphate buffer and recentrifuged.

The membrane pellet is resuspended in 10 ml cold 10 mmol/l phosphate buffer pH 7·0 and adjusted to give a final protein concentration of 10 mg/ml, as determined by the method of Lowry *et al.* (1951). Approximately 18–20 ml of membrane suspension is obtained by the above procedure, and this is dispensed into aliquots of 2·7 ml and stored at −70°C.

Penicillin-binding protein assay

Reagents

(^{14}C)-Benzylpenicillin was purchased from Amersham International Ltd. Unlabelled Benzylpenicillin G was prepared in our own laboratories. Sarkosyl NL97 (sodium lauryl sarkosinate) was a gift from Ciba-Geigy Ltd.

Method

Eleven serial dilutions of the test antibiotic are prepared in 50 mmol/l phosphate buffer pH 7·0 at 20 times the final concentration required in the assay, and 10 μl of each dilution added to a separate Eppendorf tube (Sarstedt Ltd, Beaumont Leys, Leicestershire, cat. no. 72-690) and equilibrated at 30°C. Two tubes containing 10 μl of buffer instead of antibiotic solution are used as controls. The assay is started by addition of 200 μl of pre-warmed membrane suspension and each tube vortexed and then incubated for 10 min. After this time 20 μl of (^{14}C)-benzylpenicillin (50 μCi/ml; 54 mCi/mmol/l) is then added to each tube, the mixture again vortexed and incubated a further 10 min. The reaction is terminated by addition of 5 μl of non-radioactive benzylpenicillin (120 mg/ml), followed by 20 μl of 20% (w/v) sarkosyl, the tubes vortexed and allowed to stand at room temperature for 20 min.

The sarkosyl-insoluble outer membrane and peptidoglycan are sedimented by ultracentrifugation (100,000 **g**/30 min/10°C) using adaptors designed to take the Eppendorf tubes and supplied by Whiteleaf Engineering,

Croydon, Surrey. The press-on caps of the tubes are removed prior to centrifugation as a precaution against implosion. The sarkosyl-soluble supernatants are carefully removed from the tubes and either prepared for electrophoresis as detailed later, or stored at −20°C until required.

Electrophoresis

The apparatus and discontinuous buffer system used for the vertical slab gel electrophoretic separation of the PBPs are essentially as described by Laemmli & Favre (1973).

Apparatus

Equipment. Any vertical slab gel electrophoresis equipment can be used. However, for economy, we routinely use the slab gel apparatus (20 × 20 cm) supplied by Raven Scientific, Haverhill, Suffolk and the Vokam 500-500 power pack (Shandon Southern Products Ltd, Runcorn, Cheshire). With this power pack four 'tanks' can be run simultaneously. The methodology described below is specific for these 'tanks', but can easily be modified to accommodate other makes.

Many PAGE equipment manufacturers (including Raven) supply perspex sample combs and these have been found difficult to remove from set gels. In our experience, combs made from PTFE material eliminate these problems.

Cleanliness. All glass plates, plastic formers and sample combs must be kept scrupulously clean. A good laboratory detergent such as Pyroneg (Diversay Ltd, Northampton) is excellent for this, but all traces of the detergent must be removed by extensive washing in warm running water, followed by distilled water. The plates etc. must be thoroughly dried before assembly.

Reagents

Solution A: Acrylamide/bisacrylamide. 300 g Acrylamide (BDH cat. no. 15212) and 3 g N,N^1-methylenebisacrylamide (BDH cat. no. 15213) dissolved in 1 litre distilled water and stored at 4°C in a dark bottle. Both solids are 'specially purified for electrophoresis'.

Solution B: 1·5 mol/l Tris–HCl pH 8·8. 181·5 g Tris(hydroxymethyl) methylamine (BDH Analar cat. no. 10315) dissolved in 1 litre distilled water and pH adjusted to 8·8 with concentrated hydrochloric acid.

Solution C: 10% (w/v) Sodium dodecyl sulphate. 100 g Sodium dodecyl sulphate (Sigma cat. no. L5750) dissolved in 1 litre distilled water. Far better results are achieved if the SDS is *not* 'specially purified'.

Solution D: 0·5 mol/l Tris–HCl pH 6·8. 60·5 g Tris(hydroxymethyl) methylamine dissolved in 1 litre distilled water and pH adjusted with concentrated hydrochloric acid.

Running buffer. 120 g Tris(hydroxymethyl) methylamine, 576 g glycine (Sigma) and 20 g SDS dissolved in 20 litre distilled water.

Sample buffer. Solution C (2·0 ml), Solution D (2·5 ml), glycerol (2·0 ml; BDH) and 0·5% (w/v) bromophenol blue (0·1 ml; BDH).

All other materials were obtained from either BDH—TEMED (*N*,*N*,*N*^{1},*N*^{1}-tetramethylethylenediamine) and 2-mercaptoethanol, or from Sigma—ammonium persulphate and Coomassie Brilliant Blue R (cat. no. B0630).

Preparation of gels

Separating gel. Solution A (33·3 ml), Solution B (25 ml), Solution C (1 ml) and distilled water (39·7 ml) are mixed and divided into two equal aliquots. To one portion add 0·5 ml of freshly prepared 10% (w/v) ammonium persulphate and 50 μl TEMED, mix thoroughly and use immediately, pouring as the plug at the bottom of the assembled plates. Setting time at room temperature is 5–10 min. In practice 50 ml solution is sufficient for two plugs.

When the plug is set, add ammonium persulphate and TEMED as before to the second portion, mix, and pour as the running gel between the two glass plates, so that nearly 75% of the space is filled. After pouring, the separating gel is gently overlaid, using an aerosol spray bottle, with Solution D diluted 1:4 with distilled water and containing 0·1% SDS; this allows a straight interface to form upon polymerization of the acrylamide. A sample comb is also inserted between the plates to ensure that the correct separation is achieved before the gel finally sets. Liquid remaining above the set gel is subsequently removed using filter paper.

Stacking gel. Solution A (2·0 ml), Solution C (0·1 ml), Solution D (2·5 ml) and distilled water (5·3 ml) are mixed and 50 μl freshly prepared 10% (w/v) ammonium persulphate and 10 μl TEMED added. The solution is mixed thoroughly and poured on top of the separating gel to fill the remaining gap between the plates, and the sample comb inserted.

As soon as the stacking gel has set, carefully remove the comb, wash the sample wells extensively with running buffer using a wash bottle and leave them filled with the same to prevent drying out. If the combs are left in for too long after polymerization it has been found that stray bits of polymerized material tend to be left behind in the wells and these result in irregular tracking during electrophoresis. Straighten any wells which may have been disturbed by the washing step using a syringe needle and leave them covered with the running buffer prior to loading samples.

Preparation of samples for SDS–PAGE

Aliquots (150 μl) of the sarkosyl-soluble extracts are mixed with 75 μl sample buffer and 25 μl 2-mercaptoethanol and then heated in a heating-block at 100°C for 3 min. When cool the samples can either be loaded on to the gel or stored at −20°C until required.

Separation of samples on SDS–PAGE

60–100 μl of sample (depending on the organism and the PAGE apparatus) is carefully loaded into a gel slot using a Hamilton microsyringe, so displacing the running buffer filling the sample wells. A control (see PBP assay method) is loaded at each side of the gel. The top and bottom electrolyte chambers of the apparatus are filled with running buffer, taking care not to disturb the samples in the gel slots.

The apparatus is connected to the power supply such that migration is towards the positive electrode, and electrophoresis performed at constant current. It has been found that best separations are achieved by having a different current depending on the position of the bromophenol blue tracking dye. We routinely use 40–50 mA through the stacking gel, 60–70 mA through the separating gel, and the bands are sharpened by running at 100 mA per gel for the final 20 min.

When the tracking dye has migrated a sufficient distance (14 cm into the separating gel; 3 h running time), the electrophoresis is stopped, the gel removed from the apparatus, marked to show sample orientation and the stacking gel cut off and discarded. In order to monitor the quality of the electrophoretic separation the remaining gel is immersed in warm stain [Coomassie Brilliant Blue R 0·1% (w/v), methanol 50% (v/v), glacial acetic acid 10% (v/v)] for 2 h and then destained [methanol 5% (v/v), glacial acetic acid 10% (v/v)].

Fluorography

Only very low amounts of radioactivity are bound by *E. coli* membranes, owing to the specific activity of commercially available (^{14})C-benzylpenicillin and the low numbers of PBP molecules present. This necessitates the use of fluorography as opposed to conventional autoradiography to facilitate image formation in a reasonable time.

The preparation of the gels for fluorography is as described by Bonner & Laskey (1974). The procedure, however, does introduce some errors since the image density is not proportional to the amount of radioactivity present. This problem can be largely overcome by pre-fogging the X-ray film prior to exposure to the polyacrylamide gel (Laskey & Mills 1975). This procedure also serves another purpose in that it lowers the threshold for silver halide deposition in the emulsion and therefore allows image formation to occur more rapidly.

Materials

2,5-Diphenyloxazole (PPO) chromatographically purified for scintillation was obtained from Koch Light. X-ray emulsions used were Kodak X-Omat H or RP Royal X-Omat or Fuji RX.

Method

Destained gels are completely immersed in dimethylsulphoxide (DMSO) for 1 h, followed by a second immersion in fresh DMSO for a further 1 h. They are then impregnated with the scintillation fluor by immersing in a solution of 22·2% (w/v) PPO in DMSO for 3 h. The PPO, which is soluble in DMSO but not in water, is then precipitated *in situ* in the gel by immersion in distilled water overnight (this also serves to remove DMSO), and the gel is finally dried on to Whatman No. 17 card using a slab drier. We have found the apparatus marketed by Bio-Rad Laboratories Ltd to be very satisfactory.

The dried gels are exposed to pre-fogged X-ray film by placing the emulsion directly in contact with the dried gel and enclosing the pair between two metal plates which are then held tightly together with clips. The package is wrapped in two light-proof black polythene bags, sealed with adhesive tape and stored at −70°C usually for 40 days. The X-ray emulsions are developed in Kodak liquid X-ray developer for 5 min at 20°C without agitation, washed in 3% (v/v) acetic acid and fixed for 5 min at 20°C in Kodak X-ray fixer.

The results obtained on the X-ray plates can be quantitated roughly by eye. More accurate data can be obtained by scanning the plates with a scanning microdensitometer, preferably with peak integration.

Interpretation of Results

Morphology

In *E. coli* the ability of certain β-lactams to elicit one of three morphological effects, viz.

(1) inhibition of cell division and the growth of the cells as long filaments, or
(2) rapid cell lysis and the release of cell contents as a spheroplast, or
(3) conversion of normal rod-shaped cells into large, osmotically stable spherical cells,

has been correlated with their affinities for each of the discrete 'essential' PBPs. Examples of the principal morphological effects of β-lactam antibiotics upon *E. coli* DCO are shown in Fig. 2.

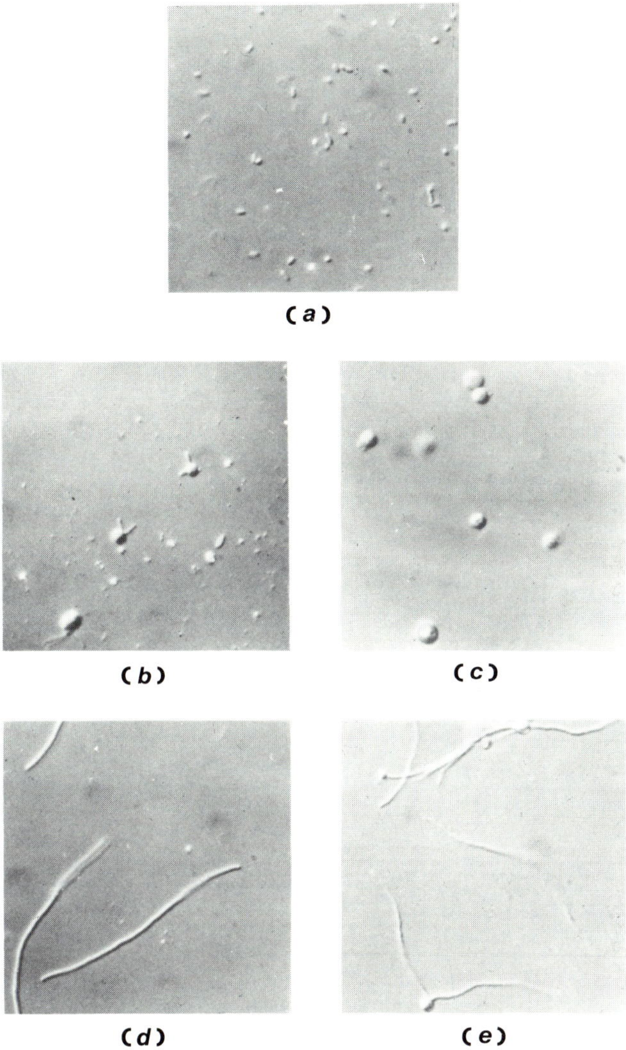

FIG. 2. Interference contrast micrographs showing the morphological responses of *Escherichia coli* DCO incubated in the presence of different β-lactam antibiotics. (*a*) Control bacteria; (*b*) 'rabbit-ear' spheroplasts induced by cephaloridine (2 μg/ml) inhibiting PBPs 1a/1bs; (*c*) 'round-forms' induced by mecillinam (1 μg/ml) inhibiting PBP 2; (*d*) filaments induced by cefuroxime (1 μg/ml) inhibiting PBP 3; (*e*) filaments showing spheroplast formation induced by a high concentration of cefuroxime (20 μg/ml) inhibiting PBPs 3 and 1a/1bs.

Cephaloridine, for example, induces spheroplast formation followed by rapid lysis at its lowest effective concentration, by competing for PBPs 1a/1bs (Curtis *et al.* 1979*b*). The formation of osmotically stable 'round-forms' has been shown to result from the binding of β-lactams to PBP 2. A well-known example of a β-lactam eliciting this effect is the amidinopenicillanic acid, mecillinam (Spratt 1977*d*). Mecillinam results in the growth of *E. coli* as spherical cells and is found to bind exclusively to PBP 2. It does not result in spheroplasting and rapid cell lysis, or filamentation at any concentration.

Many β-lactams cause filamentation without ever producing spherical cells. Rapid cell lysis may often only occur when the β-lactam is present in much higher concentrations than that required to cause filamentation (Curtis *et al.* 1979*a*, *b*). An example of such a compound is cefuroxime, which, in common with the majority of β-lactam antibiotics and in particular the aminothiazolyl cephalosporins, binds to PBP 3 thus inhibiting cell division. As with compounds which inhibit PBP 2, this proves to be lethal.

Affinity/mode of action of β-Lactams

Figure 3 is a fluorogram showing the competition of cefuroxime for the PBPs of *E. coli* DCO. It will serve as a general example to illustrate how the PBP assay can be utilized to gain knowledge of the mode of action of a particular β-lactam antibiotic.

The percentage inhibition of a PBP required to prevent its physiological function *in vivo* is unknown, and may vary for different PBPs. For the purpose of interpreting PBP affinity data, an inhibition of 50% (I_{50}) is arbitrarily taken. As the PBP assay is based on competitive binding, the I_{50} binding concentration of cefuroxime is that concentration required to inhibit subsequent binding of (^{14}C)-benzylpenicillin by 50%. The I_{50} for each of the PBPs of *E. coli* DCO was determined from the fluorogram by densitometry and the results are shown in Fig. 3.

The PBPs with highest affinity for cefuroxime are PBPs 1a and 3, both of which have an I_{50} of less than 0·25 μg/ml. More detailed experiments have given I_{50} binding concentrations of 0·12 and 0·09 μg/ml for PBPs 1a and 3 respectively. Since inhibition of PBP 1a alone is not lethal (Spratt *et al.* 1977; Tamaki *et al.* 1977) PBP 3 is the primary 'lethal' target for cefuroxime. These data correlate with its ability to induce filaments at its lowest effective concentration (Curtis *et al.* 1979*a*, *b*).

Penetration

The PBP affinity data can also be utilized to assess the ease of entry of the antibiotic under test into the intact cell. The MIC of cefuroxime against

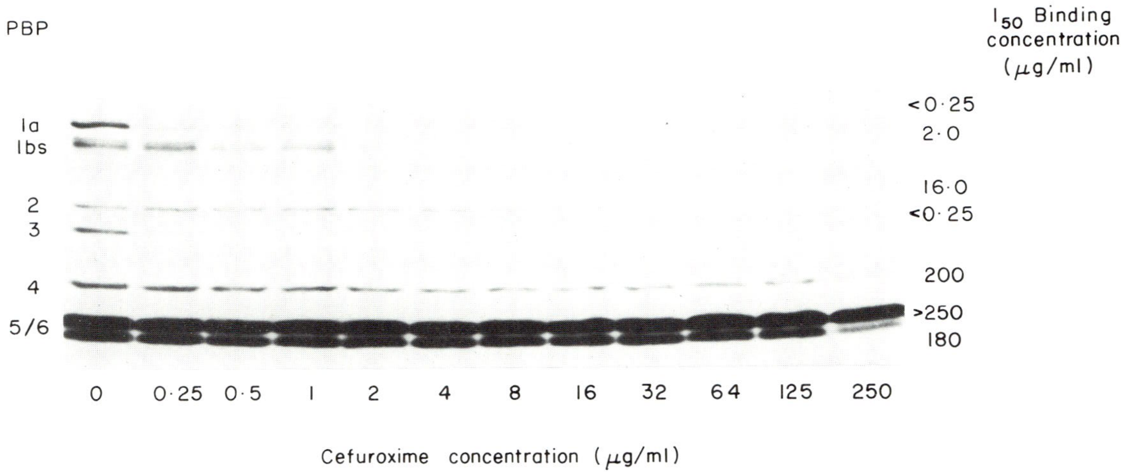

FIG. 3. Fluorogram showing the competition of cefuroxime for the penicillin-binding proteins of *Escherichia coli* DCO. I_{50} Binding concentrations were determined by densitometry.

intact *E. coli* DCO cells is found to be 2 μg/ml, whereas its affinity for PBP 3 is about 0·1 μg/ml, more than an order of magnitude lower. This suggests that cefuroxime has some difficulty in crossing the permeability barrier. This theory is supported by studies with an *E. coli* permeability mutant (*E. coli* DC2), in which the normal permeability barrier is non-functional. In this strain the I_{50} binding concentration to PBP 3 and the MIC were both found to be 0·1 μg/ml, indicating that in the wild type (*E. coli* DCO) cefuroxime is being excluded by the outer membrane barrier (Curtis *et al.* 1979*b*).

As mentioned earlier, cefuroxime has the ability to induce spheroplasting and concomitant rapid lysis at a higher concentration (20 μg/ml) than that required to cause filamentation (2 μg/ml). Study of the PBP affinity data offers an explanation for this observation. It must be remembered that the permeability barrier in *E. coli* DCO appears to reduce the external MIC concentration of cefuroxime by more than an order of magnitude by the time the compound has reached the cytoplasmic membrane target. Thus the external concentration required to produce rapid lysis *in vivo* is reduced to a concentration at the cytoplasmic membrane of approximately 2 μg/ml. From the data in Fig. 3 it can be seen that PBPs 1bs have an I_{50} binding concentration of 1·6 μg/ml and PBP 1a is inhibited at a lower level (<0·25 μg/ml). Therefore at a cytoplasmic concentration of 2 μg/ml, joint inhibition of PBPs 1a/1bs will occur leading to spheroplasting and rapid lysis.

Rational Antimicrobial Design

Correlation of PBP and MIC data not only enables one to ascertain the absolute activity of penicillins and cephalosporins against their 'essential' target PBPs, but also to assess their ease of penetration of the bacterial permeability barrier. Table 1 shows the competition of some penicillin and cephalosporin derivatives for the PBPs of *E. coli* DCO along with MIC and morphological response data.

Cephaloridine, for example, inhibits PBPs 1a/1bs (its primary 'essential' targets) at concentrations of 0·25 and 2·5 μg/ml respectively, while its MIC is 2 μg/ml. This compound therefore has no difficulty in penetrating the permeability barrier of this *E. coli* K12 strain. This is not true for the cephalosporin derivative cefsulodin. This compound, although having virtually the same affinity for PBPs 1a/1bs as cephaloridine, has an MIC more than a magnitude higher indicating difficulty in penetration. Another example of a compound possessing good affinity while demonstrating poor penetration characteristics is the penicillin derivative, methicillin. This compound has an I_{50} binding affinity for PBP 3, its primary 'essential'

Table 1

Competition of penicillin and cephalosporin derivatives for the penicillin-binding proteins of Escherichia coli *DCO*

Compound	I_{50} binding concentration (μg/ml) for protein*							MIC (μg/ml)		Primary morphological response†
	1a	1bs	2	3	4	5	6	DCO	DC2	
Ampicillin	1·4	3·9	0·7	0·9	2	140	9	3·2	0·5	F + R + S
Penicillin G	0·5	3	0·8	0·9	1	24	19	16	1·6	F + R + S
Carbenicillin	2·1	5	4	2·1	3·5	130	120	2	1	F + R + S
Methicillin	9	250	27	5·5	60	> 250	> 250	> 250	4	F(DC2)
Cloxacillin	2	23	15	3	125	8	30	> 250	4	F(DC2)
Mecillinam	> 250	> 250	< 0·25	> 250	> 250	> 250	> 250	0·05	0·01	R
Cephaloridine	0·25	2·5	50	8	17	> 250	> 250	2	2	S
Cefsulodin	0·47	3·7	> 250	> 250	> 250	> 250	> 250	25	6·4	S
Cefuroxime	0·12	1·6	13·7	0·09	200	> 250	180	2	0·1	F
Cefoxitin	0·1	3·9	> 250	5·8	7	0·6	0·9	4	2	S + F
Cefotaxime	0·05	0·7	5	< 0·05	30	> 50	> 50	0·08	0·01	F

* Values indicate the concentration of antibiotic required to reduce (^{14}C)-benzylpenicillin binding by 50%.

† (F) filamentation; (S) spheroplasting; (R) 'round-forms'. Where the primary morphological response is observed to be a mixture of more than one morphological effect, these are placed in order of dominance. Where the MIC of certain compounds has necessitated observing the morphological effects in the *E. coli* DC2 mutant rather than the parent strain, this is shown.

target, of 5·5 μg/ml. Its MIC, however, is >250 μg/ml, demonstrating that methicillin must have great difficulty in penetrating the intact permeability barrier (Curtis *et al.* 1979*a*, *b*).

The PBP assay, backed up by MIC data and studies of the effect of compounds against 'permeability' mutants, thus affords the opportunity to correlate valuable information on the effect of different structures on the permeability of β-lactam antibiotics.

The PBP assay data are also useful in the rational design of future antimicrobial agents. The most potent β-lactams should be those that have very high affinity for PBPs 1a/1bs, since the rate of 'killing' following inactivation of these targets is rapid. PBP affinity data can therefore be used to give insight into the structure/activity relationships governing affinity for the various PBPs. Compounds could thus be designed with an increased affinity for PBPs 1a/1bs, thereby eliciting a rapid lytic effect at lower and more therapeutically relevant concentrations.

Penicillin-binding Proteins of Other Gram Negative Bacteria

As mentioned earlier, a number of penicillins and cephalosporins are known which have much higher affinities for specific PBPs of *E. coli* DCO than for others. These β-lactam compounds thus elicit distinct morphological effects and can be used as probes of PBP function in other Gram negative bacteria.

We have studied the PBPs of *Enterobacter cloacae*, *Klebsiella aerogenes*, *Proteus rettgeri* and *Pseudomonas aeruginosa* using four such probes: cephaloridine (PBPs 1a/1bs), mecillinam (PBP2), cefuroxime (PBP 3) and cefoxitin (PBPs 4 and 5/6) (Curtis *et al.* 1979*c*). All the organisms used were β-lactamase non-inducible mutants.

The general pattern of their PBPs on SDS–polyacrylamide gels is similar to that of *E. coli* DCO (Fig. 4), although variations occur between species due to molecular weight differences and the relative amounts of individual PBPs. These organisms all show the same range of morphological effects when exposed to the specific β-lactam probes (spheroplasting and rapid cell lysis, spherical cells and filamentation) and the biochemical basis of the responses seems to be the same. The results indicate that the PBPs 1a/1bs, 2 and 3 of these organisms perform the same roles in elongation, shape and division respectively as has been shown for *E. coli* K12 (Noguchi *et al.* 1979; Ohya *et al.* 1979).

More detailed work, in which the binding affinities of the *Ps. aeruginosa* PBPs to α-sulfocephalosporins were studied, suggests that although the PBPs of *E. coli* DCO and *Ps. aeruginosa* may perform similar morphogenic functions, the individual binding proteins show some species-specific

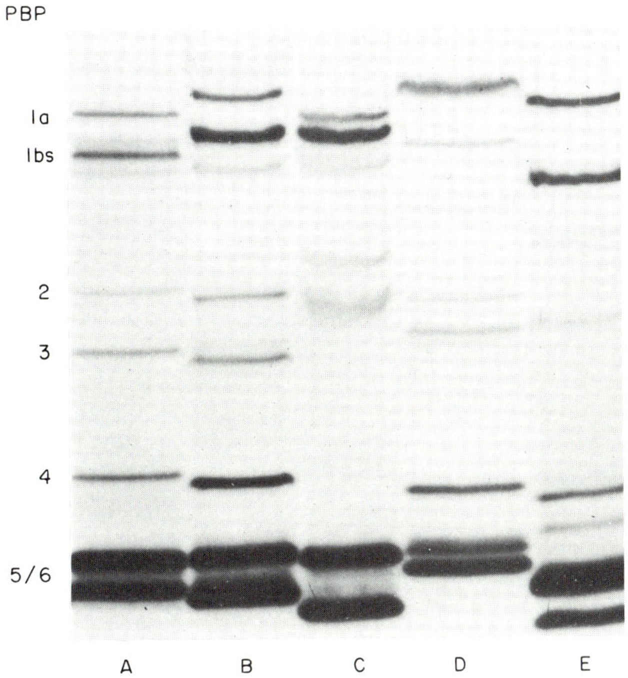

FIG. 4. Penicillin-binding protein patterns of (*a*) *Escherichia coli* DCO, (*b*) *Enterobacter cloacae*, (*c*) *Klebsiella aerogenes*, (*d*) *Proteus rettgeri* and (*e*) *Pseudomonas aeruginosa*. Taken from Curtis *et al.* (1979*c*).

variations in their stereospecific recognition of inhibitors. This is presumably due to variations in the configuration of the appropriate sites on the protein molecule (Curtis *et al.* 1980*a*).

Another observation derived from the PBP data of *Ps. aeruginosa* is the fact that its 'infamous' β-lactam resistance 'phenotype' is largely due to the permeability barrier, functional in intact cells, rather than the reduced affinity of β-lactam antibiotics for the 'essential' target PBPs (Curtis *et al.* 1980*a*, 1981).

Penicillin-binding Proteins of Gram Positive Bacteria

Although the majority of the work described here concerns the PBPs of Gram negative bacteria, and in particular *E. coli* K12 strains, the PBPs of Gram positive organisms have also been studied. As described in the methodology, the PBPs of Gram positive bacteria are visualized in the standard manner with only minor modifications of technique.

Two examples of Gram positive bacteria studied are *Bacillus megaterium* and *Staphylococcus aureus*. The cytoplasmic membrane of *B. megaterium* contains five PBPs (Chase *et al.* 1977), while four PBPs are routinely detected in the membrane of *Staph. aureus* (Curtis & Hayes 1981). Apart from PBP 4 of *Staph. aureus* which has been shown to have 'model' transpeptidase, D-alanine carboxypeptidase and β-lactamase activities *in vitro* (Kozarich & Strominger 1978), and PBP 5 of *B. megaterium* which possesses D-alanine carboxypeptidase activity (Chase 1980), no enzymic functions have been assigned to any of the remaining PBPs of either of these organisms.

In *Staph. aureus* it is not yet known which of the PBPs are essential for the 'lethal' action of β-lactam antibiotics, although viable mutants have been isolated lacking PBP 1 and PBP 4 (Curtis & Hayes 1981; Curtis *et al.* 1980*b*). It is believed, therefore, that PBPs 2 and 3 (perhaps functionally intercompensatory) represent the 'killing' targets (Hayes *et al.* 1981).

Further study of the roles of individual PBPs and PBP affinity data will afford the opportunity to design antimicrobial compounds rationally against these clinically important bacteria.

Conclusions

The antibacterial activity of β-lactam antibiotics against Gram negative bacteria depends essentially on three interacting factors:

(1) The stability of the antibiotics to periplasmically located β-lactamase.

(2) The penetration characteristics of the antibiotic through the outer membrane permeability barrier.

(3) The affinity of the antibiotic for 'essential' penicillin-binding proteins located in the cytoplasmic or inner membrane.

In the search for a new generation of β-lactam antibiotics with an improved therapeutic efficiency, it is important to understand these interacting factors that together determine the activity of these compounds against Gram negative bacteria.

A novel approach for investigating the molecular action of β-lactam antibiotics has been the development of the PBP assay, and this has led to the recognition of distinct proteins with discrete roles in bacterial morphogenesis.

Study of PBP assay data may help in clarifying structure/activity relationships governing PBP affinity of β-lactam antibiotics. This knowledge would be useful in the future rational design of molecules possessing specific affinities for certain desirable target PBPs.

A compound with this potent target activity, combined with good bacterial permeability, β-lactamase stability and favourable pharmacokinetics (especially oral absorption), could be the ideal β-lactam antibiotic.

We gratefully acknowledge the assistance of A. Wright and D. Kedgley in the development of fluorograms and for their excellent photographic services. We also thank Drs N. A. C. Curtis, M. V. Hayes and G. W. Ross for suggestions during the preparation of this paper.

References

Boman, H. G., Nordström, K. & Normark, S. 1974 Penicillin resistance in *Escherichia coli* K12: synergism between penicillinases and a barrier in the outer part of the envelope. *Annals of the New York Academy of Sciences* **235,** 569–585.

Bonner, W. M. & Laskey, R. A. 1974 A film detection method for tritium-labelled proteins and nucleic acids in polyacrylamide gels. *European Journal of Biochemistry* **46,** 83–88.

Chase, H. A. 1980 Purification of four penicillin-binding proteins from *Bacillus megaterium*. *Journal of General Microbiology* **117,** 211–224.

Chase, H. A., Shepherd, S. T. & Reynolds, P. E. 1977 Studies on the penicillin-binding components of *Bacillus megaterium*. *Federation of European Biochemical Societies, Letters* **76,** 199–203.

Curtis, N. A. C. & Hayes, M. V. 1981 A mutant of *Staphylococcus aureus* H deficient in penicillin-binding protein 1 is viable. *Federation of European Microbiological Societies Microbiology Letters* **10,** 227–229.

Curtis, N. A. C., Richmond, M. H. & Sykes, R. B. 1972 'Periplasmic' location of a β-lactamase specified either by a plasmid or a chromosomal gene in *Escherichia coli*. *Journal of Bacteriology* **112,** 1433–1434.

Curtis, N. A. C., Brown, C., Boxall, M. & Boulton, M. G. 1979*a* Inhibition of *Escherichia coli* K12 by β-lactam antibiotics with poor antibacterial activity: interaction of permeability and intrinsic activity against the penicillin-binding proteins. *Antimicrobial Agents and Chemotherapy* **15,** 332–336.

Curtis, N. A. C., Orr, D., Ross, G. W. & Boulton, M. G. 1979*b* Affinities of penicillins and cephalosporins for the penicillin-binding proteins of *Escherichia coli* K12 and their antibacterial activity. *Antimicrobial Agents and Chemotherapy* **16,** 533–539.

Curtis, N. A. C., Orr, D., Ross, G. W. & Boulton, M. G. 1979*c* Competition of β-lactam antibiotics for the penicillin-binding proteins of *Pseudomonas aeruginosa, Enterobacter cloacae, Klebsiella aerogenes, Proteus rettgeri* and *Escherichia coli:* comparison with antibacterial activity and effects upon bacterial morphology. *Antimicrobial Agents and Chemotherapy* **16,** 325–328.

Curtis, N. A. C., Boulton, M. G., Orr, D. & Ross, G. W. 1980*a* The competition of α-sulfocephalosporins for the penicillin-binding proteins of *Escherichia coli* K12 and *Pseudomonas aeruginosa*—comparison with effects upon morphology. *Journal of Antimicrobial Chemotherapy* **6,** 189–196.

Curtis, N. A. C., Hayes, M. V., Wyke, A. W. & Ward, J. B. 1980*b* A mutant of *Staphylococcus aureus* H lacking penicillin-binding protein 4 and transpeptidase activity *in vitro*. *Federation of European Microbiological Societies Microbiology Letters* **9,** 263–266.

Curtis, N. A. C., Orr, D., Boulton, M. G. & Ross, G. W. 1981 Penicillin-binding proteins of *Pseudomonas aeruginosa*. Comparison of two strains differing in their resistance to β-lactam antibiotics. *Journal of Antimicrobial Chemotherapy* **7,** 127–136.

FILIP, C., FLETCHER, G., WULFF, J. L. & EARHART, C. F. 1973 Solubilisation of the cytoplasmic membrane of *Escherichia coli* by the ionic detergent sodium lauryl sarcosinate. *Journal of Bacteriology* **115,** 717–722.

HAYES, M. V., CURTIS, N. A. C., WYKE, A. W. & WARD, J. B. 1981 Decreased affinity of a penicillin-binding protein for β-lactam antibiotics in a clinical isolate of *Staphylococcus aureus* resistant to methicillin. *Federation of European Microbiological Societies Microbiology Letters* **10,** 119–122.

ISHINO, F., MITSUI, K., TAMAKI, S. & MATSUHASHI, M. 1980 Dual enzyme activities of cell wall peptidoglycan synthesis, peptidoglycan transglycosylase and penicillin-sensitive transpeptidase, in purified preparations of *Escherichia coli* penicillin-binding protein 1a. *Biochemical and Biophysical Research Communications* **97,** 287–293.

IWAYA, M. & STROMINGER, J. L. 1977 Simultaneous deletion of D-alanine carboxypeptidase 1B-C and penicillin-binding component IV in a mutant of *Escherichia coli* K12. *Proceedings of the National Academy of Sciences of the United States of America* **74,** 2980–2984.

IZAKI, K., MATSUHASHI, M. & STROMINGER, J. L. 1968 Biosynthesis of the peptidoglycan of bacterial cell walls XIII. Peptidoglycan transpeptidase and D-alanine carboxypeptidase: penicillin-sensitive enzymatic reaction in strains of *Escherichia coli*. *Journal of Biological Chemistry* **243,** 3180–3192.

KOZARICH, J. W. & STROMINGER, J. L. 1978 A membrane enzyme from *Staphylococcus aureus* which catalyses transpeptidase, carboxypeptidase and penicillinase activities. *Journal of Biological Chemistry* **253,** 1272–1278.

LAEMMLI, U. K. & FAVRE, M. 1973 Maturation of the head of bacteriophage T4 I. DNA packaging events. *Journal of Molecular Biology* **80,** 575–599.

LASKEY, R. A. & MILLS, A. D. 1975 Quantitative film detection of ^{3}H and ^{14}C in polyacrylamide gels by fluorography. *European Journal of Biochemistry* **56,** 335–341.

LOWRY, O. H., ROSEBROUGH, N. J., FARR, A. L. & RANDALL, R. J. 1951 Protein measurement with the Folin Phenol reagent. *Journal of Biological Chemistry* **193,** 265–275.

MATSUHASHI, M., TAKAGAKI, Y., MARUYAMA, I. N., TAMAKI, S., NISHIMURA, Y., SUZUKI, H., OGINO, U. & HIROTA, Y. 1977 Mutants of *Escherichia coli* lacking in highly penicillin-sensitive D-alanine carboxypeptidase activity. *Proceedings of the National Academy of Sciences of the United States of America* **74,** 2976–2979.

MATSUHASHI, M., TAMAKI, S., CURTIS, S. J. & STROMINGER, J. L. 1979 Mutational evidence for identity of penicillin-binding protein 5 in *Escherichia coli* with the major D-alanine carboxypeptidase 1A activity. *Journal of Bacteriology* **137,** 644–647.

NGUYEN-DISTÈCHE, M., POLLOCK, J. J., GHUYSEN, J.-M., PUIG, J., REYNOLDS, P., PERKINS, H. R., COYETTE, J. & SALTON, M. R. J. 1974 Sensitivity to ampicillin and cephalothin of enzymes involved in wall peptide crosslinking in *Escherichia coli* K12, strain 44. *European Journal of Biochemistry* **41,** 457–463.

NOGUCHI, H., MATSUHASHI, M. & MITSUHASHI, S. 1979 Comparative studies of penicillin-binding proteins in *Pseudomonas aeruginosa* and *Escherichia coli*. *European Journal of Biochemistry* **100,** 41–49.

OHYA, S., YAMAZAKI, M., SUGAWARA, S. & MATSUHASHI, M. 1979 Penicillin-binding proteins in *Proteus* species. *Journal of Bacteriology* **137,** 474–479.

RICHMOND, M. H. & CURTIS, N. A. C. 1974 The interplay of β-lactamases and intrinsic factors in the resistance of Gram-negative bacteria to penicillins and cephalosporins. *Annals of the New York Academy of Sciences* **235,** 553–567.

Richmond, M. H. & Sykes, R. B. 1973 The β-lactamases of Gram-negative bacteria and their possible physiological role. *Advances in Microbial Physiology* **9**, 31–88.

Richmond, M. H., Clark, D. C. & Wotton, S. 1976 Indirect method of assessing the penetration of beta-lactamase–nonsusceptible penicillins and cephalosporins in *Escherichia coli* strains. *Antimicrobial Agents and Chemotherapy* **10**, 215–218.

Spratt, B. G. 1975 Distinct penicillin-binding proteins involved in the division, elongation, and shape of *Escherichia coli* K12. *Proceedings of the National Academy of Sciences of the United States of America* **72**, 2999–3003.

Spratt, B. G. 1977*a* Properties of the penicillin-binding proteins of *Escherichia coli* K12. *European Journal of Biochemistry* **72**, 341–352.

Spratt, B. G. 1977*b* Temperature-sensitive cell division mutants of *Escherichia coli* with thermolabile penicillin-binding proteins. *Journal of Bacteriology* **131**, 293–305.

Spratt, B. G. 1977*c* Penicillin-binding proteins of *Escherichia coli*: general properties and characterisation of mutants. *Microbiology* **1977**, 182–190.

Spratt, B. G. 1977*d* The mechanism of action of mecillinam. *Journal of Antimicrobial Chemotherapy* **3** (Supplement B), 13–19.

Spratt, B. G. 1980 Biochemical and genetic approaches to the mechanism of action of penicillin. *Philosophical Transactions of the Royal Society of London, Series B* **289**, 273–283.

Spratt, B. G. & Pardee, A. B. 1975 Penicillin-binding proteins and cell shape in *E. coli*. *Nature, London* **254**, 516–517.

Spratt, B. G. & Strominger, J. L. 1976 Identification of the major penicillin-binding proteins of *Escherichia coli* as D-alanine carboxypeptidase 1A. *Journal of Bacteriology* **127**, 660–663.

Spratt, B. G., Jobanputra, V. & Schwartz, U. 1977 Mutants of *Escherichia coli* which lack a component of penicillin-binding protein 1 are viable. *Federation of European Biochemical Societies, Letters* **79**, 374–378.

Suzuki, H., Nishimura, Y. & Hirota, Y. 1978 On the process of cellular division in *Escherichia coli*: a series of mutants of *E. coli* altered in the penicillin-binding proteins. *Proceedings of the National Academy of Sciences of the United States of America* **75**, 664–668.

Suzuki, H., Van Heijenoort, Y., Tamura, T., Mizoguchi, J., Hirota, Y. & Van Heijenoort, J. 1980 *In vitro* peptidoglycan polymerisation catalysed by penicillin-binding protein 1b of *Escherichia coli* K12. *Federation of European Biochemical Societies, Letters* **110**, 245–249.

Tamaki, S., Nakajima, S. & Matsuhashi, M. 1977 Thermosensitive mutation in *Escherichia coli* simultaneously causing defects in penicillin-binding protein 1bs and in enzyme activity for peptidoglycan synthesis *in vitro*. *Proceedings of the National Academy of Sciences of the United States of America* **74**, 5472–5476.

Tipper, D. J. & Strominger, J. L. 1965 Mechanism of action of penicillins: a proposal based on their structural similarity to acyl-D-alanyl-D-alanine. *Proceedings of the National Academy of Sciences of the United States of America* **54**, 1133–1141.

Tomasz, A. 1979 The mechanism of the irreversible antimicrobial effects of penicillins: how the beta-lactam antibiotics kill and lyse bacteria. *Annual Reviews of Microbiology* **33**, 113–137.

Zimmermann, W. & Rosselet, A. 1977 Function of the outer membrane of *Escherichia coli* as a permeability barrier to beta-lactam antibiotics. *Antimicrobial Agents and Chemotherapy* **12**, 368–372.

Detection of Aminoglycoside-modifying Strains of Bacteria

K. P. Shannon and I. Phillips

Department of Microbiology, St. Thomas's Hospital Medical School, London, UK

The antibacterial activity of aminoglycosides is thought to depend on their ability to bind to the bacterial ribosome and interfere with protein synthesis (see Gale *et al.* 1972). Bacterial resistance to aminoglycosides occurs in three ways. Firstly mutations in genes that specify ribosomal proteins may lead to diminished binding of the drug to the ribosome. The best known of these mutations occur at the *rpsL* locus (previously called *strA*) and give rise to a high level of resistance to streptomycin. Ribosomal resistance to aminoglycosides other than streptomycin is not found in clinical isolates (Price *et al.* 1974, 1977). However, ribosomal resistance to streptomycin has been reported in clinical isolates of *Pseudomonas aeruginosa* (Tseng *et al.* 1972), *Neisseria gonorrhoeae* (Maness *et al.* 1974), *Staphylococcus aureus* (Lacey & Chopra 1972) and enterococci (Zimmermann *et al.* 1971).

Secondly, the ability of the bacterial cell to take up aminoglycoside may be diminished. The mechanism of uptake of aminoglycosides is not simply one of passive diffusion, and the reasons for diminished uptake are also complex (Bryan & van den Elzen 1975, 1976, 1977; Bryan *et al.* 1976, 1980). This mechanism of resistance occurs in clinical isolates as well as in mutants produced in the laboratory and confers broad-spectrum resistance to aminoglycosides (Bryan *et al.* 1976; Phillips *et al.* 1978; Shannon *et al.* 1978; Price *et al.* 1981).

The third mechanism of resistance to aminoglycosides involves inactivation by aminoglycoside-modifying enzymes and is the main topic of this chapter.

ANTIBIOTICS
ISBN 0 12 604480 5

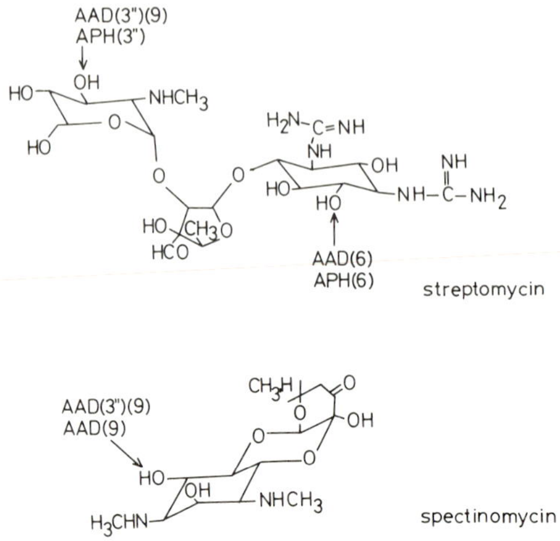

FIG. 1. Streptomycin and spectinomycin and the sites at which they can be modified.

Properties of Aminoglycoside-modifying Enzymes

Aminoglycoside-modifying enzymes have been reviewed by Davies & Smith (1978) and Reynolds & Smith (1979). Before discussing the properties of these enzymes the structures of aminoglycosides will be considered briefly. Aminoglycosides can be divided into two groups on the basis of their chemical structure. The first group contains streptomycin (Fig. 1) and its derivatives. Spectinomycin (Fig. 1), though not an aminoglycoside, is a substrate of one of the enzymes that modifies streptomycin and will, for convenience, be regarded as a member of the group. The second group consists of compounds that contain 2-deoxystreptamine and is subdivided into 4,5-substituted 2-deoxystreptamine compounds that include neomycin, ribostamycin, butirosin and lividomycin (Fig. 2), and 4,6-substituted 2-deoxystreptamine compounds that include kanamycin, amikacin, tobramycin, gentamicin, sissomicin and netilmicin (Figs 3 and 4).

There are three classes of aminoglycoside-modifying enzyme: *O*-phosphotransferases (for which the usual abbreviation is APH) which transfer a phosphate group from adenosine 5′-triphosphate (ATP) to an hydroxyl group on the aminoglycoside: *O*-adenylyltransferases (AAD) or nucleotidyltransferases (ANT) which transfer an adenylyl (or adenosine 5′-monophosphate) group from ATP to an hydroxyl group: and *N*-acetyltransferases (AAC) which transfer acetyl groups from acetyl coenzyme A to amino groups. No aminoglycoside-modifying enzymes are able to modify members of both the streptomycin and 2-deoxystreptamine groups.

The modification of aminoglycosides by these modifying enzymes is thought to prevent the binding of the aminoglycoside to the ribosome and thus prevent the inhibition of protein synthesis. On the other hand Davies & Smith (1978) argue that the mechanism of resistance should be regarded as interference with the transport of compounds into the cell. However, since modified aminoglycoside is not effective in inhibiting protein synthesis *in vitro* (Yamada *et al.* 1968) and since possession of

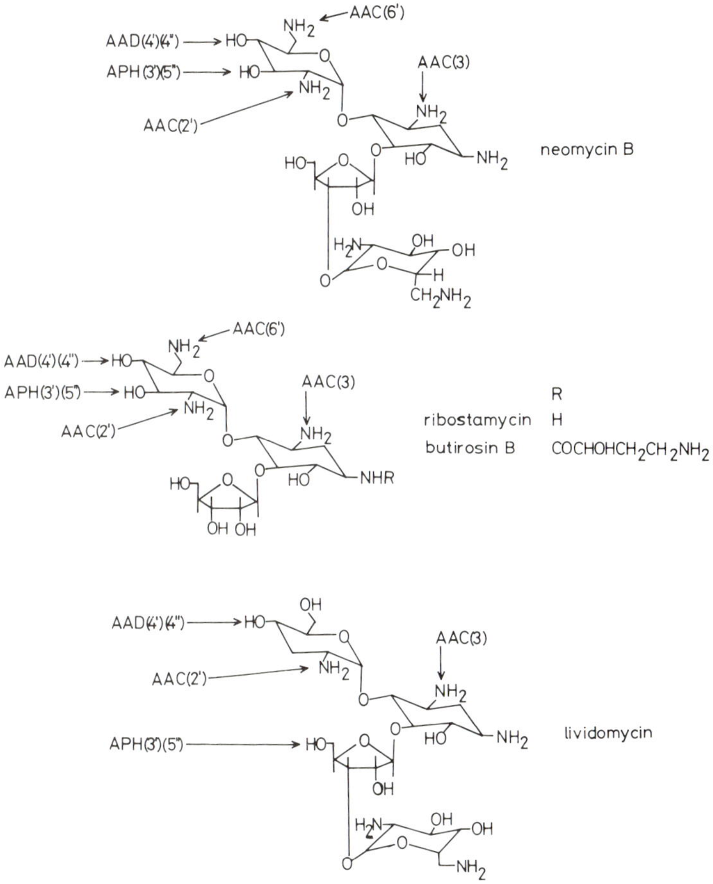

FIG. 2. Neomycin, ribostamycin, butirosin and lividomycin and the sites at which they can be modified.

modifying enzymes does not seem to prevent the first energy-dependent phase of aminoglycoside uptake (Dickie *et al.* 1978), we are reluctant to regard this mechanism of resistance as one of interference with drug transport. An important feature of aminoglycoside-modifying enzymes is

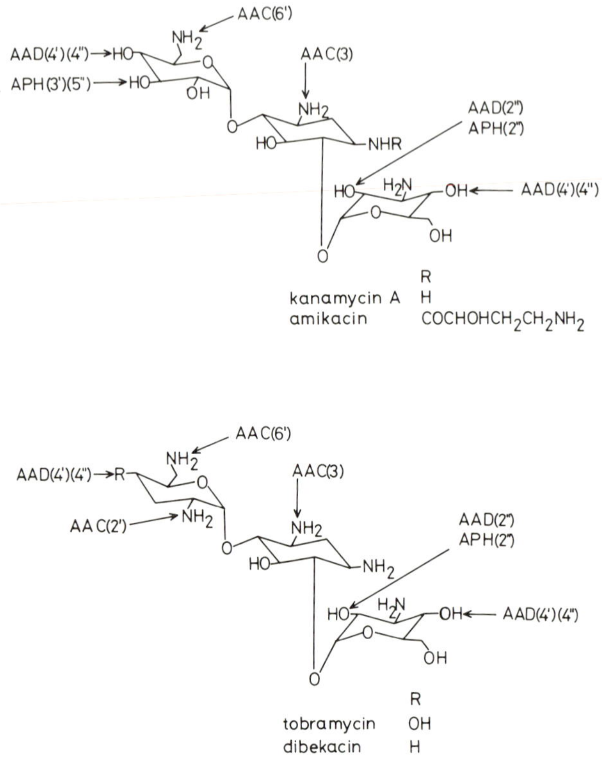

FIG. 3. Kanamycin, amikacin, tobramycin and dibekacin and the sites at which they can be modified.

that they modify aminoglycosides as the drug enters the cell, so there is essentially no change in the concentration of active aminoglycoside in the culture medium.

Aminoglycoside-modifying enzymes are further classified by the position on the aminoglycoside at which modification occurs. It is customary to write this position in brackets after the abbreviation of the modifying enzyme: thus AAC(2′) is an acetyltransferase that modifies aminoglycosides at the 2′-amino group. The sites at which aminoglycosides are modified are shown in Figs 1–4. For many enzymes the site of modification can be inferred from the substrate profile, but this is not always so. The definitive method is to determine the chemical structure of the modified aminoglycoside. This requires facilities for advanced organic chemistry, including the use of nuclear magnetic resonance, which are beyond the scope of most laboratories. However, such techniques have been used to confirm the site of modification of most modifying enzymes. For the few enzymes, notably the various forms of AAC(3), for which substrate profiles provide no clue as to the site of modification, elucidation of this site by determination of the structure of the product has allowed identification of these enzymes from their substrate profiles. Table 1 summarizes the substrate profiles of aminoglycoside-modifying enzymes.

In general, each aminoglycoside-modifying enzyme can carry out modification at only one site. There are, however, two exceptions.

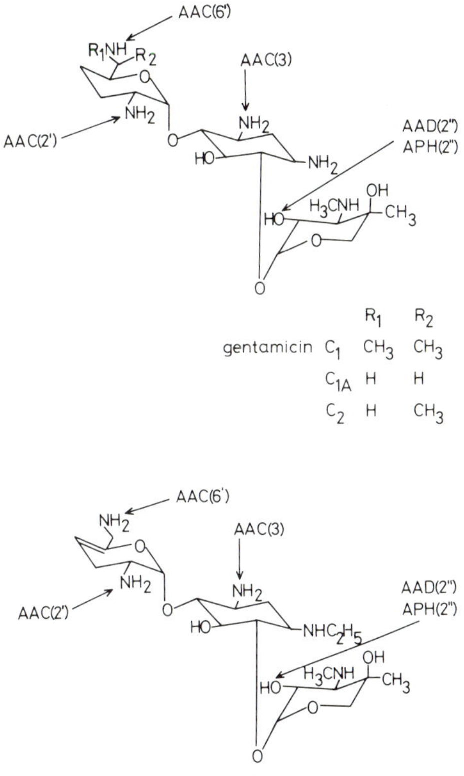

netilmicin

FIG. 4. Gentamicin and netilmicin and the sites at which they can be modified.

AAD(4′)(4″) preferentially modifies 4′-hydroxyl groups but it can also modify 4″-hydroxyl groups if the orientation of this group is equatorial, as in kanamycin, tobramycin and dibekacin, rather than polar, as in gentamicin (Santanam & Kayser 1978). APH(3′)(5″) enzymes modify most substrates at the 3′ position but some modify lividomycin, which lacks a 3′-hydroxyl group, at the 5″ position. Enzymes that phosphorylate

TABLE 1

Substrate profiles of aminoglycoside-modifying enzymes

Enzyme	Modification of									Organisms where found
	Gentamicin C	Sisomicin	Netilmicin	Tobramycin	Amikacin	Kanamycin A	Neomycin B & C	Streptomycin	Spectinomycin	
Phosphotransferases										
APH(3″)(5′)	0	0	0	0	−/+	+	+	0	0	Enterobacteria, pseudomonas, staphylococci, *Streptococcus faecalis*
APH(2″)	+	+	+	+	−	+	0	0	0	Staphylococci, *Strep. faecalis*
APH(6)	0	0	0	0	0	0	0	+	−	Pseudomonas
APH(3″)	0	0	0	0	0	0	0	+	−	Enterobacteria, pseudomonas, Gram positive organisms
Adenylyltransferases										
AAD(4′)(4″)	0	0	0	+	+	+	+	0	0	Staphylococci
AAD(2″)	+	+	±	+	−	+	0	0	0	Enterobacteria, pseudomonas
AAD(6)	0	0	0	0	0	0	0	+	−	Staphylococci
AAD(3″)(9)	0	0	0	0	0	0	0	+	+	Enterobacteria, pseudomonas
AAD(9)	0	0	0	0	0	0	0	−	+	Staphylococci
Acetyltransferases										
AAC(3)I	+	+	±	±	−	−	−	0	0	Enterobacteria, pseudomonas
AAC(3)II	+	+	?	+	−	+	−	0	0	Enterobacteria
AAC(3)III/IV	+	+	?	+	−	+	+	0	0	Pseudomonas, enterobacteria
AAC(2′)	+	+	+	+	0	0	+	0	0	*Providencia* spp.
AAC(6′)	−/+*	+	+	+	variable	+	variable	0	0	Enterobacteria, pseudomonas, staphylococci, *Strep. faecalis*

* Gentamicin C_1, 0: C_{1A} and C_2, +.

+, Modified; ±, poor modification; −, not significantly modified; 0, substituent necessary for modification absent.

lividomycin or ribostamycin at the 5″-position, with little or no activity on neomycin or kanamycin have been reported (Yamaguchi *et al.* 1972; Kida *et al.* 1974). It is not clear whether they are distinct from the APH(3′)(5″) group, but as lividomycin and ribostamycin are of little medical importance, such enzymes will not be considered further.

Three of the modifying enzymes can be subdivided. The most important differences occur with AAC(3) and are shown in Table 1. All types of the enzyme modify tobramycin if the antibiotic is present in high concentrations, but AAC(3)I has low affinity for the compound. Consequently, strains that produce AAC(3)I are susceptible to tobramycin. AAC(3)IV differs from AAC(3)III in that it acetylates apramycin (Davies & O'Connor, 1978). There are at least two conflicting suggestions for the classification of subtypes of AAC(6′). Kawabe *et al.* (1975) classify the enzymes on their ability to acetylate kanamycin, neomycin, gentamicins C_{1A} and C_2, dibekacin and amikacin. AAC(6′)I acetylates only neomycin and kanamycin. AAC(6′)II also acetylates gentamicins C_{1A} and C_2. AAC(6′)III acetylates dibekacin in addition to the substrates of AAC(6′)II. AAC(6′)IV acetylates all the compounds listed above. The broad-spectrum AAC(6′) enzyme specified by the R5 plasmid is classified as AAC(6′)IV according to this system. In contrast, in the classification proposed by Miller *et al.* (1980) it is called AAC(6′)I. In this classification AAC(6′)II enzymes have poor activity against amikacin and are associated with the gentamicin- and tobramycin-resistant, amikacin-susceptible phenotype that Haas *et al.* (1976) and Phillips *et al.* (1978) also observed. The AAC(6′) enzyme produced, in addition to APH(2″), by gentamicin-resistant staphylococci also would be called AAC(6′)II in Miller's system. APH(3′)(5″) is divided into three types on the basis of phosphorylation of butirosin and lividomycin (Table 2). APH(3′)(5″)III enzymes from *Staph. aureus* and *Streptococcus faecalis* phosphorylate amikacin, though strains that produce them show little, if any, increased resistance to the compound.

TABLE 2

Subdivisions of APH(3′)(5″)

Enzyme subtype	Modification of		
	Kanamycin and neomycin	Lividomycin	Butirosin
APH(3′)(5″)I	+	+	−
APH(3′)(5″)II	+	−	+
APH(3′)(5″)III	+	+	+

Detection of Aminoglycoside-modifying Enzymes

Enzyme preparation

The organism is grown in nutrient broth (for example Oxoid No. 2, CM67) until late logarithmic phase or early stationary phase. The cells are harvested by centrifugation in a bench centrifuge and resuspended, concentrated 10- to 20-fold, in magnesium chloride (0·5 mmol/l) and dithiotreitol (1 mmol/l), or alternatively in the buffer to be used for detection of the enzyme. It is then necessary to release the enzyme in some way. Ultrasonic disintegration of the cells is a suitable method, at least for Gram negative organisms, as small volumes (1 ml) can be treated. Other methods that can be used include disruption of the cells with a French pressure cell, lysis of the cells by lysozyme or, for *Staph. aureus*, lysostaphin and, for species for which it is effective, osmotic shock (Haas & Dowding 1975).

Assay methods

Cellulose phosphate paper binding method

The most commonly used method for the detection of aminoglycoside-modifying enzymes is the cellulose phosphate paper binding method first used by Ozanne *et al.* (1969). The method which can be used for detection of all the aminoglycoside-modifying enzymes by measurement of the transfer of [^{14}C]acetate from [^{14}C]acetyl coenzyme A, [^{14}C]AMP from [^{14}C]ATP, or [^{32}P]phosphate from [γ^{32}P]ATP to the aminoglycoside. Radiolabelled cofactors can be purchased from Amersham International, Amersham, Buckinghamshire, UK. Since the method employs radioactive materials, the advice of the Radiation Safety Officer of the institution in which the work is to be performed should be sought.

The procedure is performed in the following steps.

(1) Mix together aminoglycoside solution, radiolabelled cofactor, buffer and enzyme preparation and incubate at 37°C for 30 min.
(2) Pippette the mixture on to squares of cellulose phosphate paper.
(3) Wash the pieces of paper three times in water or buffer.
(4) Dry the squares of paper.
(5) Measure the radioactivity bound to each square of paper.

In the first step, a radiolabelled derivative of the aminoglycoside will be formed if an appropriate modifying enzyme is present. Several buffers, pH values and concentrations of aminoglycoside and cofactor have been suggested for the detection of the various modifying enzymes (see Haas & Dowding 1975; Drasar 1978). For simplicity, we prefer to use a single buffer and to prepare the cell extract in this buffer in order to achieve a higher concentration of enzyme. In our experience, acetyltransferases are much more easily detected than are adenylyltransferases or phosphotransferases. Therefore, the buffer we use is a slight modification of that suggested by Haas & Dowding (1975) for the detection of AAD(2″). It is prepared as follows: mix together 2 ml of 1 mol/l tris(hydroxymethyl)-aminomethane, 1·25 ml of 1 mol/l magnesium chloride, 6 ml of 2 mol/l ammonium chloride and 15 ml of distilled water; adjust the pH to 7·8 with 1 mol/l maleic acid and make the total volume up to 30 ml; add dithiothreitol (5 mmol/l final concentration) to as much buffer as is required just before use. For acetyltransferases we use low concentrations of both aminoglycoside and acetyl coenzyme A, whereas for adenylyltransferases higher concentrations prove more satisfactory, probably because of the lower affinity of adenylyltransferases for both aminoglycosides and ATP (Davies & Smith 1978). Therefore, the reaction mixtures we suggest are:

For acetyltranserases
- 10 μl of 20 mg/l aminoglycoside
- 10 μl of 0·2 mmol/l [1-^{14}C]acetyl coenzyme A (specific activity 5 Ci/mol)
- 20 μl of enzyme preparation in buffer.

For adenylyltransferases and phosphotransferases
- 10 μl of 200 mg/1 aminoglycoside
- 10 μl of 1 mmol/l [8-^{14}C]ATP or [γ-^{32}P]ATP (specific activity 5 Ci/mol)
- 20 μl of enzyme preparation in buffer.

For all reactions, tubes are prepared in which the aminoglycoside solution is replaced by water.

In the second step 35-μl samples of the reaction mixture are pipetted on to squares (20 × 20 mm) of Whatman P81 cellulose phosphate paper. The aminoglycosides, whether modified or not, bind to the negatively charged cellulose phosphate paper because of their positive charge. Cellulose phosphate paper is supplied in large sheets (460 × 570 mm) which can be cut into pieces of approximately 20 × 20 mm with a guillotine. For adenylylation and phosphorylation it is advisable to use paper that has been soaked in 20 mmol/l ATP in a saturated solution of sodium pyrophosphate and then allowed to dry. This reduces the non-specific binding of ATP (Drasar 1978).

In the third step, unreacted cofactor is washed off the paper while aminoglycosides remain bound. We wash the pieces of paper in tap water. Others use distilled water or, in the case of Drasar (1978), 5 mmol/l Tris–HCl buffer pH 7·4. Three washes, with gentle swirling in a large beaker, of about 1 min each are sufficient. There should be at least 10 ml of washing solution for each square of paper. If desired, the initial wash may be in water at 80°C to stop the reaction quickly, but this is not necessary unless the time course of the reaction is to be followed.

The fourth step, drying the pieces of paper, can be carried out in several ways. We blot the papers on a paper towel, then place them in an incubator at 37°C for 30–40 min. A drying oven or infrared lamp may also be used.

The final step, measurement of radioactivity, is carried out in a liquid scintillation spectrometer. We use 5–10 ml per vial of a scintillation fluid that consists of 2,5-diphenyloxazole (6 g/l) and 1,4-di[2-(5-phenyloxazolyl)]benzene (100 mg/l) in toluene/methanol (9 : 1). The radiolabelled aminoglycoside remains bound to the cellulose phosphate paper even in scintillation fluid. Consequently the paper may be removed from the scintillation vial and the latter re-used after determination of the background count.

If the radioactivity bound in the presence of an aminoglycoside is at least twice the background bound in its absence, it can be assumed that modification of the aminoglycoside has occurred. If the counts in the presence of an aminoglycoside exceed those in its absence by less than two-fold, Drasar (1978) has suggested that the dose response be tested. By her criterion, if a modifying enzyme is present the radioactivity bound should at least double when the antibiotic concentration is increased eight-fold.

TABLE 3

Compounds tested in screening isolates for the production of aminoglycoside-modifying enzymes

Reaction	Compound tested	If compound is modified, then
Acetylation	Gentamicin	Test gentamicin, gentamicin C_1, tobramycin, kanamycin, amikacin and neomycin in order to identify enzyme (see Table 1)
Adenylylation	Gentamicin	Enzyme is AAD(2″)
	Tobramycin	Enzyme is AAD(2″) or AAD(4′)(4″)
	Streptomycin	Enzyme is AAD(6) or AAD(3″) (9)
	Spectinomycin	Enzyme is AAD(3″)(9) or AAD(9)
Phosphorylation	Gentamicin	Enzyme is APH(2″)
	Neomycin	Enzyme is APH(3′)(5″)
	Streptomycin	Enzyme is APH(6) or APH(3″)

When screening strains for the production of modifying enzymes it is not necessary to test the whole range of substrates. The compounds that need to be tested in order to detect all the important enzymes are listed in Table 3. In many cases, detection of modification of a particular compound is sufficient for identification of the enzyme. However, since all the acetyltransferases modify at least some of the components of gentamicin, identification of these enzymes requires the testing of a range of compounds.

Microbiological method

This method is simpler than the cellulose phosphate paper binding method. The cell extract is mixed with aminoglycoside, buffer and cofactor. After incubation of the mixture, residual antibiotic is measured by agar diffusion. We have no experience of this method, but suggest that the same reaction mixtures as for the cellulose phosphate paper binding method be used (but with non-radioactive cofactors). This method has two drawbacks. The most important is that adenylyltransferases cannot be distinguished from phosphotransferases. Also, some modified aminoglycosides retain appreciable antibacterial activity (for example, neomycin 6′-*N*-acetate; Benveniste & Davies 1971).

Spectrophotometric methods

These methods are not as sensitive as the cellulose phosphate paper binding method and require at least partly purified enzymes (Davies & Smith 1978). Consequently they are not suitable for screening isolates for the production of modifying enzymes. However, they are useful for kinetic studies. As we have no experience of these methods, we shall do no more than briefly summarize the methods suggested by Davies & Smith (1978). For acetylation, the reduction in absorbance due to the thioester of acetyl coenzyme A can be monitored at 232 nm. For adenylylation, a pyrophosphate-dependent phosphofructokinase from *Propionibacterium shermanii* is used to form fructose 1,6-diphosphate from fructose and the pyrophosphate formed by the adenylylation reaction. The fructose 1,6-diphosphate is cleaved to glyceraldehyde 3-phosphate and dihydroxyacetone phosphate by aldolase. These two compounds are interconverted by triose phosphate isomerase. The oxidation of glyceraldehyde 3-phosphate by glyceraldehyde 3-phosphate dehydrogenase is coupled to the formation of NADH from NAD which is monitored at 340 nm. For phosphorylation, the formation of ADP is followed by coupling the oxidation of NADH (monitored at 340 nm) to an ATP-regenerating system.

Inference of Production of Aminoglycoside-modifying Enzymes from Susceptibility Patterns

Since it is easier to determine minimum inhibitory concentrations (MICs) of aminoglycosides than to prepare, detect and identify modifying enzymes, it is not surprising that there have been a number of attempts to infer the production of modifying enzymes from susceptibility patterns. Since we have discussed these methods elsewhere (Shannon & Phillips 1982) here we shall confine ourselves to a brief account of our own findings for resistance to 2-deoxystreptamine aminoglycosides (Table 4). MICs were determined by agar dilution in Oxoid Diagnostic Sensitivity Test Agar (CM261) with an inoculum of 10^3 to 10^4 c.f.u.'s. Strains that are resistant to kanamycin and neomycin may be inferred to produce APH(3′)(5″) regardless of their susceptibility to the other compounds. Enzymes that modify gentamicin are usually easily identified in enterobacteria though AAC(2′) and AAD(2″) are distinguished largely on the restriction of the former to *Providencia* spp. However, as AAC(2′) confers resistance to neomycin but not to kanamycin A, whereas the reverse is true for AAD(2″), the susceptibility pattern to these compounds may be used to distinguish between the enzymes unless the strain also produces APH(3′)(5″). MIC patterns are less useful for the identification of aminoglycoside-modifying enzymes in *Ps. aeruginosa*. The broad-spectrum 'impermeability' type of resistance to aminoglycosides, i.e. the result of diminished uptake of the compounds, may also be inferred from MIC patterns. These inferences are based on the assumption that a single strain produces only one gentamicin-modifying enzyme, though production of APH(3′)(5″) plus a gentamicin-modifying enzyme may be inferred from MIC patterns with little difficulty. Work by Kettner *et al.* (1982) and Price *et al.* (1981) suggests that two or more gentamicin-modifying enzymes may be produced by some isolates. If such isolates were to become common, inferences about modifying enzymes from MIC patterns would no longer be justified.

Detection of Aminoglycoside-modifying Enzymes in Clinical Microbiology Laboratories

In practice the study of mechanisms of resistance to aminoglycosides is divided into three stages. The first stage, which is performed routinely for clinical purposes in most clinical microbiology departments, consists of testing the susceptibility of isolates to one or two aminoglycosides by disc methods. This stage is sufficient to eliminate aminoglycoside-susceptible isolates from further study. Nowadays most clinical interest centres on gentamicin, tobramycin, netilmicin and amikacin. The testing of gentamicin alone is sufficient to detect most isolates that are resistant to the other compounds, though some producers of AAC(6′) may be missed. If an isolate is resistant to gentamicin it is worthwhile to proceed to the second stage which is to determine the MICs of gentamicin, tobramycin and amikacin for the isolate or, alternatively, to perform disc tests of

TABLE 4

*2-Deoxystreptamine aminoglycoside-modifying enzymes inferred from MIC profiles**

Organism	MIC (mg/1) of					Ratio of MICs		Inferred enzyme
	Neo-mycin	Kana-mycin	Amik-acin	Tobra-mycin	Genta-micin	Tobramycin / Gentamicin	Amikacin / Gentamicin	
Enterobacteria	⩾2	⩾32	—†	—	—	—	—	APH(3′)(5″)
Enterobacteria	—	—	1–4	0·5–4	8–32	—	—	AAC(3)I
Enterobacteria	—	—	1–4	⩾16	⩾64	0·25	—	AAC(3)II
Enterobacteria‡	—	—	1–4	⩾4	⩾4	1	—	AAD(2″)
Enterobacteria	—	—	4–64	⩾16	2–16	⩾4	—	AAC(6′)
Enterobacteria	—	—	16–64	4–16	4–16	1	⩾2	'Impermeability'
Providencia spp.	—	—	1–8	⩾2	⩾2	1	—	AAC(2′)
Pseudomonas aeruginosa	⩾2	⩾32	—	—	—	—	—	APH(3′)(5″)
Ps. aeruginosa	—	—	0·5–4	0·25–1	4–256	—	—	AAC(3)I
Ps. aeruginosa	—	—	1–4	⩾8	⩾16	—	—	AAD(2″), AAC(6′) or AAC(3)
Ps. aeruginosa	—	—	8–64	4–32	4–32	—	⩾2	'Impermeability'
Staphylococci	⩾16	⩾64	—	—	—	—	—	APH(3′)(5″)
Staphylococci	—	—	1–32	4–128	4–128	—	⩽0·5	APH(2″) + AAC(6′)
Staphylococci	—	—	16–64	4–32	4–32	—	⩾2	'Impermeability'
Streptococcus faecalis	—	⩾1024	—	—	—	—	—	APH(3′)(5″)

* Modified from Shannon & Phillips (1982).
†—: Inferences not made on the basis of MICs of these compounds.
‡ Excluding *Providencia* spp.

susceptibility to tobramycin and amikacin. This stage, also, should be within the capabilities of all laboratories. From the results it will often be possible to infer what the mechanism of resistance is likely to be and whether or not it is worthwhile to proceed to the third stage, which is to test the isolates for the production of aminoglycoside-modifying enzymes. The same stages of investigation may be carried out in investigations of resistance to other aminoglycosides.

References

BENVENISTE, R. & DAVIES, J. 1971 Enzymatic acetylation of aminoglycoside antibiotics by *Escherichia coli* carrying an R factor. *Biochemistry* **10,** 1787–1796.

BRYAN, L. E. & VAN DEN ELZEN, H. M. 1975 Gentamicin accumulation by sensitive strains of *Escherichia coli* and *Pseudomonas aeruginosa. Journal of Antibiotics, Tokyo* **28,** 696–703.

BRYAN, L. E. & VAN DEN ELZEN, H. M. 1976 Streptomycin accumulation in susceptible and resistant strains of *Escherichia coli* and *Pseudomonas aeruginosa. Antimicrobial Agents and Chemotherapy* **9,** 928–938.

BRYAN, L. E. & VAN DEN ELZEN, H. M. 1977 Effects of membrane-energy mutations and cations on streptomycin and gentamicin accumulation by bacteria: a model for the entry of streptomycin and gentamicin in susceptible and resistant bacteria. *Antimicrobial Agents and Chemotherapy* **12,** 163–177.

BRYAN, L. E., HARAPHONGSE, R. & VAN DEN ELZEN, H. M. 1976 Gentamicin resistance in clinical isolates of *Pseudomonas aeruginosa* associated with diminished gentamicin accumulation and no detectable enzymatic modification. *Journal of Antibiotics, Tokyo* **29,** 743–753.

BRYAN, L. E., NICAS, T., HOLLOWAY, B. W. & CROWTHER, C. 1980 Aminoglycoside-resistant mutation of *Pseudomonas aeruginosa* defective in cytochrome c_{552} and nitrate reductase. *Antimicrobial Agents and Chemotherapy* **17,** 71–79.

DAVIES, J. & O'CONNOR, S. 1978 Enzymatic modification of aminoglycoside antibiotics: 3-*N*-acetyltransferase with broad substrate specificity that determines resistance to the novel aminoglycoside apramycin. *Antimicrobial Agents and Chemotherapy* **14,** 69–72.

DAVIES, J. & SMITH, D. I. 1978 Plasmid-determined resistance to antimicrobial agents. *Annual Review of Microbiology* **32,** 469–518.

DICKIE, P., BRYAN, L. E. & PICKARD, M. A. 1978 Effect of enzymatic adenylylation on dihydrostreptomycin accumulation in *Escherichia coli* carrying an R-factor: model explaining aminoglycoside resistance by inactivating mechanisms. *Antimicrobial Agents and Chemotherapy* **14,** 569–580.

DRASAR, F. A. 1978 Detection of aminoglycoside degrading enzymes. In *Laboratory Methods in Antimicrobial Chemotherapy* ed. Reeves, D. S., Phillips, I., Williams, J. D. & Wise, R. pp. 70–75. Edinburgh: Churchill Livingstone.

GALE, E. F., CUNDLIFFE, E., REYNOLDS, P. E., RICHMOND, M. H. & WARING, M. J. 1972 *The Molecular Basis of Antibiotic Action* pp. 290–306. London: John Wiley & Sons.

HAAS, M. J. & DOWDING, J. E. 1975 Aminoglycoside-modifying enzymes. *Methods in Enzymology* **43,** 611–628.

HAAS, M., BIDDLECOME, S., DAVIES, J., LUCE, C. E. & DANIELS, P. J. L. 1976 Enzymatic modification of aminoglycoside antibiotics: a new 6′-*N*-acetylating enzyme from a *Pseudomonas aeruginosa* isolate. *Antimicrobial Agents and Chemotherapy* **9,** 945–950.

KAWABE, H., KONDO, S., UMEZAWA, H. & MITSUHASHI, S. 1975 R factor-mediated aminoglycoside antibiotic resistance in *Pseudomonas aeruginosa*: a new aminoglycoside 6′-*N*-acetyltransferase. *Antimicrobial Agents and Chemotherapy* **7,** 494–499.

KETTNER, M., NAVAROVA, J., RYDL, Z., KNOTHE, H., LEBEK, G. & KRCMERY, V. 1982 Occurrence of aminoglycoside-modifying enzymes in resistant strains of enterobacteria and *Pseudomonas aeruginosa* from several countries. *Journal of Antimicrobial Chemotherapy* **8,** 175–185.

KIDA, M., IGARASI, S., OKUTANI, T., ASAKO, T., HIRAGA, K. & MITSUHASHI, S. 1974 Selective phosphorylation of the 5′-hydroxyl group of ribostamycin by a new enzyme from *Pseudomonas aeruginosa*. *Antimicrobial Agents and Chemotherapy* **5,** 92–94.

LACEY, R. W. & CHOPRA, I. 1972 Evidence for mutation to streptomycin resistance in clinical strains of *Staphylococcus aureus*. *Journal of General Microbiology* **73,** 175–180.

MANESS, M. J., FOSTER, G. C. & SPARLING, P. F. 1974 Ribosomal resistance to streptomycin and spectinomycin in *Neisseria gonorrhoeae*. *Journal of Bacteriology* **120,** 1293–1299.

MILLER, G. H., SABATELLI, F. J., HARE, R. S. & WAITZ, J. A. 1980 Survey of aminoglycoside resistance patterns. *Developments in Industrial Microbiology* **21,** 91–104.

OZANNE, B., BENVENISTE, R., TIPPER, D. & DAVIES, J. 1969 Aminoglycoside antibiotics: inactivation by phosphorylation in *Escherichia coli* carrying R factors. *Journal of Bacteriology* **100,** 1144–1146.

PHILLIPS, I., KING, B. A. & SHANNON, K. P. 1978 The mechanisms of resistance to aminoglycosides in the genus *Pseudomonas*. *Journal of Antimicrobial Chemotherapy* **4,** 121–129.

PRICE, K. E., GODFREY, J. C. & KAWAGUCHI, H. 1974 Effect of structural modifications on the biological properties of aminoglycoside antibiotics containing 2-deoxystreptamine. *Advances in Applied Microbiology* **18,** 191–307.

PRICE, K. E., GODFREY, J. C. & KAWAGUCHI, H. 1977 Effect of structural modifications on the biological properties of aminoglycoside antibiotics containing 2-deoxystreptamine. (Supplement) In *Structure–Activity Relationships among the Semisynthetic Antibiotics*, ed. Perlman, D. Ch. 6, pp. 357–395, New York & London: Academic Press.

PRICE, K. E., KRESEL, P. A., FARCHIONE, L. A., SISKIN, S. B. & KARPOW, S. A. 1981 Epidemiological studies of aminoglycoside resistance in the U.S.A. *Journal of Antimicrobial Chemotherapy* **8** (Supplement A), 89–105.

REYNOLDS, A. V. & SMITH, J. T. 1979 Enzymes which modify aminoglycoside antibiotics. In *Recent Advances in Infection*, *Volume 1*, ed. Reeves, D. S. & Geddes, A. pp. 165–181. Edinburgh: Churchill Livingstone.

SANTANAM, P. & KAYSER, F. H. 1978 Purification and characterization of an aminoglycoside inactivating enzyme from *Staphylococcus epidermidis* FK109 that nucleotidylates the 4′- and 4″-hydroxyl groups of the aminoglycoside antibiotics. *Journal of Antibiotics* (*Tokyo*) **31,** 343–351.

Shannon, K. P. & Phillips, I. 1982 Mechanisms of resistance to aminoglycosides in clinical isolates. *Journal of Antimicrobial Chemotherapy* **9,** 91–102.

Shannon, K. P., Phillips, I. & King, B. A. 1978 Aminoglycoside resistance among Enterobacteriaceae and *Acinetobacter* species. *Journal of Antimicrobial Chemotherapy* **4,** 131–142.

Tseng, J. L., Bryan, L. E. & van den Elzen, H. M. 1972 Mechanisms and spectrum of streptomycin resistance in a natural population of *Pseudomonas aeruginosa*. *Antimicrobial Agents and Chemotherapy* **2,** 136–141.

Yamada, T., Tipper, D. J. & Davies, J. 1968 Enzymatic inactivation of streptomycin by R-factor resistant *Escherichia coli*. *Nature, London* **219,** 288–291.

Yamaguchi, M., Koshi, T., Kobayashi, F. & Mitsuhashi, S. 1972 Phosphorylation of lividomycin by *Escherichia coli* carrying an R factor. *Antimicrobial Agents and Chemotherapy* **2,** 142–146.

Zimmermann, R. A., Moellering, R. C. & Weinberg, A. N. 1971 Mechanism of resistance to antibiotic synergism in enterococci. *Journal of Bacteriology* **105,** 873–879.

Enzymatic Assay of Aminoglycoside Antibiotics

L. O. White and D. S. Reeves

Department of Microbiology, Southmead Hospital, Bristol, UK

The aminoglycoside antibiotics or, more correctly, since some contain no aminosugar, the aminoglycoside–aminocyclitols (AGAC), comprise a large group many of which are of clinical and veterinary importance. Some are shown in Table 1. Those of greatest clinical importance are the 4,6-disubstituted deoxystreptamines (Fig. 1) because many, e.g. amikacin, gentamicin, tobramycin and the newer derivatives sisomicin and netilmicin, are clinically active against a wide range of Gram positive and Gram negative bacterial species. AGAC antibiotics act on the bacterial ribosome and interfere with normal protein synthesis (Davies 1980; Franklin & Snow 1981).

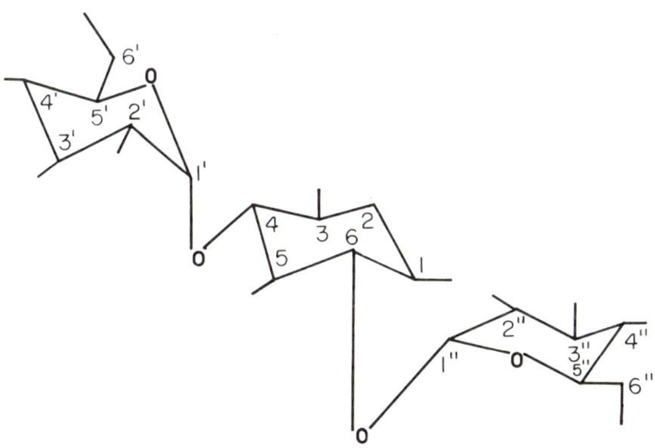

Fig. 1. Skeletal structure of a 4,6-disubstituted deoxystreptamine illustrating the numbering of the carbon atoms.

ANTIBIOTICS
ISBN 0 12 604480 5

TABLE 1

Some aminoglycoside–aminocyclitol antibiotics and enzymes suitable for assaying them

Drug name	3	6	9	2′	3′	4′	6′	2″	3″	AAC	AAD
Amikacin*	NH_2	—	—	OH	OH	OH	NH_2	OH	NH_2	(6′)	(4′)
Apramycin	NH_2	OH	—	NH_2	H	H	OH	—	—	(3)†	—
Butirosin B	NH_2	OH	—	NH_2	OH	OH	NH_2	OH	OH	(2′)(6′)	(4′)
Gentamicin C1*	NH_2	—	—	NH_2	H	H	CH_3NH	OH	CN_3NH	(2′)(3)	(2″)
Gentamicin C1a*	NH_2	—	—	NH_2	H	H	NH_2	OH	CH_3NH	(2′)(6′)(3)	(2″)
Gentamacin C2, C2a*	NH_2	—	—	NH_2	H	H	NH_2	OH	CH_3NH	(2′)(6′)(3)	(2″)
Kanamycin A*	NH_2	—	—	OH	OH	OH	NH_2	OH	NH_2	(6′)(3)	(4′)(2″)
Kanamycin B*	NH_2	—	—	NH_2	OH	OH	NH_2	OH	NH_2	(2′)(6′)(3)	(4′)(2″)
Lividomycin	NH_2	OH	—	NH_2	H	OH	OH	OH	—	(2′)(3)	(4′)
Neomycin B	NH_2	OH	—	NH_2	OH	OH	NH_2	OH	—	(2′)(6′)(3)	(4′)
Paromomycin	NH_2	OH	—	NH_2	OH	OH	OH	OH	—	(2′)(3)	(4′)
Ribostamycin	NH_2	OH	—	NH_2	OH	OH	NH_2	OH	OH	(2′)(6′)(3)	(4′)
Spectinomycin	—	—	OH	—	—	—	—	—	OH	—	(3″)(9)‡
Streptomycin	—	OH	—	—	OH	CH_3	—	$NHCH_3$	OH	—	(3″)‡
Tobramycin*	NH_2	—	—	NH_2	H	OH	NH_2	OH	NH_2	(2′)(6′)(3)	(4′)(2″)

* 4,6-Disubstituted deoxystreptamines. † Davies & O'Connor (1978). ‡ Cannon *et al.* (1978).

Sensitive bacterial species may become resistant to the action of AGACs by either (1) mutational changes to the ribosome, (2) loss of permeability to the drug or (3) the synthesis of specific enzymes which inactivate the antibiotics. The third mechanism is a common cause of resistance in clinical practice and some of the enzymes responsible have been exploited by man for the assay of those AGAC antibiotics which they inactivate.

Aminoglycoside–Aminocyclitol-modifying Enzymes

AGAC-modifying enzymes have been found in both Gram positive and Gram negative species, coded for, in many instances, by part of the DNA of a transmissible plasmid conferring resistance to several antibiotics. Three classes of enzyme have been described:

Aminoglycoside acetyltransferases (*AAC*). These enzymes transfer an acetyl group from acetyl-coenzyme A to susceptible amino groups in the AGAC.

Aminoglycoside adenylyltransferases (*AAD*). Also referred to as nucleotidyltransferase (ANT), these enzymes transfer an adenyl monophosphate (AMP) moiety from adenosine triphoshate (ATP) to susceptible hydroxyl groups.

Aminoglycoside phosphotransferases (*APH*). These phosphorylate susceptible hydroxyl groups, the source of phosphate being ATP.

The current nomenclature for these enzymes is the three-letter prefix of AAC, AAD, ANT or APH followed by (in brackets) the number of the carbon atom which bears the susceptible group. In the case of the disubstituted deoxystreptamines the carbon atoms in the deoxystreptamine ring are numbered 1 to 6, those in the sugar linked at the 4 position 1′ to 6′ and those in the residue linked at the 5 or 6 position 1″ to 6″ (see Fig. 1). If more than one distinct enzyme acting at the same site has been described then these are numbered sequentially, e.g. AAC(3)-1, AAC(3)-2.

Substrate specificity

Substrates suitable for modification must have an amino or hydroxyl group at a susceptible site (Table 1). Gentamicin, for example, is a mixture of four components three of which (C1a, C2a, C2) have an amino group at the 6′ position and are susceptible to AAC (6′). The 6′ amino group of the fourth component (C1) is methylated and is not susceptible to acetylation. The presence of a susceptible group does not, however, necessarily indicate that an AGAC will be susceptible to a particular enzyme. For example, amikacin has an amino group in the 3 position but is not acetylated by AAC(3). Some types of AAC(3) will acetylate tobramycin and some will not. One type of AAC(3) acetylates apramycin (Davies & O'Connor 1978).

Some substrates are susceptible to a large number of enzymes (e.g. kanamycin B), whereas others are susceptible to very few (e.g. amikacin).

Use of enzymes for assay of AGAC antibiotics

The AGACs used clinically have a narrow margin between toxic and effective blood concentrations and serum concentrations in patients must be monitored (Reeves & White 1981). This clinical need for rapid specific assays was probably the major reason for the tranferase enzymes being exploited for assays. The assays to be detailed in this chapter were designed to measure AGACs in serum but could with suitable modification be used for other applications (e.g. see pp. 339–348, this volume). All the assays have a common theme. A specific enzyme and a radiolabelled cofactor are used to modify the drug with a radioactive group. The radiolabelled AGAC is separated from the reaction mixture by exploiting its basicity and binding it strongly to phosphocellulose paper. The reactions are stoichiometric and hence the radioactive counts bound to the paper are directly proportional to the amount of AGAC present. A modification of the acetyltransferase assay eliminates the need for a separation step and radioactive cofactor by using a sulphydryl reagent, 5,5′-dithiobis-(2)-nitrobenzic acid (BTNB), which reacts with reduced coenzyme A as it is produced to yield a coloured product which is measured spectrophotometrically.

Several AAC and AAD enzymes have been exploited for assay purposes but theoretically any of the modifying enzymes could be. The phosphotransferases have probably received little attention because of the need to use (^{32}P)ATP. The assay methodology can be modified for the identification of enzymes on the basis of substrate specificity rather than the measurement of AGAC concentration (see pp. 183–198, this volume).

Acetyltransferase Assay using AAC(6′) (syn. Kanamycin Acetyltransferase, KAT)

(Broughall & Reeves 1975)

Materials

Substrates and cofactor

Kanamycins A and B, tobramycin, amikacin, sisomicin, netilmicin, verdamycin, neomycin, ribostamycin, butirosin, gentamicin C1a and C2. NOTE. This assay has been extensively used to measure gentamicin in serum although it does not detect the C1 component; the results obtained have correlated well with other methods (Broughall & Reeves 1975;

White *et al.* 1980, 1981). Recent work, however, using high pressure liquid chromatography (White & Reeves 1981) shows that brands of gentamicin obtained world-wide vary considerably in their C1 content (24·5–45·2%). Therefore we suggest that this enzyme is not used for gentamicin assay unless both standards and tests are known to have similar compositions.

(1-^{14}C)Acetyl coenzyme A (Amersham, specific activity approx 60 mCi/mmol), 50 μCi (*ca.* 0·75 mg) is mixed with unlabelled acetyl coenzyme A (Sigma, 1·0 mg) in distilled water (12 ml). Dispense in 250 μl aliquots, freeze dry and store at −20°C.

Source and preparation of enzyme

Escherichia coli W677/R5 (NCTC 11186), maintained on nutrient agar containing tobramycin (10 mg/l) or freeze-dried, is inoculated from overnight culture into 2·5 l nutrient broth (Oxoid CM1) and incubated with shaking overnight at 30°C. Harvest cells by centrifugation (4°C), wash twice in Tris–HCl buffer, resuspend in buffer (50 ml) and disrupt over ice by ultrasonication (osmotic shock may be used instead: see below). Centrifuge (22,000 **g**, 30 min, 4°C). Decant the supernatant aliquot and store at −20°C, at which temperature it is stable for several months.
Buffer. Tris–HCl (20 mmol/l) containing magnesium chloride (0·5 mmol/l), pH 7·5.
Assay buffer. Trisodium citrate buffer (120 mmol/l) containing magnesium chloride (12 mmol/l) and dithiothreitol (4 mmol/l), pH 5·7, aliquot and store at −20°C.

Procedure

The assay may be performed in plastic tubes or microtitre plates.

(1) Dispense 25 μl of test or standard solutions.
(2) Reconstitute the acetyl coenzyme A in 250 μl of assay buffer.
(3) Mix acetyl coenzyme A solution with enzyme (ratio 3:5) to give sufficient for 40 μl per tube. Then add 40 μl to each tube and mix gently.
(4) Cover and incubate at 37°C for 30 min.
(5) Pipette 55 μl from each tube onto pre-cut rectangles of phosphocellulose paper (Whatman P81) measuring 25 × 20 mm. NOTE. For convenience the squares may be joined along a 'backbone' (Broughall & Reeves 1975).
(6) Wash the squares in two changes of distilled water (1 litre) containing 50 ml of phosphate buffered saline (Oxoid, Dulbecco A), pH 7·5.
(7) Dry papers (60–100°C) until crisp.
(8) Place individual rectangles into 10 ml of scintillant (e.g. butyl PBD (Koch-Light) 5·6 g/l in toluene) and count for 1 min.

(9) Plot counts per min (counts/min) against standard concentration on linear graph paper. A straight line should be obtained up to 16 mg/l.

Acetyltransferase Assay using AAC(2′)
(Shannon & Phillips 1977)

Materials

Substrates and cofactor

Kanamycin B, C, gentamicin, tobramycin (possibly also netilmicin, sisomicin, neomycin, ribostamycin, butirosin, lividomycin, paromomycin).

(1-^{14}C) Acetyl coenzyme A (Amersham) 0·2 mmol/l (sp. act. 3·5–4·6 Ci/mol). May be prepared as described for AAC(6′) above.

Source and preparation of enzyme

Providencia stuartii D1017 maintained on nutrient agar containing gentamicin (20 mg/l) or freeze-dried. Inoculate 100 ml of Nutrient Broth No. 2 (Oxoid) and incubate at 37°C overnight. Harvest cells by centrifugation, wash with Tris–HCl buffer, resuspend in dithiothreitol solution (5 ml) and disrupt cells by ultrasonication. Aliquot and store at −20°C.

Buffer. Tris–HCl (10 mmol/l), NaCl (30 mmol/l), pH 7·8.

Assay buffer. Tris–HCl (200 mmol/l), magnesium chloride (32 mmol/l), pH 7·8.

Dithiothreitol solution. Dithiothreitol (10 mmol/l), magnesium chloride (0·5 mmol/l).

Procedure

(1) Dispense into plastic tubes or microtitre plates 36 μl of standard or sample, acetyl coenzyme A (14 μl), assay buffer (30 μl) and enzyme (30 μl).
(2) Incubate at 37°C, 20–30 min.
(3) Proceed as described for AAC(6′). The scintillant suggested by the original authors is 2,6-diphenyloxazole (6 g) and 1,4 di(2-(5-phenyloxazolyl)) benzene (100 mg) per litre of toluene.

Adenylyltransferase Assay using AAD(4′) (syn. Tobramycin Adenylyltransferase) and AAD(2′) (syn. Gentamicin Adenylyltransferase) (Santanam & Kayser 1976)

Materials

Substrates and cofactor

AAD(4′): kanamycin, butirosin, amikacin, ribostamycin, neomycin, tobramycin, paromomycin.

AAD(2″): gentamicin, sisomicin, tobramycin.

(8-^{14}C) adenosine triphosphate (Amersham, sp. act. 60 μCi/μmol) at the concentration specified under 'Procedure'.

Source and preparation of enzymes

Staphylococcus epidermidis 109 is the source of AAD(4′). *Escherichia coli* W677/HJR66 is the source of AAD(2″). The organisms are grown overnight in broth containing either 10 mg/l neomycin (for AAD(4′)) or gentamicin (for AAD (2″)) and then inoculated into fresh medium (100 ml) and incubated (37°C) until the late log phase is reached. The cells are centrifuged and the pellet is osmotically shocked.

Osmotic shock

This method may also be used to liberate acetylating enzymes. Suspend the cells in 10 ml of Tris–HCl buffer (33 mmol/l pH 7·8) containing EDTA (6 mmol/l) and sucrose (20% w/v). Stand for 30 min at room temperature then stir (5 min) and centrifuge (12,000 **g**, 15 min, 4°C). Discard the supernatant fluid and swab the pellet to remove all the sucrose solution. Resuspend the cells rapidly in 5 ml of ice-cold magnesium chloride solution (0·5 mmol/l). After violent agitation and mixing for 5–10 min, centrifuge (as before), decant the supernatant, add 150 μl of dithiothreitol (40 mmol/l), aliquot and store at −20 or −40°C. (See also pp. 93–110, this volume.)

Assay buffer. Tris–HCl adjusted to pH 8·3 for all AAD(4′) and AAD(2″) assays of neomycin and paromomycin; pH 7·5 for all other AGACs.

Procedure for AAD(4′)

(1) If the drug is present in a body fluid the sample should be heated to 60°C for 5 min to destroy endogenous adenosine triphosphatase (ATPase).

(2) Place into each tube
   - i. 25 μl of Tris–HCl buffer (60 mmol/l) containing magnesium chloride (40 mmol/l), dithiothreitol (2·2 mmol/l) and (^{14}C)ATP (0·8 mmol/l),
   - ii. 10 μl of standard or sample solution,
   - iii. 25 μl of enzyme.

(3) Incubate at 37°C for 35 min.

(4) Proceed as described for AAC(6′).

Procedure for AAD(2″)

The procedure is identical to that described for AAD (4′) except that 20 μl of standard or test solution is used, and only 15 min incubation is required.

Spectrophotometric Assay using AAC(6′) or AAC(3)

(Williams *et al.* 1975; Scarbrough *et al.* 1979)

Materials

Substrates

As described for AAC(6′) plus gentamicin when AAC(3) is used.

Source and preparation of enzymes

Escherichia coli JR88 C600 (AAC(3)-1) and *E. coli* CH-15 (AAC(6′)). These enzymes must be partially purified before they can be used in this assay. Details of the purification are beyond the scope of this chapter and the reader should consult the original articles (Williams & Northrop 1976; Scarbrough *et al.* 1979). The purified enzymes are available commercially (Sigma).

Procedure

The assay is performed in cuvettes of 1 cm light path.

(1) To each cuvette add
  i. 0·5 ml Tris–HCl buffer (25 mmol/l) pH 7·8 containing EDTA (0·5 mmol/l) and ammonium sulphate (25 mmol/l),
  ii. 0·5 ml of enzyme solution (0·05 international units),
  iii. 1·0 ml of sample or standard solution,
  iv. 0·25 ml of acetyl coenzyme A (0·7 mmol/l),
  v. 0·25 ml 5,5′-dithiobis-(2)-nitrobenzoic acid (DTNB; 2·5 mmol/l).

(2) Similarly set up a control tube containing drug-free sample matrix.

(3) Time the addition of the last two reagents and allow the reaction to proceed for a fixed time, e.g. 15 min.

(4) Read the optical density at 412 nm.

(5) Construct a standard curve by plotting drug concentration against optical density.

Alternatively, the reaction can be read kinetically in a reaction-rate analyser. NOTE. The reaction proceeds more slowly in serum than in buffer and DTNB appears to react with serum components. Consequently a drug-free control must be run.

Comments and Problems

All the methods detailed have been designed for the assay of aminoglycosides in serum up to approximately 16 mg/l. If it is required to measure higher concentrations then sample size should be reduced and/or the reagent concentrations should be increased such that a linear standard curve is obtained over the complete range of concentrations to be measured. Non-linearity of standard curves may be due to either depletion of cofactor or an insufficiently long incubation time and this can be determined experimentally. Also, a factor in some normal sera which inhibits the acetyltransferase reaction has been noted (Minshew *et al.* 1975).

If patients' serum contains cationic radionucleotides (e.g. ^{67}gallium) falsely elevated results will be obtained. To monitor for this a sample of serum can be spotted directly onto P81 paper, washed and counted. If ^{67}gallium is present it can be removed by solvent extraction (Bhallacharya *et al.* 1978). Chloramphenicol will interfere with the acetyltransferase assay if the organism used to prepare the enzyme also produces chloramphenicol acetyltransferase, as does *E. coli* W677/R5. This can be avoided by using an alternative organism as a source of enzyme (Phillips & Shannon 1977). Lipaemic sera or some other sample body fluids may cause problems by producing non-specific binding to P81 paper. This should be checked for. In the case of adenylyltransferases it is recommended that the P81 paper squares are pre-soaked in adenine (20 mmol/l) to prevent the non-specific binding of ATP and its metabolites (Edberg & Sabath 1980). Non-specific binding of [^{14}C] acetyl coenzyme A can be reduced by pre-soaking in sodium acetate (0·4 mmol/l) (Santanam & Kayser 1979).

Calculation of Results

For transferase assays the standard curve (drug concentration plotted against counts/min, on an arithmetic scale) should be linear and requires no mathematical manipulation. Many laboratories now have access to microcomputers (e.g. PET, APPLE). Figure 2 is a program routine (in a form of BASIC) which takes data for any number of standards, computes the best straight line and then uses this to back-compute a value for the standards from their counts/min. This technique allows a rapid appraisal of a standard curve without the need for manual plotting by comparing the back-computed values of the standards with their actual values.

A typical output from this program is shown in Table 2.

```
1      STANDARD
10     X=Y=D=E=0
20     T=5               !T is the number of standards
30     FOR N=1 TO T
40     DISP "Enter Concentration of STD ";N;
50     INPUT C(N)        !C(N) = concentration of standard N
60     X=X+C(N)
70     NEXT N
80     FOR N=1 TO T
90     DISP "Enter the Counts/min of STD";N;
100    INPUT V(N)       !V(N) = counts/min of standard N
110    Y=Y+V(N)
120    NEXT N
130    X1=X/T
140    Y1=Y/T
150    FOR N=1 TO T
160    D=D+(C(N)-X1)*V(N)
170    E=E+(C(N)-X1)^2
180    NEXT N
190    B=D/F
200    F=Y1-B*X1
210    PRINT "No.                    STD Conc              Counts/min            Back-c
omputed conc."
220    FIXFD 2
230    FOR N=1 TO T
240    Z(N)=(V(N)-F)/B  !Z(N) = back-computed result for standard N
250    PRINT N,C(N),V(N),Z(N)!Prints STD No,Conc,Counts,Calculated Conc
260    NEXT N
261    STANDARD
270    DISP "Enter the number of Tests";
280    INPUT S
290    FOR N=1 TO S
300    DISP "Enter the counts/min of test ";N;
310    INPUT A
311    FIXED 2
320    PRINT "The Result of test ";N;" is ";(A-F)/B
321    STANDARD
330    NEXT N
340    END
```

FIG. 2. Program routine in a form of BASIC for computing transferase curves.

TABLE 2

Computer program output

No.	STD Conc	Counts/min	Back-computed conc.
1.00	1.00	1257.00	.65
2.00	2.00	2876.00	2.32
3.00	4.00	4278.00	3.78
4.00	8.00	8765.00	8.43
5.00	16.00	15900.00	15.82

References

BHALLACHARYA, I., SELIGSOHN, R. & LERNER, S. A. 1978 Effects of radio pharmaceuticals on radioenzymatic assays of aminoglycoside antibiotics: interference by Gallium-67 and its elimination. *Antimicrobial Agents and Chemotherapy* **14,** 448–453.

BROUGHALL, J. M. & REEVES, D. S. 1975 The acetyl transferase method for the assay of serum gentamicin concentration and a comparison with other methods. *Journal of Clinical Pathology* **28,** 140–145.

CANNON, J. G., MORAN, C. P. & BOTT, K. F. 1978 Improved radioenzyme assay for spectinomycin. *Antimicrobial Agents and Chemotherapy* **14,** 168–171.

DAVIES, J. 1980 In *Antibiotics in Laboratory Medicine* ed. Lorian, V. pp. 474–490. Baltimore: Williams & Wilkins.

DAVIES, J. & O'CONNOR, S. 1978 Enzymatic modification of aminoglycoside antibiotics: 3-*N*-Acetyltransferase with broad specificity that determines resistance to the novel aminoglycoside apramycin. *Antimicrobial Agents and Chemotherapy* **14,** 69–72.

EDBERG, S. C. & SABATH, L. D. 1980 In *Antibiotics in Laboratory Medicine* ed. Lorian, V. pp. 206–264. Baltimore: Williams & Wilkins.

FRANKLIN, T. J. & SNOW, G. A. 1981 *Biochemistry of Antimicrobial Action,* 3rd edn. London: Chapman & Hall.

MINSHEW, B. H., HOLMES, R. K. & BAXTER, C. R. 1975 Comparison of radioimmunoassay with an enzymatic assay for gentamicin. *Antimicrobial Agents and Chemotherapy* **7,** 107–109.

PHILLIPS, I. & SHANNON, K. P. 1977 Gentamicin assay in the presence of chloramphenicol. *Journal of Antimicrobial Chemotherapy* **3,** 624–625.

REEVES, D. S. & WHITE, L. O. 1981 In *Therapeutic Drug Monitoring* ed. Richiens, A. & Marks, V. pp. 445–456. Edinburgh: Churchill Livingstone.

SANTANAM, P. & KAYSER, F. H. 1976 Enzymatic adenylylation by aminoglycoside 4′-adenylyltransferase and 2″-adenylyltransferase as a means of determining concentrations of aminoglycoside antibiotics in serum. *Antimicrobial Agents and Chemotherapy* **10,** 664–667.

SANTANAM, P. & KAYSER, F. H. 1979 An improved radioenzymatic assay of aminoglycoside antibiotics in human serum by aminoglycoside 6′-*N*-acetyltransferase [AAC(6′)]. *Journal of Antimicrobial Chemotherapy* **5,** 477–479.

SCARBROUGH, E., WILLIAMS, J. W. & NORTHROP, D. B. 1979 Spectrophotometric assay for amikacin using purified kanamycin acetyl transferase. *Antimicrobial Agents and Chemotherapy* **16,** 221–224.

SHANNON, K. P. & PHILLIPS, I. 1977 The use of aminoglycoside 2′-*N*-acetyl transferase for the assay of gentamicin in serum, plasma and urine. *Journal of Antimicrobial Chemotherapy* **3,** 25–33.

WHITE, L. O. & REEVES, D. S. 1981 HPLC analysis of the C component ratios in some brands of gentamicin used clinically. *Proceedings of the 12th International Congress of Chemotherapy, Florence* p. 146.

WHITE, L. O., SCAMMELL, L. M. & REEVES, D. S. 1980 Evaluation of a gentamicin fluoroimmunoassay kit: correlation with radioimmunoassay acetyl transferase and microbiological assay. *Journal of Antimicrobial Chemotherapy* **6,** 267–273.

White, L. O., Scammell, L. M. & Reeves, D. S. 1981 Serum aminoglycoside assay by enzyme-mediated immunoassay (EMIT): correlation with radioimmunoassay, fluoroimmunoassay, and acetyl transferase and microbiological assays. *Antimicrobial Agents and Chemotherapy* **19,** 1064–1066.

Williams, J. W., Langer, J. S. & Northrop, D. B. 1975 A spectrophotometric assay for gentamicin. *Journal of Antibiotics* **28,** 982–987.

Williams, J. W. & Northrop, D. B. 1976 Purification and properties of gentamicin acetyl transferase 1. *Biochemistry* **15,** 125–131.

Aminoglycoside Antibiotic Assay by Fluoroimmunoassay Methods

ELIZABETH J. SHAW

Department of Medical Microbiology, St. Bartholomew's Hospital, London, UK

A. MUNRO AND D. S. SMITH

Department of Chemical Pathology, St. Bartholomew's Hospital, London, UK

Therapeutic monitoring of aminoglycoside therapy is frequently performed because toxic side effects occur at antibiotic levels only slightly higher than those required for therapeutic success. A reliable assay which is specific (measuring the antibiotic but not inactive metabolites or any other drug being given concurrently) is required. Furthermore, it is extremely advantageous if the result can be obtained in time to determine the next dose. The classical microbiological assay requires long incubation and has limited specificity. Work has therefore been directed at developing rapid, specific assays.

Immunoassays for Aminoglycosides

Immunoassays are based on the competitive binding of labelled and unlabelled analyte for a fixed, limited amount of antibody, and many such methods have been developed for aminoglycosides (Munro *et al.* 1982*a*). To produce antisera, the antibiotics must be rendered immunogenic by covalent linkage to protein carriers such as bovine serum albumin or thyroglobulin (Lewis *et al.* 1972; Watson *et al.* 1976*b*). Many types of label have been used. In the earliest assays, the beta-emitting radioisotope tritium was incorporated (Lewis *et al.* 1972; Watson *et al.* 1976*b*). Later, the antibiotics were labelled indirectly with the gamma-emitter ^{125}iodine (Broughton & Strong 1976; Watson *et al.* 1979) and such radioimmunoassays (RIA) were produced in kit form by a number of companies and

ANTIBIOTICS
ISBN 0 12 604480 5

were used widely, especially in North America. However, RIA has a number of disadvantages. Preparation of ^{125}iodine-labelled materials (in contrast to their routine use) is not without health hazard; the labelled antibiotic has a relatively short shelf-life (owing chiefly to radioactive decay) and it is invariably necessary to separate antibody-bound and free fractions. Hence there has been much investigation of alternative, non-isotopic labels. Three different types of label have been used: fluorescent molecules (such as fluorescein), enzymes and particles (Munro *et al.* 1982*a*). This report will describe the use of fluorescent labels in the fluoroimmunoassay (FIA) of aminoglycosides.

The aminoglycosides are easily labelled by reaction with fluorescein isothiocyanate (FITC), and the products purified on a Sephadex G-15 column to give a safe tracer with a stability of several years (Watson *et al.* 1976*a*). Binding of fluorescein-labelled aminoglycoside (FTC-aminoglycoside) to specific antibody can be demonstrated by several different techniques and it is these that have led to the development of FIA suitable for use in the clinical laboratory. Some FIA require no separation of antibody-bound and free tracer, while in others a separation step is necessary.

Non-separation Fluoroimmunoassays

Polarization fluoroimmunoassay

When a fluorescent molecule is excited with polarized light, the degree of polarization of the emitted light is related to the molecular size. FTC-gentamicin, when bound to specific antibody, emits light with a considerable degree of residual polarization whereas the small FTC-gentamicin emits light with a low degree of polarization. This is illustrated diagrammatically in Fig. 1. The overall polarization signal observed from an unseparated immunoassay mixture serves to indicate the extent of antibody binding of the FTC-gentamicin. The polarization fluoroimmunoassay (PIA) method (Watson *et al.* 1976*a*) requires only the mixing of FTC-gentamicin with a suitably diluted serum sample (for example 50 μl of a 40-fold dilution) or assay standard, addition of antiserum, incubation for a few minutes and measurement of polarization. Until recently, suitable fluorimeters were expensive, complex and not readily available, but Abbott (Diagnostics Division, North Chicago, Illinois, USA) have introduced a simple instrument designed for routine PIA use (Popelka *et al.* 1981) and described its application in the assay of aminoglycosides (Jolley *et al.* 1981).

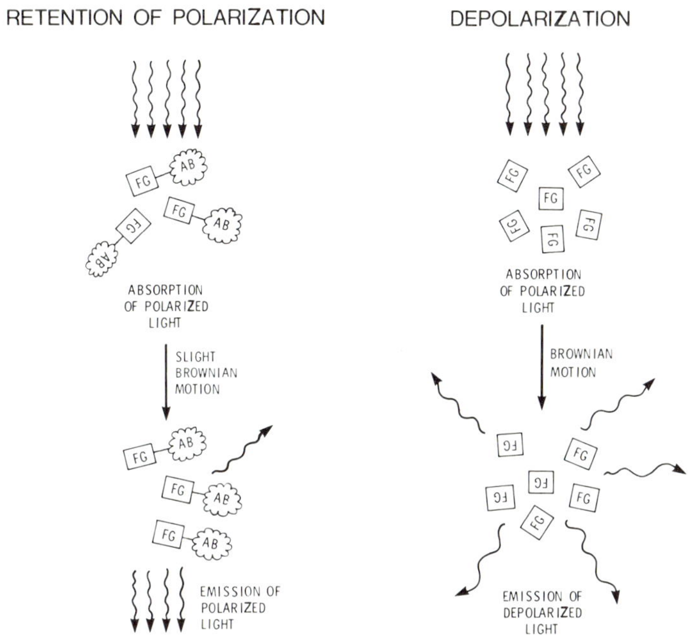

FIG. 1. Diagram showing the principle of polarization fluoroimmunoassay (PIA). Polarized exciting light is depolarized by FTC-gentamicin to a greater extent than by FTC-gentamicin–antibody complex. FG: fluoresceinthiocarbamyl gentamicin; AB: gentamicin antibody.

Quenching fluoroimmunoassay

When FTC-gentamicin is bound by some anti-gentamicin sera, a partial quenching is observed (see Fig. 2). Antibody binding of FTC-gentamicin may therefore be assessed by conventional fluorimetry of unseparated immunoassay mixtures. This gives a very simple non-separation technique (Shaw *et al.* 1977; Munro *et al.* 1982*b*). 20 μl of sample or standard is dispensed together with 2 ml of FTC-gentamicin (using a sampler-diluter) into a disposable polystyrene fluorimeter cuvette and the fluorescence of the mixture measured (blank reading). Anti-gentamicin serum (50 μl) is then added, the mixture incubated for 15 min or longer, and fluorescence measured again (test reading). The 'quenching' value for each sample is obtained by subtraction of the test from the blank reading. This quenching fluoroimmunoassay (QIA) involves only two pipetting steps and the entire procedure can be performed in the cuvette used for measurement of fluorescence. The technique has been automated using standard Technicon AutoAnalyzer equipment (Shaw *et al.* 1979).

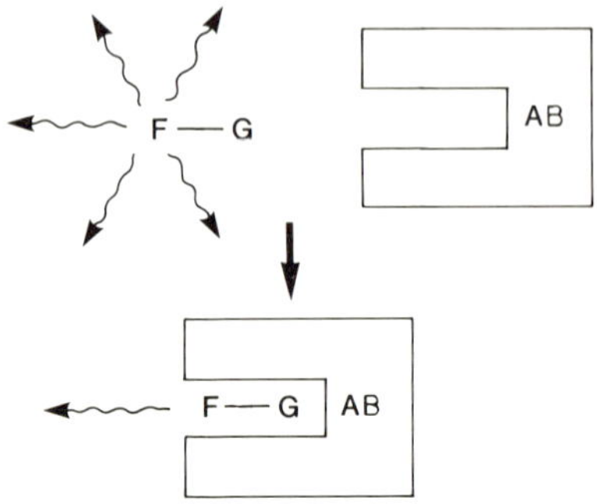

FIG. 2. Diagram showing the principle of quenching fluoroimmunoassay (QIA). Fluorescence of FTC-gentamicin is reduced when it is bound to gentamicin antibody. F-G: fluoresceinthiocarbamyl gentamicin; AB: gentamicin antibody.

Substrate-labelled fluoroimmunoassay

In this technique, developed by Burd and his colleagues (1977) and in commercial production by Ames (Elkhart, Indiana, USA), the drug is labelled with umbelliferyl-β-galactoside to give a non-fluorescent conjugate. The free labelled drug may be split by a bacterial β-galactosidase with liberation of a fluorescent product, but when bound by antibody the action of the enzyme is inhibited. Good correlations are obtained with RIA results for assay of gentamicin (Burd *et al.* 1977), tobramycin (Burd *et al.* 1978) and amikacin (Thompson & Burd 1980).

Separation Fluoroimmunoassays

The assays described above can all be performed in a single reaction tube with no separation procedure, which makes for technical simplicity. However, all substances present in the serum sample are also present when fluorescence is measured. Thus, if any of these substances are fluorescent, they can contribute to the measured signal. Other substances may reduce the fluorescence by quenching. In practice these effects have been shown to be of clinical significance in samples from severely jaundiced patients when assayed by PIA (Jolley *et al.* 1981) or QIA (Munro *et al.* 1982*b*). However, as aminoglycosides are used most frequently in patients who are seriously ill, many variable and unknown abnormalities might be present and lead to interference. In the classical RIA it is necessary to separate the antibody-bound and antibody-free fractions of the tracer and the separation procedure may be used to ensure that interfering factors are also discarded. There are many methods of separation but almost all involve centrifugation which is tedious and time-consuming and does not lend itself to automation.

Second-antibody separation

Antibody-bound tracer may be precipitated by the addition of a second antiserum directed against the immunoglobulins of the specific anti-aminoglycoside serum. The resulting immuno-precipitate may be separated by centrifugation. Methods for the assay of gentamicin (O'Donnell *et al.* 1980) and tobramycin (Karnes *et al.* 1981) have been described. However, they involve multiple reagent-addition, incubation and transfer steps and are relatively impractical as compared with other techniques described here.

Dipstick technique

Antibodies may be immobilized on a disc that is attached to the end of a dipstick. This allows easy separation by manual removal of the dipstick from the assay tube containing the incubation mixture. By insertion of the dipstick into a purpose-designed fluorimeter with front-face geometry, the bound tracer on the disc may be quantitated. This is the commercially available FIAX system (I.D.T., Santa Clara, California, USA). Assays of gentamicin (Tsay *et al.* 1980) and tobramycin (Tsay & Palmer 1981) have been reported.

Magnetizable solid-phase separation

If antibodies are coupled covalently to magnetizable particles, bound tracer may be separated readily from the free fraction by placing the immunoassay incubation mixture on a magnet. The supernatant fluid, which will contain not only the free tracer but also the other components of the serum sample, may be removed by aspiration or decantation. The principle of the assay is shown in Fig. 3. Suitable solid-phase particles may be prepared by the incorporation of magnetizable iron oxide in a cellulose matrix (Kamel *et al.* 1980).

Magnetizable solid-phase FIA of aminoglycosides may be performed entirely within disposable polystyrene test tubes (No. 484, 55 × 12 mm, from Sarstedt, Leicester, UK). To 5 µl of sample or standard is added 100 µl of FTC-aminoglycoside followed by 100 µl of a suspension of antiserum coupled to magnetizable particles. After vortexing, the tubes are placed in a polystyrene rack and left for a least 10 min at room temperature. Next 1·5 ml of water is added with sufficient force to mix the particles. The rack is then placed into a magnet separator unit to sediment the particles (Fig. 4), and the supernatant fluids decanted to waste by inversion of the unit (the particles being securely retained in the tubes by magnetic attraction). Elution reagent (1·5 ml of a mixture of methanol and 100 mmol/l aqueous sodium hydroxide in proportions 2:1 by volume, containing 10 ml/l Triton X-100 detergent) is then added, the tubes vortexed, and the rack returned to the magnet. Fluorescence of the eluted supernatants is measured by placing the test tubes directly in a fluorimeter. The measured signal (from the eluted bound fraction of the tracer) is inversely related to the sample (or standard) gentamicin concentration.

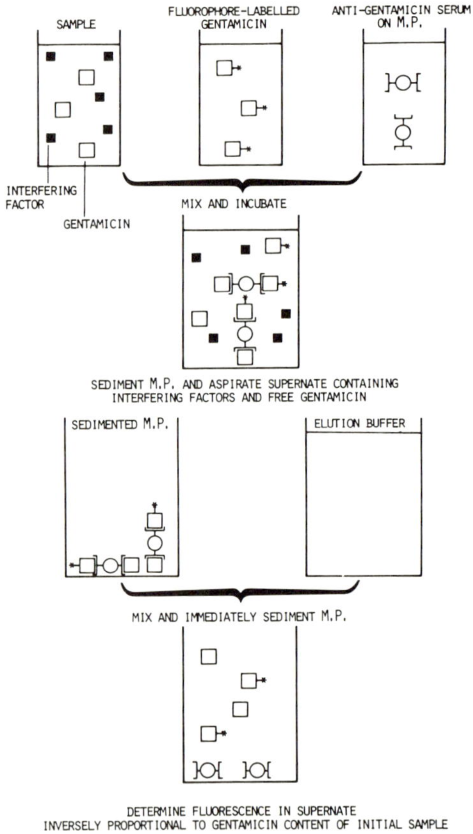

FIG. 3. Representation of a separation fluoroimmunoassay in which the separation step is also employed to remove endogenous fluorophores and interfering factors. The antibody is covalently coupled to magnetizable particles (M.P.). Bound antigen is then sedimented on a magnet allowing the supernatant containing free antigen, endogenous fluorophores and interfering factors to be discarded.

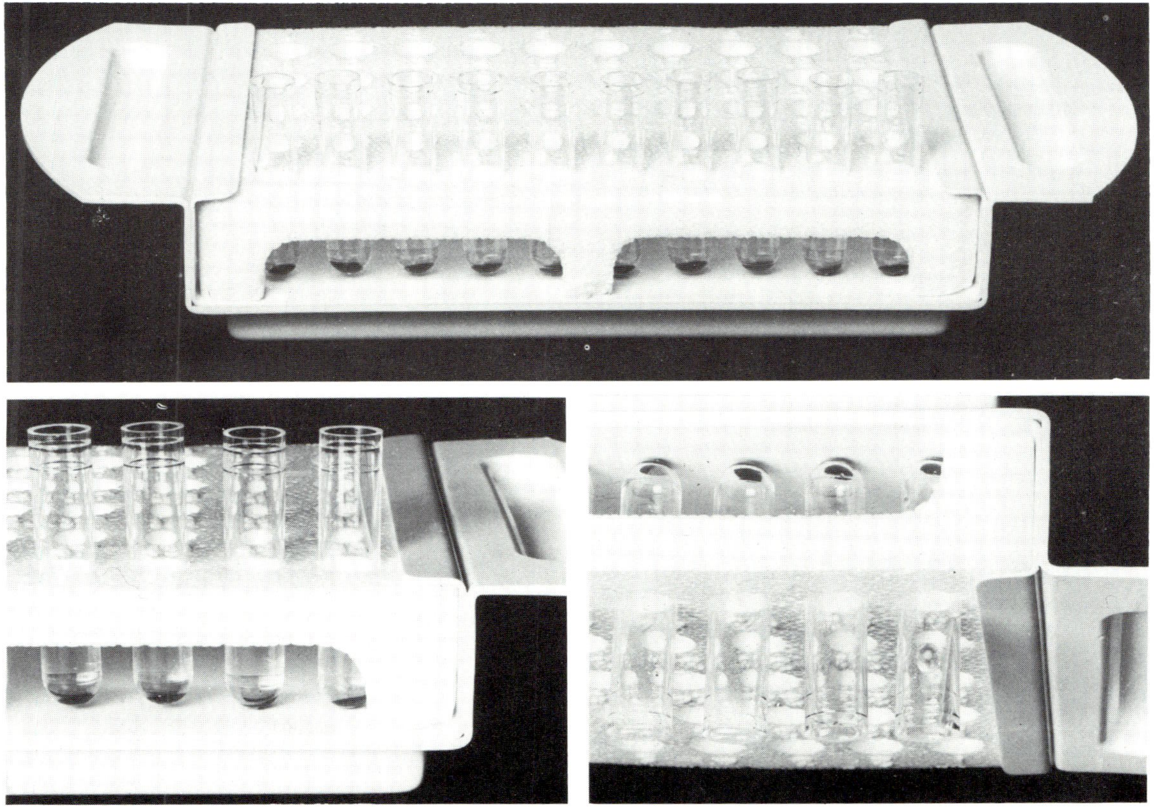

FIG. 4. Magnetic separation showing sedimentation of magnetizable particles allowing supernatant containing free antibiotic and any interfering substance present to be discarded.

A suitable magnet separator (Fig. 4) contains 50 individual rare-earth magnets. When the polystyrene test tube rack is positioned in the separator, each tube is directly above one of the magnets. The rack is gripped firmly by the casing of the separator unit, allowing it to be inverted so as to discard the supernatant fluids with retention of the magnetizable particles (Fig. 4).

Most of the work described above was performed using a Perkin-Elmer Model 1000 ratio-recording filter fluorimeter with two FITC-495-X interference filters (Fish-Schurman, New Rochelle, New York, USA) in the excitation light path, and a 520 nm cut-off filter (Technicon, Basingstoke, Hants., UK) in the emission path. The excitation filters transmitted a broad band of light (*ca.* 390–500 nm) from the continuous-spectrum xenon lamp source, and to avoid overloading the reference detector it was necessary to limit the excitation beam by means of a plate with an 8 mm diam. central aperture in the excitation filter holder. The continuous-wavelength emission filter of the Model 1000 fluorimeter was wound out of the emission beam and not used. To facilitate the measurement of fluorescence in the disposable test tubes, an adapter (Kamel *et al.* 1980) was constructed from a 45 mm length of half-inch square aluminium rod.

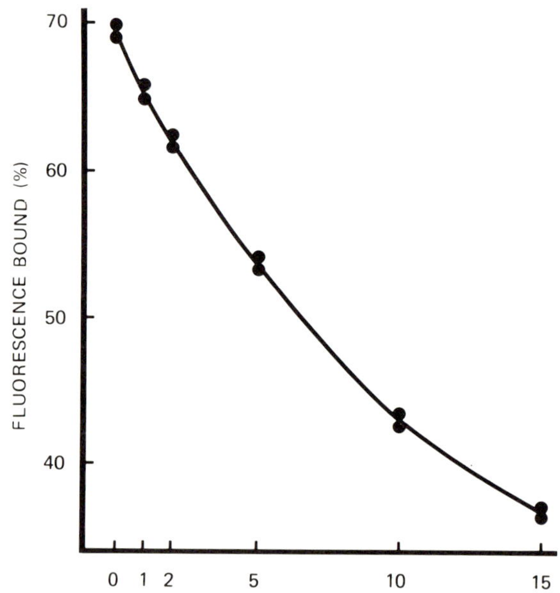

FIG. 5. Standard curve for tobramycin separation fluoroimmunoassay. Standard curves are constructed by plotting the percentage of total tracer bound by solid phase against aminoglycoside concentration.

The rod was drilled out to 12 mm diam. down its long axis and slits cut in the sides to allow passage of light beams. Finally, a matt black anodized finish was applied. The adapter was placed permanently in the sample compartment of the fluorimeter, in the position normally occupied by a conventional square-section fluorimeter cuvette. Adapters of this type are available from I.L.S., Newbury Street, London EC1, UK.

More recently a Fluoroflex ratio-recording fluorimeter has been used (Wild International, Ashford, Kent, UK). This microprocessor-controlled instrument has facilities for complete immunoassay data reduction, with curve-fitting and print-out for results.

TABLE 1

The precision of the separation fluoroimmunoassay was determined by assay of clinical samples in duplicate ten times (within assay) and ten separate occasions (between assay)

Within assay precision		Between assay precision	
Mean concentration (mg/l)	Coefficient of variation (%)	Mean concentration (mg/l)	Coefficient of variation (%)
	Gentamicin		
1·2	4·8	1·3	10·4
2·9	3·6	2·2	6·3
6·2	1·8	5·0	3·2
10·6	2·4	10·0	3·4
	Tobramycin		
1·1	9·4	3·7	8·5
3·8	4·7	6·1	6·3
5·8	1·9	8·7	4·0
8·6	2·1		
	Amikacin		
8·3	3·6	8·7	5·3
17·2	1·5	17·6	3·2
27·7	1·4	27·9	3·0
46·0	3·0	47·1	3·1

Antisera raised against three aminoglycosides (gentamicin, tobramycin and amikacin) have been coupled to magnetizable particles and used in the development of FIA employing the corresponding fluorescein-labelled antibiotic as tracer. Similar standard curves have been obtained in all three cases, and that obtained for tobramycin is shown in Fig. 5 as representative. The results of precision studies are given in Table 1. The comparison of results obtained by magnetizable solid-phase FIA of patients' samples with those obtained when the same samples were assayed by established techniques (RIA, EMIT enzymoimmunoassay and QIA) is shown in Table 2. The solid-phase assays have been shown to be unaffected by severe lipaemia, haemolysis (10%) and jaundice (800 μmol/l bilirubin), confirming the efficiency of the separation system.

TABLE 2

Correlation of aminoglycoside levels in patients' samples determined by separation fluoroimmunoassay (y *values*) *and plate diffusion bioassay, radioimmunoassay, enzymoimmunoassay or quenching fluoroimmunoassay* (x *values in each case*) *showing regression equation and correlation coefficients*

Method	Number of samples	Regression equation	Correlation coefficient
	Gentamicin		
Plate diffusion bioassay	55	$y = 0{\cdot}93x + 0{\cdot}3$	0·96
Coated-tube radioimmunoassay (Clinical Assays)	35	$y = 1{\cdot}03x - 0{\cdot}1$	0·99
Second-antibody radioimmunoassay (Diagnostic Products Corporation)	33	$y = 0{\cdot}86x + 0{\cdot}1$	0·98
Enzymoimmunoassay (EMIT; Syva)	48	$y = 1{\cdot}08x - 0{\cdot}7$	0·96
Quenching fluoroimmunoassay	41	$y = 0{\cdot}97x - 0{\cdot}2$	0·96
	Tobramycin		
Coated-tube radioimmunoassay (Clinical Assays)	30	$y = 0{\cdot}93x - 0{\cdot}1$	0·98

Summary

Non-isotopic immunoassays that incorporate a separation step are more reliable than non-separation techniques, as potentially interfering factors may be discarded. The coupling of antiserum to magnetizable particles allows simple and rapid separation, and has proved suitable for the development of aminoglycoside assays using fluorescein as label. These separation fluoroimmunoassays employ stable and safe reagents and require only a simple, relatively inexpensive fluorimeter.

References

BROUGHTON, A. & STRONG, J. E. 1976 Radioimmunoassay of iodinated gentamicin. *Clinica Chimica Acta* **66**, 125–129.

BURD, J. F., WONG, R. C., FEENEY, J. E., CARRICO, R. J. & BOGUSLASKI, R. C. 1977 Homogeneous reactant-labelled fluorescent immunoassay for therapeutic drugs exemplified by gentamicin determination in human serum. *Clinical Chemistry* **23**, 1402–1408.

BURD, J. F., CARRICO, R. J., KRAMER, H. M. & DENNING, C. E. 1978 Homogeneous substrate-labelled fluorescent immunoassay for determining tobramycin concentrations in human serum. In *Enzyme Labelled Immunoassay of Hormones and Drugs*, ed. Pal, S. B. pp. 387–403. Berlin: Walter de Gruyter.

JOLLEY, M. E., STROUPE, S. D., WANG, C. J., PANAS, H. N., KEEGAN, C. L., SCHMIDT, R. L. & SCHWENZER, K. S. 1981 Fluorescence polarisation immunoassay I. Monitoring aminoglycoside antibiotics in serum and plasma. *Clinical Chemistry* **27,** 1190–1197.

KAMEL, R. S., LANDON, J. & SMITH, D. S. 1980 Magnetisable solid-phase fluoroimmunoassay of phenytoin in disposable test tubes. *Clinical Chemistry* **26,** 1281–1284.

KARNES, H. T., GUDAT, J. C., O'DONNELL, C. & WINEFORDNER, J. D. 1981 Double-antibody fluorescence immunoassay of tobramycin. *Clinical Chemistry* **27,** 249–252.

LEWIS, J. E., NELSON, J. C. & ELDER, H. A. 1972 Radioimmunoassay of an antibiotic: gentamicin. *Nature, London* **239,** 214–216.

MUNRO, A., LANDON, J. & SHAW, E. J. 1982*a* The basis of immunoassays for antibiotics. *Journal of Antimicrobial Chemotherapy* **9,** 423–432.

MUNRO, A. J., SMITH, D. S. & SHAW, E. J. 1982*b* A simplified quenching fluoroimmunoassay for gentamicin and the effects of some potential interfering factors. *Journal of Antimicrobial Chemotherapy* **9,** 47–51.

O'DONNELL, C. M., MCBRIDE, J., SUFFIN, S. & BROUGHTON, A. 1980 A heterogeneous fluorescence immunoassay for gentamicin using a second antibody separation. *Journal of Immunoassay* **1,** 375–383.

POPELKA, S. R., MILLER, D. M., HOLEN, J. T. & KELSO, D. M. 1981 Fluorescence polarisation immunoassay II. Analyser for rapid, precise measurement of fluorescence polarisation with use of disposable cuvettes. *Clinical Chemistry* **27,** 1198–1201.

SHAW, E. J., WATSON, R. A. A., LANDON, J. & SMITH, D. S. 1977 Estimation of serum gentamicin by quenching fluoroimmunoassay. *Journal of Clinical Pathology* **30**, 526–531.

SHAW, E. J., WATSON, R. A. A. & SMITH, D. S. 1979 Continuous-flow fluoroimmunoassay of serum gentamicin, with automatic sample blank correction. *Clinical Chemistry* **25,** 322–324.

THOMPSON, S. G. & BURD, J. F. 1980 Substrate-labelled fluorescent immunoassay for amikacin in human serum. *Antimicrobial Agents and Chemotherapy* **18,** 264–268.

TSAY, Y. & PALMER, R. J. 1981 A solid-phase fluoroimmunoassay of tobramycin. *Clinica Chimica Acta* **109,** 151–157.

TSAY, Y., WILSON, L. & KEEFE, E. 1980 Quantitation of serum gentamicin concentration by a solid-phase immunofluorescence method. *Clinical Chemistry* **26,** 1610–1612.

WATSON, R. A. A., LANDON, J., SHAW, E. J. & SMITH, D. S. 1976*a* Polarisation fluoroimmunoassay of gentamicin. *Clinica Chimica Acta* **73,** 51–55.

WATSON, R. A. A., SHAW, E. J. & EDWARDS, C. R. W. 1976*b* A ^{125}I-based radioimmunoassay for serum gentamicin. In *Chemotherapy* Vol. 2, ed. Williams, J. D. & Geddes, A. M. pp. 107–110. New York: Plenum.

WATSON, R. A. A., LANDON, J., EDWARDS, C. R. W. & SHAW, E. J. 1979 Improved ^{125}I-ligands for gentamicin radioimmunoassay. *Journal of Antimicrobial Chemotherapy* **5,** 673–680.

Methods of Studying Plasmid-determined Resistance to Tetracyclines

I. Chopra, P. R. Ball and S. W. Shales

Department of Microbiology, Medical School, University of Bristol, Bristol, UK

Tetracycline resistance genes in many bacteria are located on plasmids. Details of those species from which tetracycline resistance plasmids had been isolated by the mid-1970s have been collated by several authors (Jacob *et al.* 1977*a*, *b*; Jacoby & Shapiro 1977; Novick *et al.* 1977). Since then tetracycline resistance plasmids have also been found in a number of other species and the current situation is summarized in Table 1.

Table 1

Natural bacterial isolates that contain tetracycline resistance plasmids

Achromobacter liquefaciens	*Providencia* sp.
Enterobacter cloacae	*Salmonella panama*
Bacillus cereus	*Salm. paratyphi* B
B. stearothermophilus	*Salm. typhi*
Bacteroides fragilis	*Salm. typhimurium*
Campylobacter fetus sub sp. *jejuni*	*Shigella dysenteriae*
Escherichia coli	*Sh. flexneri*
Haemophilus influenzae	*Sh. sonnei*
Klebsiella pneumoniae	*Staphylococcus aureus*
Pseudomonas aeruginosa	*Streptococcus agalactiae*
Proteus mirabilis	*Strep. faecalis*
Pr. morganii	*Strep. faecalis* sub sp. *zymogenes*
Pr. rettgeri	*Vibrio cholerae*

From Chopra (1983).

ANTIBIOTICS
ISBN 0 12 604480 5

Despite the widespread occurrence of resistance amongst different bacteria, the molecular basis of tetracycline resistance is poorly understood when contrasted with current knowledge of plasmid-determined resistance to aminoglycosides or β-lactams (Davies & Smith, 1978). Nevertheless, within the past two or three years advances have been made in the study of tetracycline resistance. This chapter describes three methods which we have recently used in studies on plasmid-determined tetracycline resistance in *Escherichia coli*, viz. fluorescence spectroscopy to measure accumulation of tetracyclines by bacteria, two-dimensional electrophoresis and crossed immunoelectrophoresis to identify a membrane protein concerned with expression of resistance.

A complete discussion of bacterial resistance to the tetracyclines is out of place here, but readers requiring a wider background can consult a number of review articles on the subject (Levy *et al.* 1977; Chopra & Howe 1978; Levy 1981; Chopra *et al.* 1981; Chopra 1983).

Fluorescence Spectroscopy to Measure Accumulation of Tetracyclines by Bacteria

It is well established that tetracycline can be used as a fluorescent probe of its own transport into bacteria (Dockter & Magnuson 1974, 1975; Weckesser & Magnuson 1976, 1979; Samra *et al.* 1979; Ball *et al.* 1980; Shales *et al.* 1980). The method depends upon the large increase in the quantum yield of fluorescence when tetracycline enters the bacterial cell. Tetracycline accumulation has also been measured using radiolabelled (^3H) antibiotic (e.g. see McMurry & Levy 1978). However, fluorescence spectroscopy offers two major advantages over methods employing labelled tetracycline.

(1) Self-radiolysis of labelled tetracycline produces degradation products that bind to bacteria (Levy *et al.* 1977), a problem clearly not encountered with the spectrofluorimetric method.

(2) Spectrofluorimetry can be applied to several members of the tetracycline series (Samra *et al.* 1979; Shales *et al.* 1980), whereas only tetracycline itself is readily available in a labelled form.

Experimental details (Ball *et al.* 1980; Shales *et al.* 1980)

The experimental protocol we have adopted for studies on tetracycline uptake by *E. coli* is simple and could easily be adapted for other bacterial species. Cultures (usually 500 ml) of late log phase bacteria (5×10^8 cells/ml) are harvested by centrifugation (30°C, 12,000 **g**, 10 min) washed and resuspended (5×10^9 cells/ml) in a Tris–HCl buffer (10 mol/l pH 8) containing glucose (0·4% w/v). Tetracyclines (usually 100 μg/ml) are added and fluorescence enhancement monitored at 37°C, e.g. using a Perkin-Elmer 3000 spectrofluorimeter. Bacteria are aerated throughout the course of each experiment by circulating the cell suspension through a flow cell. For the majority of tetracyclines, excitation is performed at 400 nm with emission at 520 nm (Samra *et al.* 1979; Shales *et al.* 1980).

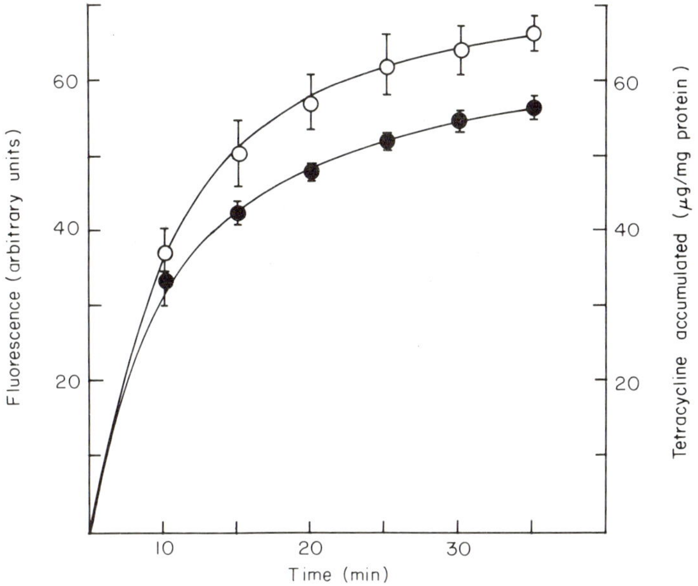

FIG. 1. Comparison of time-dependent fluorescence enhancement (●) and uptake (○) of tetracycline by strain JC3272. Bacteria (5 × 10^9/ml) were incubated with tetracycline as described in 'Experimental details'. Simultaneous fluorescence enhancement and uptake of tetracycline were measured as described by Shales *et al.* (1980). Indicated values are the means of four replicates and the error bars represent ±1 SD. Reproduced from Shales *et al.* (1980).

Results and discussion

In *E. coli* (Fig. 1) and other species (Dockter & Magnuson, 1974, 1975: Weckesser & Magnuson, 1976, 1979) time-dependent fluorescence enhancement and uptake of tetracycline are directly correlated. Uptake (fluorescence enhancement) into *E. coli* (Figs 1, 2*a*) apparently follows Michaelis–Menten kinetics (Chopra & Ball 1982). The rate and extent of tetracycline accumulation (fluorescence enhancement) is markedly reduced in resistant cells (Fig. 2*b*).

Use of the spectrofluorimetric assay permitted us to define three phenotypic mechanisms of plasmid-determined resistance in *E. coli* (Table 2) (Shales *et al.* 1980). Further studies, also using spectrofluorimetry, have confirmed the independent nature of resistance mechanisms

TABLE 2

Three phenotypes associated with expression of plasmid-mediated tetracycline and minocycline resistance in Escherichia coli*

Mechanism	Resistance pattern†	Level of resistance conferred	Decrease in uptake of antibiotic	Regulation	Encoded by resistance determinant in‡
1	Tc	10–20 fold	—	Constitutive in all cases apart from pSC101 when expression is inducible	pSC101, RP1, pIP7, pIP69, R100-1
2	Tc	4–7 fold	+	Usually inducible	RP1, pIP7, pIP69, R100-1
3	Tc, Min	2–3 fold	—	Inducible or constitutive	pIP69, R100-1

* Based on Shales *et al.* (1980).
† Tc, tetracycline; Min, minocycline.
‡ The tetracycline resistance genes in pIP69 and R100-1 are contained within the transposon Tn10 (Shales *et al.* 1980; Mendez *et al.* 1980). DNA–DNA hybridization studies (Mendez *et al.* 1980) show that the tetracycline resistance determinants belong to different classes: RP1 and pIP7 contain a TetA determinant, Tn10 contains a TetB determinant and pSC101 a TetC determinant.

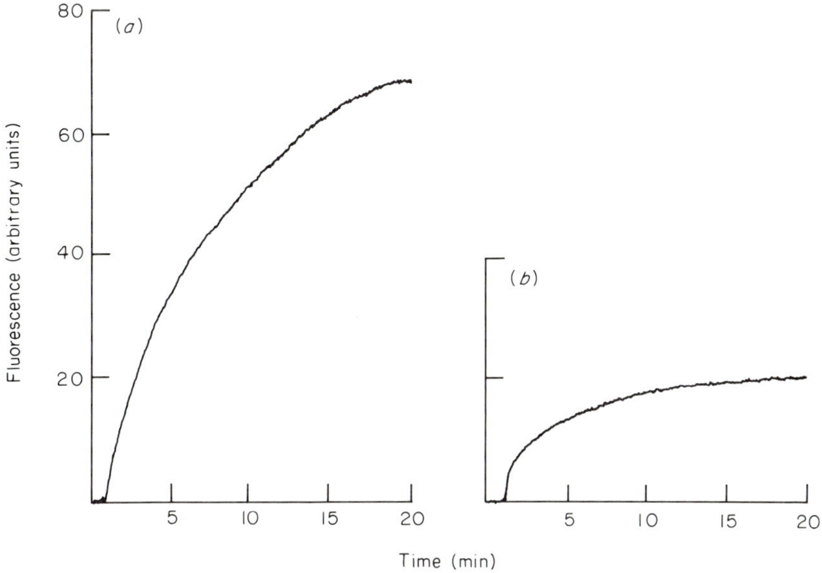

FIG. 2. Time-dependent fluorescence enhancement of suspensions of strains JC3272 (*a*) and JC3272 (pIP7) induced with tetracycline (0·5 μg/ml) during growth (*b*). Bacteria (5 × 10^9/ml) suspended in a Tris buffer containing glucose were incubated aerobically at 37°C with tetracycline (100 μg/ml) and fluorescence enhancement was determined as described in experimental details. Reproduced from Shales *et al.* (1980).

1 and 2. Plasmid pUB905 (probably containing a TetA determinant) encodes inducible resistance to tetracycline, but expression of resistance is temperature conditional (Ball *et al.* 1980; Table 3). The mutation in this determinant appears to reside in the region conferring resistance mechanism 2 because at 42°C the plasmid fails to confer decreased tetracycline uptake (Table 3). Nevertheless, bacteria harbouring pUB905 do express resistance at 42°C (Table 3). We believe that this reflects expression of mechanism 1 because the level of protection conferred is about 10-fold and expression of resistance is constitutive (Table 3). Spectrofluorimetry has also allowed characterization of the resistance mechanism 2 mediating decreased tetracycline accumulation. In each case decreased accumulation results both from reduced influx and accelerated efflux of tetracycline from the cell (Table 4). A similar mechanism operates during expression of plasmid-determined resistance in *Bacillus subtilis* (Table 4).

In summary, use of the spectrofluorimetric assay for tetracycline accumulation provides a rapid means to determine whether or not expression of resistance results from decreased accumulation of antibiotic. In

TABLE 3

Accumulation of tetracycline and expression of resistance by Escherichia coli *K-12 JC6310 containing the plasmid pUB905*

Strain	Tetracycline accumulated after 20 min (μg/mg protein)* at (°C)			Resistance level (IC_{50}) to tetracycline (μg/ml)† at (°C)		
	30	35	42	30	35	42
JC6310	67·1 ± 1·1	66·0 ± 2·6	66·0 ± 5·2	0·23 ± 0·03	0·19 ± 0·00	0·18 ± 0·02
JC6310 (pUB905)	55·2 ± 2·1	59·7 ± 3·6	70·5 ± 2·6	2·55 ± 0·15	1·68 ± 0·02	1·36 ± 0·05
JC6310 (pUB905) +Tc‡	5·2 ± 0·9	38·7 ± 2·4	63·6 ± 5·4	25·3 ± 2·3	7·0 ± 1·5	1·65 ± 0·10

* Values (±1 standard deviation) from Ball *et al.* (1980). Accumulation determined by spectrofluorimetry.

† Concentrations of tetracycline causing a 50% reduction in growth rate (IC_{50}) were determined as described (Shales *et al.* 1980). Values are the means of at least two separate determinations for each culture (±1 standard deviation).

‡ Grown for several generations at the indicated temperature in the presence of tetracycline (0·5 μg/ml).

TABLE 4

Kinetic constants for tetracycline accumulation in strains of Escherichia coli *and* Bacillus subtilis*

Strain†	Classification of resistance determinant‡	Kinetic constants§	
		Influx k_1(/min)	Efflux k_{-1}(/min)
Escherichia coli			
JC3272	—	0·130	0·072
JC3272(pIP7)	*Tet*A	0·106	0·064
JC3272(pIP7) +TC	*Tet*A	0·026	0·159
JC3272(pDU301)	*Tet*B	0·012	0·135
Bacillus subtilis			
NCIB10106	—	0·139	0·049
NCIB10106(pUB1659)	?	0·054	0·032
NCIB10106(pUB1659) +TC	?	0·003	0·078

* Data from Ball *et al.* (1980) and Eccles *et al.* (1981).

† Strains followed by +TC were grown in the presence of tetracycline prior to kinetic analysis to induce resistance. Expression of resistance in pDU301 (a mutant of R100-1) is constitutive.

‡ According to the scheme of Mendez *et al.* (1980).

§ $[TC]_{out} \underset{k_{-1}}{\overset{k_1}{\rightleftharpoons}} [TC]_{in}$ where $[TC]_{out}$ is the concentration of tetracycline outside the cell, $[TC]_{in}$ the concentration inside the cell, k_1 the rate constant for tetracycline influx (initial velocity of uptake ÷ initial $[TC]_{out}$), and k_{-1} the rate constant for tetracycline efflux (initial velocity of uptake ÷ initial $[TC]_{in}$.)

E. coli K-12, reduced accumulation of antibiotic in strains possessing resistance levels above 5 μg/ml (minimum inhibitory concentration on nutrient agar) can be taken as presumptive evidence for the presence of a resistance plasmid, since the most frequent chromosomal mutation to resistance (Omp F), although resulting in decreased uptake of tetracycline, does not confer high-level resistance (Chopra & Eccles, 1978). In Gram negative species it is clear that tetracycline resistance determinants are heterogeneous (Mendez *et al.* 1980; Levy 1981). This may reflect differences in the ability of the determinants to mediate reduced accumulation of the various tetracycline analogues in clinical use. The spectrofluorimetric assay described here could permit investigation of this hypothesis.

Detection of a Membrane Protein Concerned with Expression of Tn10-determined Tetracycline Resistance

As already discussed, expression of tetracycline resistance by wild-type

Tn10 determinants is inducible and associated with reduced accumulation of the antibiotic arising both from decreased influx and energy-dependent efflux of the drug. An inducible protein of mol. wt 36,000 (synonym 'TET' protein) known to be encoded by Tn10 and required for resistance (Jorgensen & Reznikoff 1979; Zupancic *et al.* 1980) could be responsible for decreased accumulation, but direct evidence for this hypothesis is lacking.

Clearly, studies on the cellular location of a protein can provide information relating to its function. The 'TET' protein was first detected in the envelope of *E. coli* minicells (Levy & McMurry 1974) and subsequently shown to be located in the cytoplasmic membrane of minicells (Levy *et al.* 1977). However, expression of Tn10-determined resistance is defective in minicells (Levy 1975) which raises the possibility that the 'TET' protein is not located in the cytoplasmic membrane of whole bacteria. Indeed, at least two proteins synthesized in *E. coli* minicells have different locations in whole bacteria (Ferraza & Levy 1980; Subramanian & Reeve, 1978). Early attempts to visualize the 'TET' protein in whole bacteria under normal growth conditions failed (Levy & McMurry 1974), but more recently, Levy *et al.* (1977) reported that the protein could be detected in the cytoplasmic membrane of whole bacteria inhibited with rifamycin. The studies conducted by Levy's group have relied upon separation of proteins by one-dimensional electrophoresis, but the introduction of alternative electrophoresis procedures permits, in principle, the detection of minor proteins in cells grown under physiological conditions. We have used two of these techniques to detect the 'TET' protein in the cytoplasmic membrane of *E. coli* whole cells.

Two-dimensional electrophoresis

Polyacrylamide gel electrophoresis has proved to be an extremely useful method for the separation and characterization of soluble proteins, but before it can be applied to membranes it is necessary to solubilize the proteins. Many methods rely upon the detergent sodium dodecyl sulphate (SDS) to solubilize the proteins and maintain their separation during electrophoresis. However, it is well established (e.g. see Weber & Osborn 1969) that electrophoresis in SDS separates proteins as a function of molecular weight so that different proteins may co-migrate and are not resolved from one another.

A two-dimensional method (O'Farrell 1975) in which proteins are separated by two unrelated parameters has achieved very high resolution of protein mixtures. In this procedure proteins are separated according to isoelectric point and then according to molecular weight. However, many membrane proteins are not adequately solubilized even by the very high concentrations of urea used in this method (Ames & Nikaido 1976). Ames & Nikaido (1976) adapted O'Farrell's method specifically for the separation of membrane proteins. Their procedure takes advantage of the good solubilizing properties of hot SDS followed by isoelectric focusing of proteins in gels containing a non-ionic detergent. After isoelectric focusing the proteins are separated on the basis of size by SDS slab gel electrophoresis. The details that follow are based on Ames and Nikaido's method.

Experimental details

Preparation of isoelectric focusing gels. The gel formula described in Table 5 is sufficient to prepare ten isoelectric focusing gels each of 10 cm length. The reagents are added to a small side-arm flask and the urea (ultra-pure) dissolved by warming the flask to 37°C. Ammonium persulphate (10 μl of a 10% w/v solution) is added and the gel mixture de-aerated by attachement of a vacuum line to the flask. Next, tetramethylethylendiamine (7 μl) is added and mixed gently with the other gel components. This mixture is applied to glass tubes (12 × 0·3 cm i.d.) to a depth of 10 cm and then overlaid with urea (8 mol/l). After polymerization (1–2 h) the stoppers are removed from the ends of the tubes and replaced by dialysis membrane held in place by rubber O-rings. Attachment of the dialysis membrane is most conveniently performed by locating the gel tube, O-ring and membrane in a beaker containing the anode solution (0·01 mol/l H_3PO_4). This method prevents the trapping of air bubbles between the end of the gel and the dialysis membrane. After attachment of the dialysis membrane, the tubes can be assembled in an electrophoresis apparatus (e.g. a Shandon analytical tube gel apparatus).

Sample preparation. Lyophilized protein (3 mg) is dissolved in the sample solubilization buffer (Table 5) and then heated at 100°C for 5 min. Insoluble material is removed by centrifugation (e.g. using an Eppendorff bench centrifuge for 3–5 min) and the supernatant fluid diluted with 2 vols of sample dilution buffer (Table 5). At this stage it is useful to add ultra-pure sucrose (10–20%) to facilitate overlaying of the sample. The sample is now ready for electrophoresis.

Application of sample to isoelectric focusing gel. The urea (8 mol/l) used to overlay the gels is removed and replaced with the sample (10–100 μl) as prepared above. The sample is then overlaid with about 20 μl of sample overlay solution (Table 5) to protect it from the electrode solution. In order to quantify the protein applied to the gels a protein determination (Zaman & Verwilghen 1979) may be performed at this stage.

Table 5

Materials used in two-dimensional electrophoresis

Solution for isoelectric focusing gel (10)		*Sample solubilization buffer (for 3 mg protein)*		*Sample dilution buffer (store at −20°C)*	
Urea	5·5 g	Tris–HCl (0·25 mol/l pH 6·8)	40 μl	Urea	5·7 g
Acrylamide solution*	1·33 ml	Sodium dodecyl sulphate (10% w/v)	40 μl	pH 3·5–10 ampholytes (40%)	0·5 ml
pH 3·5–10 ampholytes (40%)	0·5 ml	$MgCl_2$ (1 mmol/l)	100 μl	Mercaptoethanol	0·5 ml
Water	1·97 ml	Water	20 μl	Triton X100 (10% v/v)	0·8 ml
				Water	to 10 ml
*Acrylamide	28·38 g				
N,*N′*-methylene bis acrylamide	1·62 g				
Water	to 100 ml				
Sample overlay solution (store at −20°)		*Equilibration buffer*			
Urea	5·41 g	Tris–HCl (0·0625 mol/l pH 6·8)	85 ml		
pH 3·5–10 ampholytes (40%)	0·25 ml	Glycerol	10 ml		
		Mercaptoethanol	5 ml		
Water	to 10 ml	Sodium dodecyl sulphate	2 g		

Electrolysis of isoelectric focusing gels. The disc gel apparatus is set up with degassed NaOH (0·02 mol/l) in the cathode compartment (top) and H_3PO_4 (0·01 mol/l) in the anode compartment. Electrophoresis is performed (usually at room temperature) at 400 V for 15–18 h. The pH gradient formed is approximately linear ranging from *ca.* 7–4.

Treatment of isoelectric focusing gels prior to slab gel electrophoresis. For proteins that will be detected subsequently by staining it is wise to remove the ampholytes from the isoelectric focusing gels. This can be achieved by following the method of Jackle (1979) in which gels are treated with

(1) 0·1% Coomassie Brilliant Blue R250 in 50% methanol, 10% acetic acid (10–15 min);
(2) 50% methanol, 10% acetic acid (45–60 min);
(3) 0·005% Coomassie Brilliant Blue R250 in 5% methanol, 7% acetic acid (indefinite period).

In addition to removing ampholytes, the method will also visualize the proteins separated by isoelectric focusing. Prior to separation of proteins in the second dimension, the stained gels are immersed in equilibration buffer (Table 5) for 1·5 h, with the buffer changed twice during this period (at 30 and 60 min). O'Farrell (1975) gives details for processing gels containing radioactive proteins.

Preparation of slab gels. Separation in the second dimension is best achieved using the gel system described by Laemmli (1970) to which the reader is referred for experimental details. We routinely use 15% separating gels but variations including gradient gels (e.g. see O'Farrell 1975) are also possible. Gels (1·5 mm thick) are cast between glass plates to produce a separating gel about 17 cm wide × 12 cm long, covered by a stacking gel about 1·5 cm long. A simple slab gel apparatus (e.g. produced by Shandon, Raven, Bethesda) is adequate but the upper edge of the glass plates should be ground at an angle so that the isoelectric focusing gel effectively sits in a groove during separation of proteins in the second dimension.

Loading the isoelectric focusing gel on to the slab gel. A 1% agarose gel is used to attach the cylindrical isoelectric focusing gel to the slab stacking gel. The agarose gel mixture is prepared by melting 1 g of agarose in 100 ml of equilibration buffer (Table 5) and approximately 1 ml of this solution (held at about 70°C) is poured on top of the acrylamide slab gel surface. The cylindrical gel (placed on a piece of Parafilm) is transferred rapidly to the surface containing the molten agarose and care taken to prevent the formation of air bubbles. Further hot agarose is pipetted on top of the cylindrical gel.

Electrophoresis in the second dimension. Using the system developed by Laemmli (1970), gels 1·5 mm thick are run at 30 mA constant current for about 4 h. During this time the Coomassie Blue contained in the isoelectric focusing gel will migrate into the slab system.

Staining and de-staining of slab gels. See Ames & Nikaido (1976) for details of these steps.

TABLE 6

*Bacterial strains used for analysis of cytoplasmic membrane proteins**

Strain	Strain description	Resistance level (IC_{50}) to tetracycline (μg/ml)†	
		−Tc	+Tc
JC3272	*his trp lys rpsL*	0·29 ± 0·02	
DU3091	Transposition of Tn10 from R100-1 to the chromosome of JC3272	11·8 ± 0·4	58·0 ± 8·5
DU-1200	Transposition of Tn10 from pDU300 to the chromosome of JC3272	71·5 ± 3·5	73·0 ± 2·0

* Shales *et al.* (1980).
† Concentrations of tetracycline causing a 50% reduction in growth rate (IC_{50}) were determined as described (Shales *et al.* 1980). Values are the means of at least two separate determinations for each culture ±1 standard deviation. '+Tc': strains grown in the presence of 0·5 μg tetracycline/ml for at least 4 generations before the determination of resistance levels.

Results and discussion

Various strains of *E. coli* K-12 (Table 6) were fractionated (Chopra & Shales 1980) to produce samples containing cytoplasmic membrane proteins. Analysis of the proteins by two-dimensional electrophoresis showed the presence of the 'TET' protein (Figs 3 and 4) both in DU1200, which shows constitutive expression of Tn10-determined tetracycline resistance, and in induced cultures of DU3091. The molecular weight of the protein (36,000) was identical to that reported by Levy *et al.* (1977) and it had an isoelectric point of about 6·4 (pH gradients in isoelectric focusing gels were determined as described by Ames & Nikaido 1976). The content of the 'TET' protein in the cytoplasmic membrane was correlated with the ability of the cultures to prevent accumulation of tetracycline (Fig. 4). The 'TET' protein was not found in other cell fractions (data not shown). A normal host product (mol. wt *ca.* 34,000, pI *ca.* 6·5) was also enriched in the cytoplasmic membranes of those bacteria which express high-level resistance (Fig. 4), but the significance of this change is unknown.

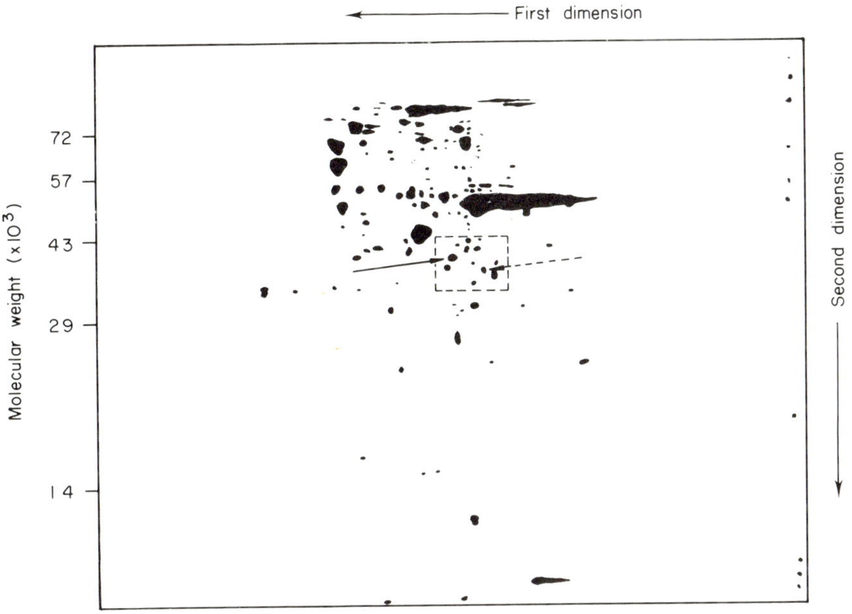

FIG. 3. Diagrammatic representation of proteins from the cytoplasmic membrane of DU1200 separated by two-dimensional electrophoresis. Membrane proteins were isolated using Sarkosyl and the polypeptides analysed as described by Chopra & Shales (1980). Basic proteins are located to the right, acidic proteins to the left. The solid line within the boxed area shows the 36 kilodalton 'TET' protein and the broken line shows a normal host product that is enriched in cells expressing high-level resistance to tetracycline (see Fig. 4 and text).

The studies described here show that the 'TET' protein has the same cellular location in minicells and whole cells. The content of the 'TET' protein was correlated with reduced drug uptake (Fig. 4) and its presence in the cytoplasmic membrane is consistent with a role in mediating energy-dependent efflux of tetracycline from the cell.

Crossed immunoelectrophoresis (*CIE*)

Crossed immunoelectrophoresis comprises electrophoretic separation of proteins in an agarose gel followed by a second (perpendicular) electrophoresis into an antibody-containing gel. The technique has been widely used in biomedical research including analysis of bacterial membrane proteins (Salton 1978). The method is useful for studies on membrane proteins because it permits analysis of the surface exposure and distribution of antigens within membranes.

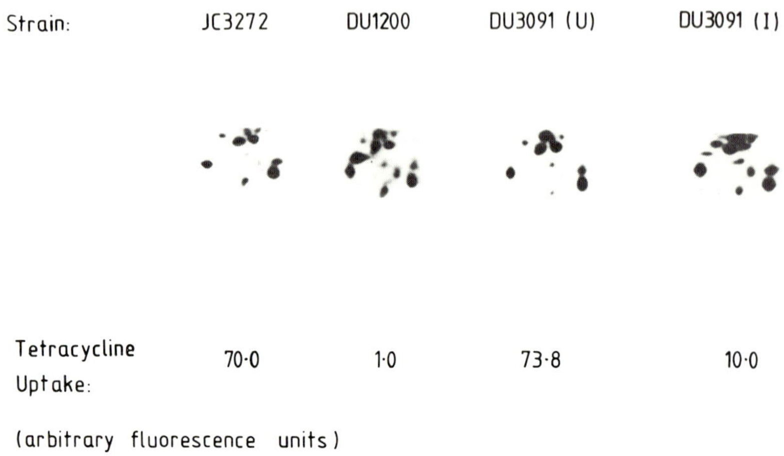

FIG. 4. Cytoplasmic membrane proteins (molecular weights 32,000–43,000, isoelectric points 6·0–6·6) from *Escherichia coli* strains described in Table 6. Gel regions corresponding to that shown in the boxed area of Fig. 3 are presented. Values for tetracycline uptake (fluorescence spectroscopy) are taken from Shales *et al.* (1980). U, uninduced; I, induced.

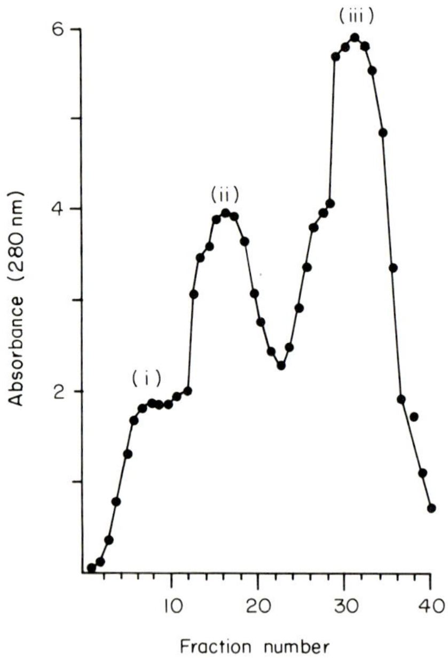

FIG. 5. Fractionation of serum using Sephacryl S200.
Peak (i) IgA, peak (ii) IgG, peak (iii) albumin.

Experimental details

Preparation of antiserum. We raised antiserum to whole cell lysates of *E. coli* K-12 DU1200 by immunizing rabbits (4 mg per injection) according to the protocol of Smyth *et al.* (1978). Immunoglobulin G (IgG) is purified by ammonium sulphate precipitation followed by gel filtration using Sephacryl S-200 (column 40 × 4 cm; elution buffer 0·5 mol/l NaCl, 0·1 mol/l Tris–HCl, 15 mmol/l NaN_3, pH 8·0; flow rate 10 ml/h). Initial fractions containing immunoglobulins M (IgM) and A (IgA) (Fig. 5) are discarded and the IgG concentrated by ultrafiltration (Amicon PM-10) to about one-fifth the original serum volume.

Electrophoresis. Because detailed descriptions of the method can be found in other articles (e.g. Laurell 1965; Weeke 1973; Smyth *et al.* 1978) only a brief account is presented here. Reagents required (apart from IgG and antigens) are listed in Table 7. The procedure is as follows:

(1) Wash four 5 × 5 cm glass slides in detergent, rinse thoroughly and dry. Engrave identifying numbers on one side of each slide.
(2) Ensure slides are dust-free by using a soft brush to sweep them. Apply a thin coat of agarose to one side of each slide using a paint-brush. Dry to a thin film in a drying cabinet.
(3) Place slides on a levelling table and apply 3·3 ml of agarose solution to each slide. Rapidly remove air bubbles with a red-hot inoculating loop and then allow the agarose to set.
(4) Using a template (Fig. 6) punch out wells for application of antigens.

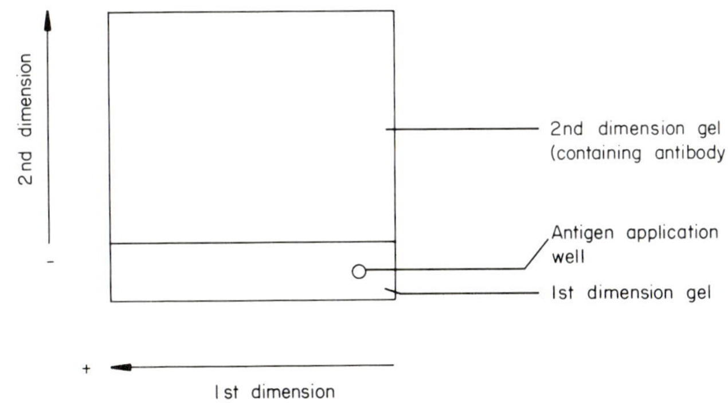

FIG. 6. Template used in crossed immunoelectrophoresis.

(5) Place the gels on the cooling labyrinth of an electrophoresis apparatus (e.g. Behring Diagnostics) and line them up centrally with the sample application wells at the top left as viewed from above (anode to right).

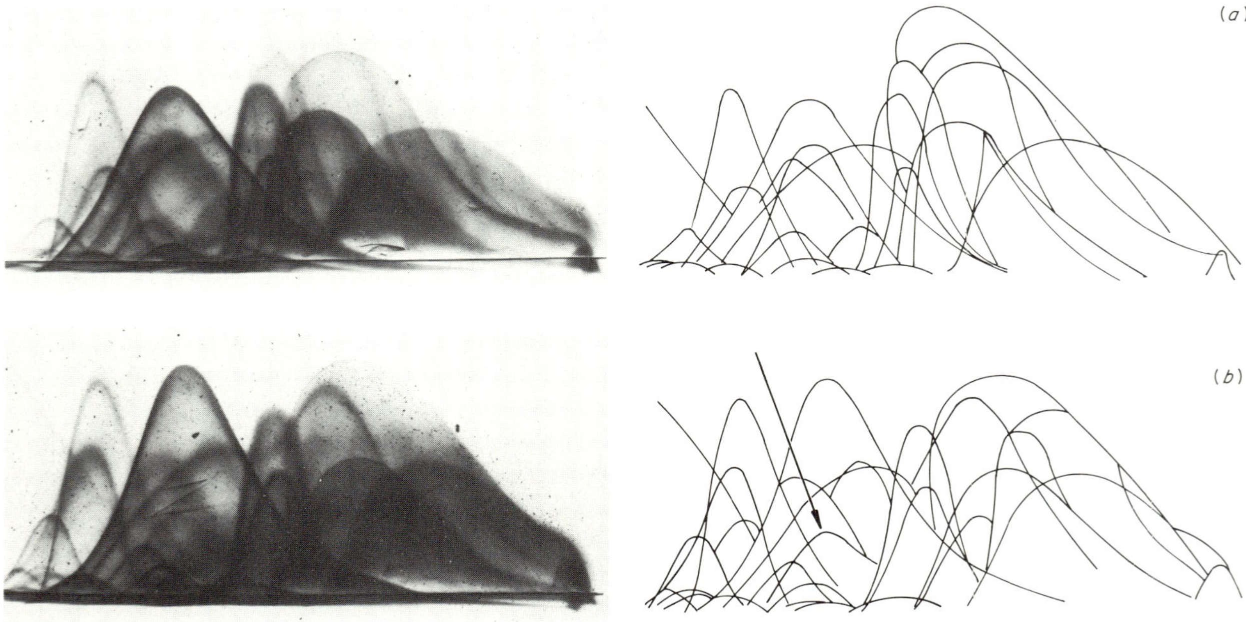

(a)

(b)

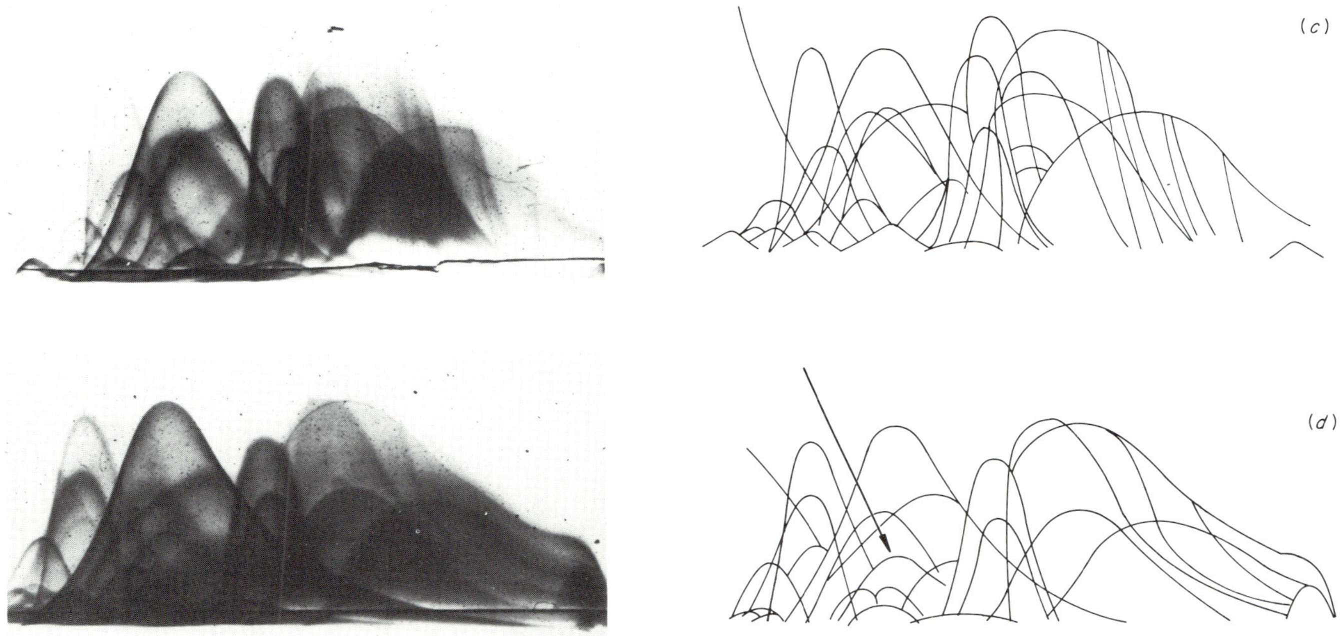

FIG. 7. Immunoprecipitate profile from analysis of cytoplasmic membranes by crossed immunoelectrophoresis. Antigens (100 μg protein) were resolved by first dimension electrophoresis into 1% agarose gels (anode at left above) followed by second dimension electrophoresis (anode at top above) into 1% agarose gels containing IgG (3 mg/cm^3 gel) raised to cell lysates of strain DU1200 (Table 6). Strains analysed were: (*a*) JC3272, (*b*) DU1200, (*c*) DU3091, (*d*) DU3091 grown for several generations in the presence of tetracycline (0·5 μg/ml). Arrows denote the presence of a novel antigen in strains expressing high-level resistance to tetracycline (see text).

Leave a gap of about 5 mm between the slides and ensure that they are approximately parallel to each other. Attach wicks (made from absorbent cloths) and fill electrode tanks with barbital buffer. Ensure that the buffer levels in the tanks are equivalent and then load the wells with antigen (we have used 100 μg protein in a volume of 4 μl).

(6) Switch on power supply and adjust the voltage to 5 V/cm. Electrophoresis is now performed for about 1 h.

(7) After 1 h the gels are removed. Wash the sample application wells and cut away the upper portion of the gel (Fig. 6). Place the gels on a levelling table and apply 2·7 ml of agarose containing IgG (3 mg/cm^3 gel). Allow the gels to set and then re-position them on the cooling labyrinth with application wells at the bottom left as viewed from above (anode to right). Mix the buffer in the electrode tanks, re-connect the wicks and commence electrophoresis (2 V/cm) for about 20 h.

(8) After electrophoresis the gels are soaked in saline for about 30 min. They are then pressed under saline-wetted filter paper covered with several layers of paper towel (plus an additional weight of approximately 1 kg) for 5 min. The process is repeated 2–5 times. Pressed gels are rinsed with distilled water and dried (50–60°C) for 30–60 min.

TABLE 7

Reagents used in crossed immunoelectrophoresis (CIE)

Reagent	Composition
Barbital buffer	Sodium barbitone (5·2 g/litre) adjusted to pH 8·6 with HCl and containing Triton X-100 (1% w/v)
Agarose	Miles HGT agarose (1% w/v) in barbital buffer (fresh solution used to prepare each batch of gels)
Saline	0·1 mol/l NaCl
Stain	Coomassie Brilliant Blue G-250 (0·5% w/v) in ethanol–acetic acid–water (45:10:45). The solution is filtered prior to use
Destain	Ethanol–acetic acid–water (45:10:45)

Gels are stained (5–10 min) and destained using several changes of the solution described in Table 7. The gels are finally dried (50–60°C) and can be stored in this form.

Results and discussion

Figure 7 shows the immunoprecipitate profile when cytoplasmic membranes from JC3272 (*a*) and DU1200 (*b*) were analysed by CIE. An immunoprecipitate detected using cytoplasmic membranes from DU1200 (arrowed in Fig. 7*b*) was absent from JC3272 (Fig. 7*a*). A similar immunoprecipitate was detected using cytoplasmic membranes from induced cultures of DU3091 (Fig. 7*d*), but this was not detected in the cytoplasmic membrane of DU3091 grown in the absence of tetracycline (Fig. 7*c*). The immunoprecipitate was not detected when other cell fractions were analysed (data not shown).

The novel antigen detected by CIE (Fig. 7*b*, *d*) is most probably identical to the protein (mol. wt 36,000, pI 6·4) already detected by two-dimensional electrophoresis (Fig. 4). To confirm this, radiolabelled membrane proteins could be used in conjunction with non-radioactive antisera. The relevant immunoprecipitate would then be excised, subjected to two-dimensional electrophoresis (leading to dissociation of the antibody–antigen complex) and radioactive protein detected by autoradiography or fluorography. This would provide the molecular weight and isoelectric point of the labelled antigen.

References

AMES, G. F-L. & NIKAIDO, K. 1976 Two-dimensional gel electrophoresis of membrane proteins. *Biochemistry* **15,** 616–623.

BALL, P. R., SHALES, S. W. & CHOPRA, I. 1980 Plasmid-mediated tetracycline resistance in *Escherichia coli* involves increased efflux of the antibiotic. *Biochemical and Biophysical Research Communications* **93,** 74–81

CHOPRA, I. 1983 Mode of action of the tetracyclines and the nature of bacterial resistance to them. In *Handbook of Experimental Pharmacology* ed. Boothe, J. H. & Hlavka, J. H. Berlin, Stuttgart and New York: Springer-Verlag. (In press.)

CHOPRA, I. & BALL, P. R. 1982 Transport of antibiotics into bacteria. *Advances in Microbial Physiology* **23,** 183–240.

CHOPRA, I. & ECCLES, S. J. 1978 Diffusion of tetracycline across the outer membrane of *Escherichia coli* K-12: involvement of protein Ia. *Biochemical and Biophysical Research Communications* **83,** 550–557.

CHOPRA, I. & HOWE, T. G. B. 1978 Bacterial resistance to the tetracyclines. *Microbiological Reviews* **42,** 707–724.

CHOPRA, I. & SHALES, S. W. 1980 Comparison of the polypeptide composition of *Escherichia coli* outer membranes prepared by two methods. *Journal of Bacteriology* **144,** 425–427.

CHOPRA, I., HOWE, T. G. B., LINTON, A. H., LINTON, K. B., RICHMOND, M. H. & SPELLER, D. C. E. 1981 The tetracyclines: propsects at the beginning of the 1980s. *Journal of Antimicrobial Chemotherapy* **8,** 5–21.

DAVIES, J. & SMITH, D. I. 1978 Plasmid-determined resistance to antimicrobial agents. *Annual Review of Microbiology* **32,** 469–518.

DOCKTER, M. E. & MAGNUSON, J. A. 1974 Characterisation of the active transport of chlorotetracycline in *Staphylococcus aureus* by a fluorescence technique. *Journal of Supramolecular Structure* **2,** 32–44.

DOCKTER, M. E. & MAGNUSON, J. A. 1975 Membrane phase transitions and the transport of chlorotetracycline. *Archives of Biochemistry and Biophysics* **168,** 81–88.

ECCLES, S., DOCHERTY, A., CHOPRA, I., SHALES, S. W. & BALL, P. 1981 Tetracycline resistance genes from *Bacillus* plasmid pAB124 confer decreased accumulation of the antibiotic in *Bacillus subtilis* but not in *Escherichia coli. Journal of Bacteriology* **145,** 1417–1420.

FERRAZZA, D. & LEVY, S. B. 1980 Biochemical and immunological characterization of an R plasmid-encoded protein with properties resembling those of major cellular outer membrane proteins. *Journal of Bacteriology* **144,** 149–158.

JACKLE, H. 1979 Visualization of proteins after isoelectric focusing during two-dimensional gel electrophoresis. *Analytical Biochemistry* **98,** 81–84.

JACOB, A. E., SHAPIRO, J. A., YAMAMOTO, L., SMITH, D. I., COHEN, S. N. & BERG, D. 1977*a* Plasmids studied in *Escherichia coli* and other enteric bacteria. In *DNA Insertion Elements, Plasmids and Episomes*, ed. Bukhari, A. I., Shapiro, J. A. & Adhya, S. L. pp. 607–638. Cold Spring Harbor Laboratory.

JACOB, A. E., SHAPIRO, J. A. & YAMAMOTO, L. 1977*b* Plasmids of other Gram-positive bacteria. In *DNA Insertion Elements, Plasmids and Episomes*, ed. Bukhari, A. I., Shapiro, J. A. & Adhya, S. L. pp. 663–664. Cold Spring Harbor Laboratory.

JACOBY, G. A. & SHAPIRO, J. A. 1977 Plasmids studied in *Pseudomonas aeruginosa* and other Pseudomonads. In *DNA Insertion Elements, Plasmids and Episomes*. ed. Bukhari, A. I., Shapiro, J. A. & Adhya, S. L. pp. 639–656. Cold Spring Harbor Laboratory.

JORGENSEN, R. A. & REZNIKOFF, W. S. 1979 Organization of structural and regulatory genes that mediate tetracycline resistance in transposon 10. *Journal of Bacteriology* **138,** 705–714.

LAEMLLI, U. K. 1970 Cleavage of structural proteins during the assembly of the head of bacteriophage T4. *Nature, London* **227,** 680–685.

LAURELL, C. B. 1965 Antigen-antibody crossed immunoelectrophoresis. *Analytical Biochemistry* **10,** 358–361.

LEVY, S. B. 1975 The relation of a tetracycline-induced R factor membrane protein to tetracycline resistance. In *Drug Inactivating Enzymes and Antibiotic Resistance*, ed. Mitsuhashi, S. pp. 215–225, Prague: Avecinum.

LEVY, S. B. 1981 The tetracyclines: microbial sensitivity and resistance. In *New Trends in Antibiotics: Research and Therapy*, ed. Grassi, G. G. & Sabath, L. D. pp. 27–44, Amsterdam: Elsevier/North Holland Biomedical Press.

LEVY, S. B. & MCMURRY, L. 1974 Detection of an inducible membrane protein associated with R-factor-mediated tetracycline resistance. *Biochemical and Biophysical Research Communications* **56,** 1060–1068.

LEVY, S. B., MCMURRY, L., ONIGMAN, P. & SAUNDERS, R. M. 1977 Plasmid-mediated tetracycline resistance in *Escherichia coli.* In *Topics in Infectious Diseases,* Vol. 2, ed. Drews, J. & Hogenauer, G. pp. 181–203, New York: Springer-Verlag.

MENDEZ, B., TACHIBANA, C. & LEVY, S. B. 1980 Heterogeneity of tetracycline resistance determinants. *Plasmid* **3,** 99–108.

MCMURRY, L. & LEVY, S. B. 1978 Two transport systems for tetracycline in sensitive *Escherichia coli*: critical role for an initial rapid uptake system insensitive to energy inhibitors. *Antimicrobial Agents and Chemotherapy* **14,** 201–209.

NOVICK, R. P., COHEN, S., YAMAMOTO, L. & SHAPIRO, J. A. 1977. Plasmids of *Staphylococcus aureus*. In *DNA Insertion Elements, Plasmids and Episomes*. ed. Bukhari, A. I., Shapiro, J. A. & Adhya, S. L. pp. 657–662. Cold Spring Harbor Laboratory.

O'FARRELL, P. H. 1975 High-resolution two-dimensional electrophoresis of proteins. *Journal of Biological Chemistry* **250,** 4007–4021.

SALTON, M. R. J. 1978 Structure and function of bacterial plasma membranes. In *Relations between Structure and Function in the Prokaryotic Cell*, ed. Rogers, H. J. & Ward, J. B. pp. 201–223, Twenty-Eighth Symposium of the Society for General Microbiology. Cambridge: University Press.

SAMRA, Z., KRAUSZSTEINMETZ, J. & SOMPOLINSKY, D. 1979 Transport of tetracyclines through the bacterial cell membrane assayed by fluorescence-study with susceptible and resistant strains of *Escherichia coli* and *Staphylococcus aureus*. *Microbios* **21,** 7–22.

SHALES, S. W., CHOPRA, I. & BALL, P. R. 1980 Evidence for more than one mechanism of plasmid-determined tetracycline resistance in *Escherichia coli*. *Journal of General Microbiology* **121,** 221–229.

SMYTH, C. J., SIEGEL, J., SALTON, M. R. J. & OWEN, P. 1978 Immunochemical analysis of inner and outer membranes of *Escherichia coli* by crossed immunoelectrophoresis. *Journal of Bacteriology* **133,** 306–319.

SUBRAMANIAN, A. P. & REEVE, J. N. 1978 Synthesis of ribosomal proteins in λrif^d infected minicells of *Escherichia coli* and selective incorporation into ribosomes. *Federation of European Biochemical Societies, Letters* **95,** 265–269.

WEBER, K. & OSBORN, M. J. 1969 The reliability of molecular weight determinations by dodecyl sulphate-polyacrylamide gel electrophoresis. *Journal of Biological Chemistry* **244,** 4406–4412.

WECKESSER, J. & MAGNUSON, J. A. 1976 Light-induced tetracycline accumulation by *Rhodopseudomonas sphaeroides*. *Journal of Supramolecular Structure* **4,** 515–520.

WECKESSER, J. & MAGNUSON, J. A. 1979 Light-induced, carrier mediated transport of tetracycline by *Rhodopseudomonas sphaeroides*. *Journal of Bacteriology* **138,** 678–683.

WEEKE, B. 1973 Crossed immunoelectrophoresis. *Scandinavian Journal of Immunology* **2** (Supplement 1), 47–56.

ZAMAN, Z. & VERWILGHEN, R. L. 1979 Quantitation of proteins solubilized in sodium dodecyl sulphate-mercaptoethanol-tris electrophoresis buffer. *Analytical Biochemistry* **100,** 64–69.

ZUPANCIC, T. J., KING, S. R., POGUE-GEILE, K. L. & JASKUNAS, S. R. 1980 Identification of a second tetracycline-inducible polypeptide encoded by Tn10. *Journal of Bacteriology* **144,** 346–355.

Note added in proof

Since this article was written important studies on the fluorescence assay for tetracycline transport have been completed (Smith & Chopra 1983). The section dealing with the fluorescence assay (pp. 224–229) reports that fluorescence enhancement and uptake of tetracycline are directly correlated. Although this is true for tetracycline added at concentrations up to 100 μg/ml, deviation occurs above this level (Smith & Chopra 1983). Furthermore, tetracycline uptake is not saturable as implied by the fluorescence assay (Smith & Chopra 1983).

Within the last 18 months major advances have also been made in the field of plasmid-determined tetracycline resistance. These developments will be considered in a further review article (Chopra 1984).

CHOPRA, I. 1984 Bacterial resistance to antibiotics resulting from decreased drug accumulation. In *Antibiotic Resistance in Bacteria*, ed. Datta, N. British Medical Bulletin **40** (in press).

SMITH, M. C. M. & CHOPRA, I. 1983 Limitations of a fluorescence assay for studies on tetracycline transport into *Escherichia coli*. *Antimicrobial Agents and Chemotherapy* **23** (in press).

Methods of Studying Inhibitors of Bacterial Folate Metabolism

D. F. BROAD AND J. T. SMITH

The Microbiology Section, Department of Pharmaceutics, The School of Pharmacy, Brunswick Square, London, UK

Tetrahydrofolic acid (THFA) and its derivatives play a vital role in cellular metabolism as they are the source of one carbon units for protein and purine biosyntheses (Smith 1979). In addition one derivative, N^5,N^{10}-methylene THFA is the sole source of reduction potential for the enzyme thymidylate synthetase in the unique pathway for the production of thymidylate. Thus any depletion of the cell's THFA pool will have extremely deleterious effects upon cellular metabolism, particularly DNA synthesis.

THFA is produced in both bacterial and mammalian cells by the reduction of dihydrofolic acid (DHFA) by the enzyme dihydrofolate reductase (DHFR; 5,6,7,8-tetrahydrofolate: $NADP^+$ oxidoreductase; E.C.1.5.1.3). Thus inhibitors of DHFR are very useful in chemotherapy because they cause such a depletion in the cell's THFA pool with ensuing damage to cellular metabolism. However, to be of use in antibacterial chemotherapy they must be considerably more active against bacterial than mammalian DHFR.

Only one such inhibitor, trimethoprim (Tp), which is 80,000 times more active against the *Escherichia coli* chromosomal DHFR than against mammalian DHFR (Burchall 1979) has been in widespread use, both on its own, but mainly in combination with, the sulphonamide sulphamethoxazole, with considerable success in the treatment of bacterial infection, particularly urinary tract infections. Although another bacterial DHFR inhibitor, tetroxoprim, which is some 50,000 times more active against the *E. coli* chromosomal DHFR than the mammalian DHFR (Aschoff & Vergin 1979) has been introduced it is no more active than Tp against *E. coli* that are either sensitive or resistant to Tp (Broad & Smith 1980).

ANTIBIOTICS
ISBN 0 12 604480 5

Bacteria can resist Tp when they possess R-plasmids that mediate the production of a Tp-resistant DHFR thus allowing the cell to by-pass the action of Tp on the chromosomal Tp-sensitive DHFR (Amyes & Smith 1974). We are interested in monitoring the spread of such R-plasmid-mediated Tp-resistant DHFRs in clinical and veterinary bacterial isolates. However, before this could be undertaken a satisfactory system for classifying these enzymes had to be devised. R-plasmid-mediated Tp-resistant DHFRs have been divided into two types (types I and II) on the basis of their sensitivities to folate inhibitors, with type II DHFRs being considerably more resistant than type I enzymes (Pattishall *et al.* 1977). The first R-plasmid-mediated Tp resistant DHFR discovered, that mediated by R388, appeared to be a type I DHFR on this classification (Amyes & Smith 1974, 1976), as did all the Tp-resistant DHFRs described by Amyes & Smith (1978). These authors also studied the temperature sensitivity of these enzymes and found them all to be extremely labile at 45°C.

Tennhammar-Ekman & Skold (1979) also studied some of the DHFRs described by Amyes & Smith (1978) and concluded on the basis of their inhibitor and temperature sensitivities that the R388 DHFR described by Amyes & Smith (1978), was a type II enzyme (type II DHFRs are resistant to heating at 45°C) and that the DHFR mediated by R751 was a novel type. The situation is further confused by the results obtained by Fling & Elwell (1980) who classified the R751 DHFR as a type II enzyme on the basis of its sub-unit structure and antibody cross-reactivity. Because of the confusion in the classification of these enzymes we have developed a new method for distinguishing between different types of Tp-resistant DHFR by analytical isoelectric focusing. This method is described here with various other methods for classifying these enzymes.

Materials and Methods

Reagents

Dihydrofolic acid and 3-(4,5-dimethylthiazolyl-2)-2,5-diphenyl tetrazolium bromide (MTT) were obtained from Sigma Ltd. NADPH was obtained from P-L Biochemicals Ltd, DEAE-cellulose from Whatman Ltd and bovine serum albumin from Arrow Pharmaceuticals Ltd. Trimethoprim lactate was a generous gift from Wellcome Research Laboratories. Streptomycin sulphate was a generous gift from Glaxo Laboratories.

R-plasmids

All R-plasmids studied were available in this laboratory; R-plasmids

R483, R721, R388 and R751 have been described previously (Amyes & Smith 1978) as have R-plasmids R67bis and R27 (Pattishall *et al.* 1977). The host strain for these R-plasmids was *E. coli* K12 strain J62 which is F^-, *lac*$^-$ and requires proline, tryptophan and histidine (Clowes & Rowley 1954).

Enzyme preparations made from 50-litre bacterial cultures

Bacteria were grown for 18 h at 37°C with aeration in 50 litre minimal medium (Davis & Mingioli 1950) containing 0·28% (w/v) D-glucose and 40 μg/ml of the appropriate L-amino acids. Cells in the stationary phase of growth were then harvested using a Griffin Christ continuous flow centrifuge at 12,000 r/min with a flow rate of 200 ml/min. The pellet was resuspended in 1000 ml of minimal medium without supplements and centrifuged at 5000 **g** for 20 min at 4°C. This constituted the washing process and was repeated as required. The cells were then resuspended in 100 ml of cold 40 mmol/l $Na_2HPO_4.NaH_2PO_4$ buffer pH 7·4 + 1 mmol/l EDTA + 10 mmol/l mercaptoethanol (buffer A). This suspension was ultrasonically disrupted using an M.S.E. ultrasonic disintegrator set at 6 μm peak to peak for 3 × 1 min bursts in a container surrounded by crushed ice and water. The disrupted cell suspension was centrifuged at 32,000 **g** for 60 min at 4°C to remove cell debris. The supernatant was kept as the crude enzyme sample and can be stored at −20°C for at least 1 week. Subsequent operations were performed between 0 and 4°C. Contaminant NADPH oxidase activity was removed by ammonium sulphate precipitation (Amyes & Smith 1974) and nucleic acid was removed by streptomycin precipitation as follows. All centrifugations were at 12,000 **g** for 20 min at 4°C. 0·1 vol. of 10% (w/v) streptomycin sulphate solution was slowly added to the crude enzyme preparation with stirring for 5 min. The mixture was centrifuged and the supernatant fluid made up to 50% saturation by slowly adding solid ammonium sulphate with stirring for 30 min; it was then centrifuged. The pellet, which contained the bulk of the NADPH oxidase activity, was discarded and the supernatant, which contains the DHFR activity, was made up to 80% saturation by slowly adding solid ammonium sulphate with stirring for 30 min, and then centrifuged. The pellet was resuspended in 10 ml of 10 mmol/l Tris–HCl buffer pH 8·5 + 1 mmol/l EDTA + 10 mmol/l 2-mercaptoethanol (buffer B) and dialysed for 18 h at 4°C against 100 volumes of buffer B.

The enzyme sample was then loaded onto a cooled column (30 cm × 2 cm^2) containing DEAE-cellulose (DE52, Whatman Ltd) equilibrated with buffer B. Buffer B was pumped downwards at a flow rate of 60 ml/h until all unbound protein had been eluted (this was monitored by absorbtion at 280 nm). This unbound protein was collected as 10 ml fractions in a cooled fraction collector. A 0–1 mol/l NaCl gradient in buffer B (400 ml) was then applied and 10 ml fractions collected and assayed for DHFR activity and protein content. Fractions containing peak DHFR activity were stored at −20°C for up to several months.

Enzyme preparations made from 5-litre bacterial cultures

The method is essentially the same as that described above for 50-litre bacterial cultures except that bacteria were grown in 2 × 2·5 litre amounts of the medium used for the 50-litre cultures containing additionally 0·18% (w/v) yeast extract in 5-litre flasks for 18 h at 37°C without aeration. The cells were harvested, washed and ultrasonically disrupted as described above, except that they were resuspended in 20 ml of buffer A and ultrasonically disrupted for 2 × 1 min. Streptomycin and ammonium sulphate precipitations were carried out as above with the 80% saturation ammonium sulphate precipitate being resuspended in 3 ml of buffer B. After dialysis the samples were loaded onto a DEAE-cellulose column (20 cm × 2 cm^2) equilibrated with buffer B. Buffer was passed downwards at 60 ml/h and 2·5 ml fractions collected before and after the application of a 0–1 mol/l NaCl gradient in buffer B (100 ml). Fractions were assayed for DHFR activity and those with peak activity stored at −20°C.

Protein determinations

Protein was determined spectrophotometrically by the difference in absorbtion at 225 and 215 nm in 40 mmol/l $Na_2HPO_4.NaH_2PO_4$ buffer pH 7·4 as described by Waddell (1956). Bovine serum albumin was used as a standard.

Dihydrofolate reductase assays

DHFR activity was measured by the method of Osborn & Heunnekens (1958) as described by Amyes & Smith (1976). Assays were performed at 30°C in a Pye Unicam SP30 spectrophotometer fitted with a water jacket maintained at 30°C. The assay mixture contained 50 mmol/l $Na_2HPO_4.NaH_2PO_4$ buffer pH 6·0 + 10 mmol/l 2-mercaptoethanol, 0·08 mmol/l NADPH (stock solution made fresh daily at a concentration of 1 mmol/l in water), the required amount of enzyme solution, and trimethoprim if required, made to a final volume of 2·3 ml with water. The blank was as for the assay mixture except that the NADPH was replaced by water. A 4-min equilibration period was allowed during which time any DHFA-independent NADPH oxidase activity could be measured by the decrease in absorbance at 340 nm and could be allowed for in the calculation of DHFR activity. At the fourth minute 0·2 ml aliquots of a 1 mmol/l solution of DHFA in 50 mmol/l $Na_2HPO_4.NaH_2PO_4$ buffer pH 7·4 + 50 mmol/l 2-mercaptoethanol (which can be stored in separate aliquots at −20°C for up to 1 week) were added to both the blank and the assay mixture, and the rate of conversion of DHFA to THFA followed by the decrease in absorbance at 340 nm. By reference to standard curves, the DHFR activity could be calculated after making allowance for any DHFA-independent NADPH oxidase activity and for the contribution of the oxidation of NADPH involved in the production of THFA from DHFA to the overall decrease in absorbance at 340 nm. DHFR activity is expressed as nmol DHFA reduced/min/ml (Units/ml).

Temperature sensitivity tests

These tests were performed at 45°C by heating the enzyme preparations eluted after DEAE-cellulose chromatography which were in buffer B to which, unlike other workers (Zolg *et al.* 1978), NADPH was not added, for the required amount of time. The enzyme preparations were then rapidly cooled by immersion in ice and assayed for DHFR activity.

Trimethoprim sensitivity tests

These were performed by adding the required amount of Tp, in the form of Tp lactate (as opposed to pure Tp dissolved in 96% ethanol as used by Amyes and Smith (1978)) to the assay mixture and incubated at 30°C for 4 min prior to the addition of the substrate, DHFA.

Preparation of DHFR samples for isoelectric focusing

Fractions in 10 mmol/l Tris–HCl buffer pH 8·5 + 10 mmol/l 2-mercaptoethanol + 1 mmol/l EDTA containing peak DHFR activities after ion-exchange chromatography were pooled and used as a source of enzyme for isoelectric focusing. Samples were dialysed against 100 vols of water for 6 h with stirring at 4°C to reduce the concentration of any ions present that might interfere with the isoelectric focusing. These samples were concentrated, if necessary, by rapidly shell-freezing them in liquid nitrogen followed by freeze-drying. The lyophilized samples were then resuspended in ice-cold water prior to isoelectric focusing.

It was found that fractions containing the peak DHFR activities mediated by R-plasmids R483 and R721 also contained protein(s) that precipitated in acid conditions, giving heavy precipitates during isoelectric focusing and such precipitates took up stain non-specifically. Most of this protein could be removed prior to dialysis by lowering the pH of the sample to pH 6·0 with 0·1 mol/l HCl. This caused heavy precipitation. The resultant precipitate was separated and discarded by centrifugation at 12,000 **g** for 20 min at 4°C. The enzymes were then found to be stabilized by the addition of 1 mg/ml bovine serum albumin (to replace protein that had been precipitated) and by then increasing the pH to 8·5 by the addition of 0·1 mol/l NaOH. These samples were then dialysed as described above prior to isoelectric focusing. This treatment did not alter the pI of any of the DHFRs studied and was therefore used routinely for all enzyme samples.

Isoelectric focusing

Isoelectric focusing was carried out using an LKB 2103 power supply and LKB 2117 Multiphor apparatus. Pre-packed ampholine PAG plates (pH range 3·5–9·5) were obtained from LKB. These plates were used according to the manufacturer's instructions with 1 mol/l H_3PO_4 as the anode solution and 1 mol/l NaOH as the cathode solution. The gels were cooled during electrophoresis by pumping iced water through the base plate of the Multiphor apparatus.

Isoelectric focusing was performed using constant power of 15 W/gel. Prior to loading the samples, current was passed through the gel for 20 min to allow the pH gradient to form. Samples (15 μl of suitably diluted enzyme loaded onto 3 MM Whatman Paratex filters obtained from LKB) were then placed onto the gel. Because of the problem of acid precipitable protein in the R483 and R721 enzyme samples it was found that better results were obtained if these samples were loaded at the acidic (anode) end of the gel (although the position of applying the samples on the gels did not affect the pI of any of the enzymes studied).

Isoelectric focusing was allowed to progress for a further 45 min when the sample filter papers were removed. Isoelectric focusing was then continued until there was no further decrease in current (usually 45 min). If focusing was allowed to occur for longer periods no alteration in pI occurred although the enzyme activity decreased with time.

The pH gradient in the gel was then measured using a Pye Unicam surface pH electrode at 1-cm intervals along the gel. As it was possible that during these measurements of the pH values the bands of focused proteins could have broadened due to diffusion they were refocused for 15 min prior to removal of each gel for staining.

Enzymic staining of gels

Bands of DHFR activity were located on the gels using the zymographic stain described previously (Tennhammar-Ekman & Skold 1979). The tetrazolium salt MTT is reduced by THFA, which is produced by DHFR from the substrate DHFA, to form an insoluble blue precipitate at the site of DHFR activity. Non-specific reduction of MTT was monitored for by incubating control gels containing enzyme with staining mixture that lacked DHFA. Trimethoprim (10^{-5} mol/l) was included routinely in the staining mixture except when *E. coli* K12 strain J62 chromosomal DHFR samples were being used, in which case the staining was done both in the presence and absence of 10^{-5} mol/l trimethoprim.

Results and Discussion

R-plasmid-mediated DHFRs studied

The Tp-resistant DHFRs mediated by R-plasmids R483 and R721 have been classified as type I DHFRs (Amyes & Smith 1978; Tennhammar-Ekman & Skold 1979). Those mediated by R-plasmids R67bis and R27 are prototype type II DHFRs (Pattishall *et al.* 1977) and as discussed above there is some confusion as to the classification of the DHFRs mediated by the R-plasmids R388 and R751.

Before these Tp-resistant DHFRs can be studied they must first be separated from the host chromosomal Tp-sensitive DHFR. This is achieved using DEAE–cellulose ion-exchange chromatography.

Purification of DHFRs by ion-exchange chromatography

After ion-exchange chromatography the host strain *E. coli* K12 J62 showed a single peak of DHFR activity, which was eluted at an NaCl concentration of 0·37 mol/l (Fig. 1*a*, Table 1). The activity of this peak was abolished completely in the presence of 4×10^{-6} mol/l Tp. All the R-plasmid containing strains, however, exhibited two peaks of DHFR activity (Fig. 1*b* to *g*), one of which corresponded to the host chromosomal, Tp-sensitive DHFR, and the other to the R-plasmid-mediated Tp-resistant enzyme, which retained its activity in the presence of 4×10^{-6} mol/l Tp. The DHFRs coded for by R-plasmids R483 and R721 were eluted with 0·21 mol/l NaCl (Fig. 1*b*, *c*; Table 1) whereas the DHFRs mediated by R67bis, R27 and by R388 were eluted with a significantly lower NaCl concentration of 0·16 mol/l NaCl (Fig. 1*d*, *e*, *f*; Table 1). Thus the type I and type II DHFRs can be clearly distinguished even by ion-exchange chromatography, with the R388 mediated DHFR eluting as a type II enzyme.

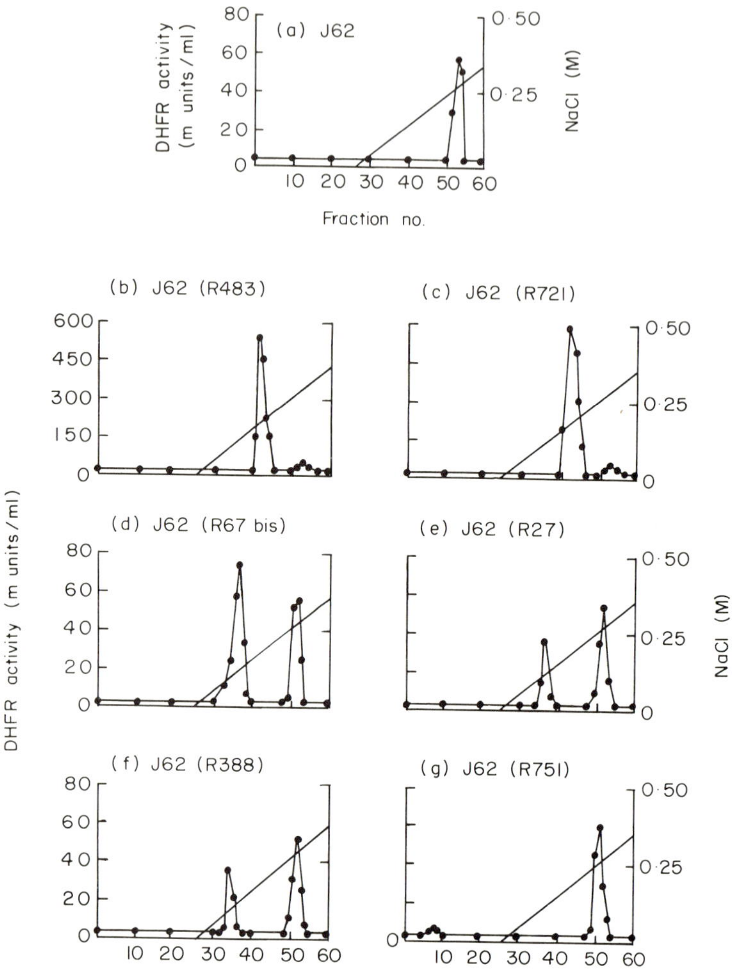

FIG. 1. Elution of DHFR activity after ion-exchange chromatography using DEAE–cellulose.——NaCl gradient; ●——● DHFR activity.

The R751 Tp-resistant DHFR did not bind to the column (Fig. 1*g*), but was eluted with unbound protein prior to application of the NaCl gradient, indicating that it differs from both type I and type II DHFRs.

These results clearly indicate that the type I, type II and R751 DHFRs have different overall charges and thus could possibly be separated by isoelectric focusing. The amount of each type of R-plasmid Tp-sensitive chromosomal DHFR, relative to the amount of Tp-sensitive chromosomal DHFR produced is also different for each type (Table 1). In agreement

TABLE 1

Properties of dihydrofolate reductases

DHFR source	Ratio of R-plasmid to chromosomal DHFR*	NaCl concentration to elute DHFR activity (mol/l)†	pI	ID_{50} for Tp (mol/l)	Time to inhibit 50% activity at 45°C (min)
R483	11·5	0·21	6·4	$3·0 \times 10^{-4}$	0·5
R721	11·9	0·21	6·4	$3·0 \times 10^{-4}$	0·5
R67bis	1·49	0·16	5·5	$2·0 \times 10^{-2}$	>15
R27	0·46	0·16	5·5	$4·0 \times 10^{-2}$	>15
R388	0·56	0·16	5·5	$8·0 \times 10^{-2}$	>15
R751	0·07	0‡	7·2	$2·0 \times 10^{-2}$	>15
E. coli K12 strain J62 chromosomal	—	0·37	4·4 and 4·0	$2·0 \times 10^{-8}$	>15

* Taken from enzyme activities eluted after DEAE–cellulose ion-exchange chromatography (Fig. 1).

† Taken from DEAE–cellulose ion-exchange chromatography results (Fig. 1). In the case of the R-plasmid-mediated DHFRs the NaCl concentration refers to these and not to the *E. coli* K12 strain J62 DHFR which was also eluted during this process.

‡ Did not bind to the DEAE–cellulose resin.

with previous studies (Pattishall *et al.* 1977; Amyes & Smith 1978; Tennhammar-Ekman & Skold 1979) considerably more (approximately ten times more) type I DHFR than chromosomal enzyme is produced, whereas there were approximately equal amounts of type II DHFR and chromosomal enzyme. With the DHFRs mediated by R388 and by R751, both Amyes & Smith (1978) and Tennhammar-Ekman & Skold (1979) found that considerably smaller amounts of these enzymes than the host chromosomal DHFR were produced, although in this study it was found that this was the case only for the R751-mediated DHFR, with the R388-mediated enzyme behaving as a typical type II DHFR (Table 1).

Classification of Tp-resistant DHFRs

If a classification system is to be devised for epidemiological studies for these enzymes it must be relatively simple and unambiguous because of the large numbers of isolates involved in such studies. Below are discussed some criteria which have been used for the classification of Tp-resistant DHFRs and which might satisfy these requirements.

Enzymic properties—Trimethoprim and heat sensitivity of DHFRs

Amyes & Smith (1978) studied the DHFRs mediated by R388, R751, R483 and R721 and found that on the basis of their M_rs, heat sensitivities and trimethoprim sensitivities, they were all similar, having properties characteristic of type I DHFRs. They found that they all had M_rs of between 33,000 and 38,000, ID_{50} values for Tp of $1{\cdot}0 \times 10^{-4}$ mol/l and were extremely sensitive to heating at 45°C, losing more than half their activity in less than 2 min at this temperature. The type II DHFRs described by Pattishall *et al.* (1977) had similar molecular weights to type I enzymes, but were considerably more resistant to Tp, having ID_{50} values of between 6·0 and $7{\cdot}0 \times 10^{-2}$ mol/l. These authors did not study the heat sensitivities of these enzymes. Tennhammar-Ekman & Skold (1979) also studied the Tp and heat sensitivities of the DHFRs mediated by R-plasmids R483, R388, R721 and R751 and found, in agreement with Aymes & Smith (1978), that the ID_{50} values for Tp against the R483- and R721-mediated DHFRs were about 1×10^{-4} mol/l and that these enzymes were extremely labile at 45°C.

However, they found that the R388- and R751-mediated DHFRs and ID_{50} values for Tp were similar to those obtained for type II DHFRs, being 1×10^{-2} to 1×10^{-3} mol/l and 1×10^{-1} to 1×10^{-2} mol/l, respectively. They also found that these enzymes were extremely resistant to heating at 45°C, losing little activity after 15 min at this temperature. Thus the only difference between the classification of the R388- and

R751-mediated DHFRs by Amyes & Smith (1978) and other workers appears to be on the basis of the heat and Tp sensitivities of these enzymes, both of which are enzymic techniques and as such may vary with different assay conditions used in different laboratories.

For instance, the DHFR enzyme co-factor NADPH is known to protect Tp-resistant DHFR against heat inactivation. It was found (Zolg *et al.* 1978) that the R388-mediated DHFR retained its activity for at least 20 min at 100°C when heated in the presence of 0·75 mmol/l NADPH. We have also found (unpublished results) that this concentration of NADPH protects the R483- and R721-mediated DHFRs (which have a half-life of 0·5 min at 45°C (Table 1)) against inactivation at 45°C.

Furthermore, the form of Tp used for inhibition studies varies from laboratory to laboratory. Because pure Tp base is too insoluble in aqueous solution to use at the high concentrations required for inhibition studies, some workers (Tennhammar-Ekman & Skold 1979) use Tp-lactate which is more soluble than Tp base, while others (Amyes & Smith 1978) solubilize pure Tp in 96% ethanol. In this study the ID_{50} values for Tp were determined using Tp-lactate and the temperature sensitivities were determined in the absence of added NADPH.

The temperature and Tp sensitivities of the R483, R721, R67bis, R27, R388 and R751 R-plasmid-mediated DHFRs and the *E. coli* K12 J62 host chromosomal DHFR, which was included as a control, were therefore studied to determine whether they could provide a basis for classification. The ID_{50} values for Tp were determined using Tp-lactate and the temperature sensitivities were determined at 45°C in the absence of added NADPH.

In agreement with previous authors (Pattishall *et al.* 1977; Amyes & Smith 1978; Tennhammar-Ekman & Skold 1979) the ID_{50} values for Tp against the R483- and R721-mediated DHFRs were both found to be $3{\cdot}0 \times 10^{-4}$ mol/l (Table 1) and are typical of type I DHFRs. The DHFRs mediated by R67bis and R27 had considerably higher ID_{50} values against Tp, i.e. between $1{\cdot}0 \times 10^{-2}$ and $1{\cdot}0 \times 10^{-1}$ mol/l (Table 1) and are therefore in agreement with the ID_{50} values for type II DHFRs described by Pattishall *et al.* (1977). We found that the R388- and R751-mediated DHFRs also have 'type II ID_{50}s' of between $1{\cdot}0 \times 10^{-2}$ and $1{\cdot}0 \times 10^{-1}$ mol/l for Tp (Table 1) and are therefore in contrast to those results obtained by Amyes & Smith (1978). As expected, the *E. coli* K12 strain J62 chromosomal DHFR was considerably more sensitive to Tp, having an ID_{50} value of $2{\cdot}0 \times 10^{-8}$ mol/l (Table 1).

The DHFRs mediated by R483 and R721 also showed temperature sensitivities at 45°C typical of type I enzymes, losing over 90% of their activity within 2 min at this temperature (Table 1), whereas the DHFRs mediated by R67bis, R27, R388 and R751, like the *E. coli* K12 strain J62 chromosomal DHFR, were all stable at 45°C, retaining more than 90% of their activity after 15 min at this temperature (Table 1). Thus the R388- and R751-mediated DHFRs appear not to be type I enzymes even when classified on the basis of heat and Tp sensititivity.

Thus the R388- and R751-mediated DHFRs appear to be of type II by these criteria which is in contrast with the results obtained by Amyes and Smith (1978). Also Tennhammar-Ekman & Skold (1979) suggested that the R751 had enzymic properties different to those of both type I and type II DHFRs. It is in fact probable that the R751 DHFR is a variant type II enzyme (see 'Isoelectric focusing'). Hence the use of Tp and temperature sensitivities of these DHFRs did not appear to be a sufficiently sensitive method of classifying these enzymes.

Serology

It was hoped to raise serum in rabbits against type I (R483) and type II (R67bis) DHFRs, which would allow the differentiation of these two groups of enzymes and also possibly facilitate the discovery of any new groups of Tp-resistant DHFRs.

DHFR preparations obtained after DEAE–cellulose chromatography were used to immunize the rabbits; however, because these preparations were not pure (no method of purifying these enzymes had been developed at the time) immunoprecipitation techniques could not be used to test for immunological cross-reactivity. Instead enzymes and serum samples were mixed in equal proportions and incubated for 18 h at 4 or 20°C (it was necessary to include 0·75 mmol/l NADPH in these mixtures to stabilize the type I DHFRs; 0·75 mmol/l NADPH was in fact included in all DHFR samples for both immunization and enzyme inhibition tests) and assayed for remaining DHFR activity. In some experiments immune precipitates were removed by centrifugation and the supernatants assayed for DHFR activity. These remaining activities were then compared to those in control samples containing enzyme and serum from non-immunized rabbits.

It was found that serum from rabbits that had been immunized with R483 DHFR inhibited not only this enzyme but also the R721 DHFR (this inhibition was not improved by removing immune precipitates). However, this serum did not inhibit the *E. coli* K12 J62 chromosomal, R67bis, R27, R388 and R751 DHFRs. This confirms that the R483 and R721 enzymes are similar (type I) DHFRs, whereas the R388 and R751 DHFRs are not.

Attempts to raise serum in rabbits that were immunized with the R67bis DHFR, however, proved unsuccessful. During the course of these studies Fling & Elwell (1980) reported that they had raised serum against another type II DHFR, that mediated by R-plasmid R67 (which is thought to be identical to that mediated by R-plasmid R67bis (Pattishall *et al.* 1977)). However, these authors did not measure antibody inhibition of enzyme activity but used *Staphylococcus aureus* cells which contain protein A (which binds to IgG and IgG–antigen complexes (Kessler 1975)) to precipitate complexes formed between anti-R67 DHFR antibodies and enzymes. Using this technique they found that their anti-R67 DHFR serum showed no cross-reactivity with the R483 DHFR protein, whereas it did cross-react with both the R388 and R751 DHFR proteins.

Attempts to use *Staph. aureus* NCTC 8530 cells to precipitate antibody–enzyme complexes formed between our putative anti-R67bis serum and R67bis DHFR, however, proved unsuccessful, as did the use of anti-rabbit IgG serum produced in sheep, extended incubation periods of the serum/enzyme mixture and high speed (60,000 **g** for 60 min) centrifugation to precipitate any antibody–enzyme complexes.

The reasons for our failure to produce serum active against type II DHFR remain unclear but it could be that Fling & Elwell (1980) used pure R67 DHFR to immunize their rabbits whereas in our study impure enzyme was used. Fling & Elwell (1980) were able to utilize facilities at the Wellcome Research Laboratories, North Carolina, to produce large numbers of R-plasmid-containing cells for the purification of DHFR whereas such facilities were unavailable at our, and indeed most, university research laboratories.

It may, however, be fortuitous that we were unable to raise serum against type II DHFRs because, as mentioned above, the anti-type II DHFR serum raised by Fling & Elwell (1980) showed immunological cross-reactivity with the R751 DHFR whereas our isoelectric focusing results (see next section) indicate that the R751 is not a type II DHFR but a variant of this type. Hence, it would appear that serology is not a sensitive enough technique to be used for epidemiological studies of R-plasmid-mediated Tp-resistant DHFRs.

Analytical isoelectric focusing

The results obtained during the separation of DHFRs by DEAE–cellulose chromatography (Fig. 1; Table 1) indicated that the type I, type II and R751 DHFRs had different overall charges and thus could possibly be separated by analytical isoelectric focusing. Rcsults obtained by Tennhammar-Ekman & Skold (1979) with normal polyacrylamide gel electrophoresis reinforced this view.

Initially enzyme fractions with peak DHFR activity obtained from 50 litre bacterial cultures after DEAE–cellulose ion-exchange chromatography were pooled, subjected to analytical isoelectric focusing and stained for DHFR activity.

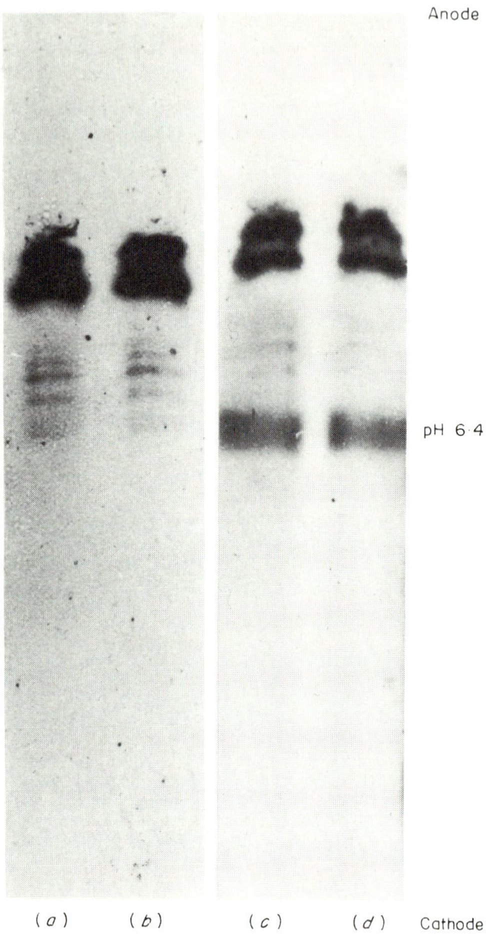

FIG. 2. Isoelectric focusing of R483 and R721 DHFRs. R483 samples contained, in 15 μl, 94·1 mUnits of DHFR activity and 945 μg of protein. R721 samples contained, in 15 μl, 84·1 mUnits of DHFR activity and 1008 μg of protein. Tracks (*a*) and (*b*) are the R483 and R721 DHFR samples respectively, stained in the absence of substrate dihydrofolic acid. Tracks (*c*) and (*d*) are the R483 and R721 DHFR samples respectively, stained in the presence of dihydrofolic acid.

The R483 and R721 preparations showed heavy staining even in the absence of the substrate DHFA (Fig. 2, tracks *a* and *b*). However, when DHFA was included in the assay mixture an extra band with a pI of 6·4 was seen in both the R483 and R721 enzyme samples (Fig. 2 tracks *c* and *d*; Table 1). These correspond to the R-plasmid-mediated DHFRs and, in agreement with the ion-exhange chromatography results, indicate that these two type I DHFRs have the same overall charge.

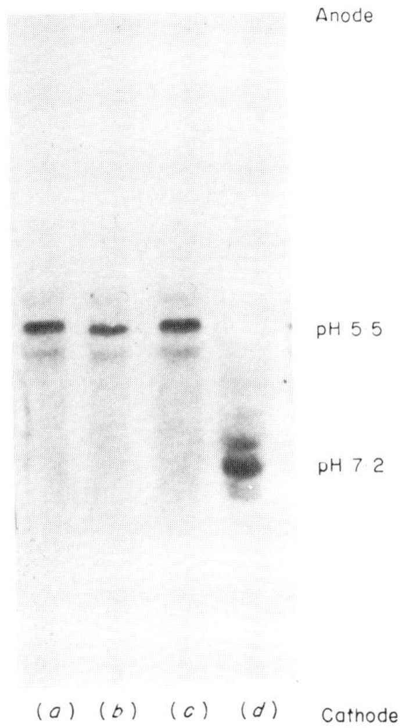

FIG. 3. Isoelectric focusing of the R388, R751, R67bis and R27 DHFRs. All samples were stained in the presence of substrate dihydrofolic acid. Track (*a*) R67bis sample containing 0·18 mUnit DHFR activity and 43·5 μg of protein. Track (*b*) R27 sample containing 0·27 mUnit DHFR activity and 45·1 μg of protein. Track (*c*) R388 sample containing 0·15 mUnit DHFR activity and 42·0 μg of protein. Track (*d*) R751 sample containing 0·33 mUnit DHFR activity and 60·2 μg of protein. All samples were in a volume of 15 μl.

When the R27, R67bis, R388 and R751 DHFR preparations were subjected to isoelectric focusing and stained in the absence of dihydrofolic acid no bands were seen, indicating that no non-specific staining occurred. When DHFA was included in the assay mixture a major band of pI 5·5 was seen in the R67bis, R27 and R388 preparations and of pI 7·2 in the R751 DHFR preparation (Fig. 3 tracks *a*, *b*, *c* and *d*; Table 1). This confirms that the R388-mediated DHFR is indeed a type II DHFR, whereas the R751 enzyme is different from both type I and type II DHFRs. Minor bands of pI 5·1 and 6·0 were seen occasionally in the R67bis, R27 and R388 samples stained in the presence of DHFA, but not in corresponding samples stained in the absence of the substrate. Similarly minor bands of pI 6·9, 7·8 and 7·9 were seen occasionally in R751 preparations. These could correspond to isoenzymic forms of these enzymes (multiple bands of protein are often seen during isoelectric focusing) or they could represent multimeric forms of these enzymes, which have been observed previously (Zolg *et al.* 1978; Smith *et al.* 1979).

When the *E. coli* K12 strain J62 Tp-sensitive chromosomal DHFR preparation was examined by isoelectric focusing two bands, of pI 4·0 and pI 4·4, were seen in the samples stained in the presence of DHFA (Table 1); these bands did not stain, however, if 1×10^{-5} mol/l Tp was added to, or DHFA was omitted from the staining mixture. These bands, therefore, correspond to the chromosomal DHFR and their pIs are in good agreement with those obtained elsewhere (Baccanari *et al.* 1977) where two isoenzymic forms of the *E. coli* B chromosomal DHFR were also observed. Because of the low pI of these bands it proved very difficult to stain them zymographically to a degree of resolution which would facilitate the production of reasonable photographs. No such photographs are therefore included.

These results were, however, obtained using enzyme samples prepared from 50-litre bacterial cultures, which do not lend themselves to epidemiological studies. A 'scale down' technique using 5-litre bacterial cultures was therefore developed. This technique is essentially the same as that used for 50-litre bacterial cultures except that because the level of enzyme and protein present in these DHFR samples is less the need to remove acid-precipitable protein from these samples is obviated. However, type I DHFRs are extremely labile and considerable activity is lost in the dialysis procedure used to remove ions present in the enzyme samples prior to analytical isoelectric focusing. This can be overcome largely by including 0·75 mmol/l NADPH in the enzyme samples prior to dialysis. This treatment does not alter the pI values of the type I DHFRs or indeed of any other DHFR studied and was therefore used routinely. Also, considerable amounts of heat are generated during analytical isoelectric focusing and thus great care must be taken to ensure adequate cooling of the gels. This problem should be eased by the use of recently developed gels thinner than those used in this study, which have a consequent decrease in power required for, and thus heat generated during, analytical isoelectric focusing.

This 'scale-down' technique allows the type I and type II DHFRs to be studied by analytical isoelectric focusing, although it cannot be used for the R751 DHFR because only minute amounts of Tp-resistant DHFR are produced by cells harbouring this R-plasmid. Therefore 50-litre bacterial cultures must be used to study this type of DHFR. This is not, however, such a major problem as it would appear because the majority of R-plasmid-mediated Tp-resistant DHFRs found in this country so far appear to be of type I (unpublished results), a situation analogous to that observed with R-plasmid-mediated β-lactamases where the TEM-type enzymes preponderate (Hedges *et al.* 1974).

Summary

An analytical isoelectric focusing method has been developed which clearly separates three distinct groups of Tp-resistant R-plasmid-mediated DHFRs from each other and from the *E. coli* K12 strain J62 Tp-sensitive, chromosomal DHFR using enzyme samples prepared from 50 litre bacterial cultures. This has been scaled down successfully to using 5 litre bacterial cultures which facilitates the use of analytical isoelectric focusing for epidemiological studies.

This separation by analytical isoelectric focusing is in agreement with the results obtained by ion-exchange chromatography which also separated three distinct types of R-plasmid-mediated Tp-resistant DHFRs. However, the elution profiles of these enzymes by an NaCl gradient during ion-exchange chromatography, using an anion exchange resin at pH 8·5, would appear to indicate that the *E. coli* K12 strain J62 chromosomal DHFR would have the lowest pI value followed by the type I R-plasmid DHFRs (R483 and R721), then the type II R-plasmid-mediated DHFRs (R67bis, R27 and R388) with the R751-mediated DHFR having the highest pI value. Whilst the *E. coli* K12 strain J62 chromosomal DHFR had the lowest pI value (pH 4·0 and 4·4) and the R751-mediated DHFR had the highest (pH 7·2), the position is reversed for the type I and type II DHFRs, with the type I enzymes having pI values of pH 6·4 and that of the type II DHFRs being pH 5·5. One reason for this could be that a type II DHFR was purified using hydrophobic interaction chromatography (Smith *et al.* 1979), indicating that this enzyme was relatively hydrophobic. This hydrophobicity could result in decreased binding of type II DHFRs to the hydrophilic matrix used during ion-exchange chromatography than would be expected from their pI values. Similarly it would have been expected that the R751-mediated DHFR with a pI of 7·2 would have bound to the anion-exchange resin at pH 8·5, whereas it did not bind to the column, eluting with the unbound protein. It could be that this DHFR is also relatively hydrophobic. Probably the DHFR mediated by R751 is a variant type II enzyme because it has a similar sub-unit structure to other type II DHFRs and also shows immunological cross-reaction with serum raised against type II DHFRs (Fling & Elwell 1980). Also, in our laboratory it could not be separated enzymically, only on the basis of charge, i.e. by ion-exchange chromatography and by isoelectric focusing, from type II DHFRs.

Analytical isoelectric focusing appears to be superior to other techniques used to identify R-plasmid-mediated, Tp-resistant DHFRs in that enzymic studies have indicated that the R388 DHFR is both a type I (Amyes & Smith 1978) and a type II DHFR (Tennhammar-Ekman & Skold 1979; this study), with the R751 DHFR being classified as a type I DHFR (Amyes & Smith 1978), type II DHFR (this study) and a type III DHFR (Tennhammar-Ekman & Skold 1979). Serological studies indicated that the R388 and R751 DHFRs are type II enzymes (Fling & Elwell 1980), whereas analytical isoelectric focusing indicates that the R751 DHFR is neither a type I nor a type II DHFR although the R388 DHFR appears to be type II.

D. F. B. is grateful to the Medical Research Council for financial support. J. T. S. is grateful to the Royal Society for an equipment grant to purchase analytical isoelectric focusing equipment.

References

AMYES, S. G. B. & SMITH, J. T. 1974 R-factor trimethoprim resistance mechanism: an insusceptible target site. *Biochemical and Biophysical Research Communications* **58,** 412–418.

AMYES, S. G. B. & SMITH, J. T. 1976 The purification and properties of the trimethoprim-resistant dihydrofolate reductase mediated by the R-factor, R388. *European Journal of Biochemistry* **61,** 597–603.

AMYES, S. G. B. & SMITH, J. T. 1978 R-factor mediated dihydrofolate reductases which confer trimethoprim resistance. *Journal of General Microbiology* **107,** 263–271.

ASCHOFF, H. S. & VERGIN, H. 1979 Tetroxoprim—a new inhibitor of dihydrofolate reductase. *Journal of Antimicrobial Chemotherapy* **5** (Supplement B), 19–25.

BACCANARI, D. P., AVERETT, D., BRIGGS, C. & BURCHALL, J. 1977 *Escherichia coli* dihydrofolate reductase: isolation and characterization of two isozymes. *Biochemistry* **16,** 3566–3572.

BROAD, D. F. & SMITH, J. T. 1980 Activity of tetroxoprim against R-factor mediated trimethoprim resistant bacteria. *Journal of Pharmacy and Pharmacology* **32,** 29P.

BURCHALL, J. J. 1979 The development of diaminopyrimidines. *Journal of Antimicrobial Chemotherapy* **5** (Supplement B), 3–14.

CLOWES, R. C. & ROWLEY, D. 1954 Some observations on linkage effects in genetic recombination in *Escherichia coli* K12. *Journal of General Microbiology* **11,** 250–260.

DAVIS, B. D. & MINGIOLI, E. S. 1950. Mutants of *Escherichia coli* requiring methionine or vitamin B12. *Journal of Bacteriology* **60,** 17–28.

FLING, M. E. & ELWELL, L. P. 1980 Protein expression in *Escherichia coli* minicells containing recombinant plasmids specifying trimethoprim-resistant dihydrofolate reductases. *Journal of Bacteriology* **141,** 779–785.

HEDGES, R. W., DATTA, N., KONTOMICHALOU, P. & SMITH, J. T. 1974 Molecular specificities of R-factor determined β-lactamases: correlation with plasmid compatibility. *Journal of Bacteriology* **117,** 56–62.

KESSLER, S. W. 1975 Rapid isolation of antigens from cells with a staphylococcus protein A-antibody absorbant: parameter for interaction of antibody–antigen complexes with protein A. *Journal of Immunology* **115,** 1617–1624.

OSBORN, M. J. & HUENNEKENS, F. M. 1958 Enzymic reduction of dihydrofolic acid. *Journal of Biological Chemistry* **233,** 964–974.

PATTISHALL, K. H., ACAR, J., BURCHALL, J. J., GOLDSTEIN, F. W. & HARVEY, R. J. 1977 Two distinct types of trimethoprim-resistant dihydrofolate reductase specified by R-plasmids of different compatibility groups. *Journal of Biological Chemistry* **252,** 2319–2323.

SMITH, J. T. 1979 In *Antibiotic Interactions* ed. Williams, J. D. pp. 87–98. London & New York: Academic Press.

SMITH, S. S., STONE, D., NOVAK, P., BACCANARI, D. P. & BURCHALL, J. J. 1979 R-plasmid dihydrofolate reductase with sub-unit structure. *Journal of Biological Chemistry* **254,** 6222–6225.

TENNHAMMAR-EKMAN, B. & SKOLD, O. 1979 Trimethoprim resistance plasmids of different origin encode different drug-resistant dihydrofolate reductases. *Plasmid* **2,** 334–346.

WADDELL, W. J. 1956 A simple ultraviolet spectrophotometric method for the determination of protein. *Journal of Laboratory and Clinical Medicine* **48,** 311–314.

ZOLG, J. W., HANGGI, U. J. & ZACHAU, H. G. 1978 Isolation of a small DNA fragment carrying the gene for a dihydrofolate reductase from a trimethoprim resistance factor. *Molecular and General Genetics* **164,** 15–29.

Methods of Studying Transferable Resistance To Antibiotics *In Vitro*

J. A. FROST, E. J. THRELFALL AND G. A. WILLSHAW

Division of Enteric Pathogens, Central Public Health Laboratory, Colindale, London, UK

Transferable drug resistance was first demonstrated in shigellae isolated in Japan in 1959 (Ochiai *et al.* 1959; Akiba *et al.* 1960). The first evidence for plasmid-determined resistance in the UK was provided by N. Datta, who described an epidemic strain of drug-resistant *Salmonella typhimurium* in 1962 (Datta 1962). Since then, plasmid-determined resistance has been shown to be of considerable importance in many organisms throughout the world.

The most dramatic incident to date was an epidemic of Shiga dysentery which started in Guatemala in 1969 (Gangarosa *et al.* 1970) and spread through Central America causing many thousands of deaths. The strain of *Shigella dysenteriae* 1 involved was resistant to chloramphenicol, streptomycin, sulphonamides and tetracyclines; these resistances were shown to be plasmid-determined. This epidemic was closely followed by a typhoid epidemic which started in Mexico in 1972 causing over 10,000 infections and many deaths (Anderson 1975). Since both the *Salm. typhi* and *Sh. dysenteriae* 1 strains involved were resistant to the same drugs it was initially thought that the same resistance plasmid might have been present in both the shigella and the *Salm. typhi*. Genetic studies showed that the two plasmids belonged to different compatibility groups; H in the *Salm. typhi* and B in the *Sh. dysenteriae*, and were therefore completely unrelated (Grindley *et al.* 1972).

Since 1970 the Enteric Reference Laboratory, now part of the Division of Enteric Pathogens, has studied resistance plasmids in enteric bacteria, particularly *Salm. typhimurium*, from many parts of the world. It has been shown that many plasmid types have distinctive distribution patterns both in the host bacteria in which they are most frequently encountered and in the geographical areas in which they predominate (Anderson 1977).

ANTIBIOTICS
ISBN 0 12 604480 5

Thus, the identification of the plasmids present in the strain may provide valuable information as to the possible source of the infection.

The value of plasmid characterization in epidemiological studies has been further demonstrated in the tracing of multiresistant strains of *Salm. typhimurium* which have become epizootic in cattle in Britain and subsequently appeared in human infections. This epidemiological pattern first emerged in *Salm. typhimurium* phage type 29 between 1963 and 1970 (Anderson 1968) and more recently in *Salm. typhimurium* phage types 204 and 193 between 1974 and the present. The latter example is discussed in some detail in this volume, pp. 285–297.

Plasmid Classification

Historically, plasmids were first differentiated by the ability of some plasmids to restrict the fertility of the sex factor F (Watanabe *et al.* 1964). Further discrimination was provided by the observation that closely related plasmids cannot coexist stably in the same cell. This incompatibility has led to the definition of at least 30 different compatibility groups and forms the basis of resistance plasmid classification.

Different compatibility groups can be distinguished by a number of characteristics such as transfer kinetics, plasmid-specific phage propagation and typing phage restriction, as well as incompatibility. Plasmids belonging to the same compatibility group often have a relatively narrow range of molecular weights and a high level of DNA homology (Grindley *et al.* 1973). In recent years, relatively simple, quick and inexpensive methods have been devised to prepare plasmid DNA from bacterial strains and to separate and visualize it by agarose gel electrophoresis. These techniques are used together with genetic studies to identify and characterize plasmids coding for drug resistance or other properties. The results obtained with three representative *Salm. typhimurium* strains are given as an example of their use.

The methods used for plasmid characterization have been summarized by Anderson & Threlfall (1974). Although these have been developed specifically in relation to enterobacterial plasmids, the principles can be applied to plasmids from other groups of micro-organisms. By exploiting differences in transfer kinetics and interactions with various bacteriophages, it has been possible to develop a pattern of investigation which, in the more straightforward examples, results in the identification of the compatibility group with the minimum number of tests. This system is shown schematically in Fig. 1.

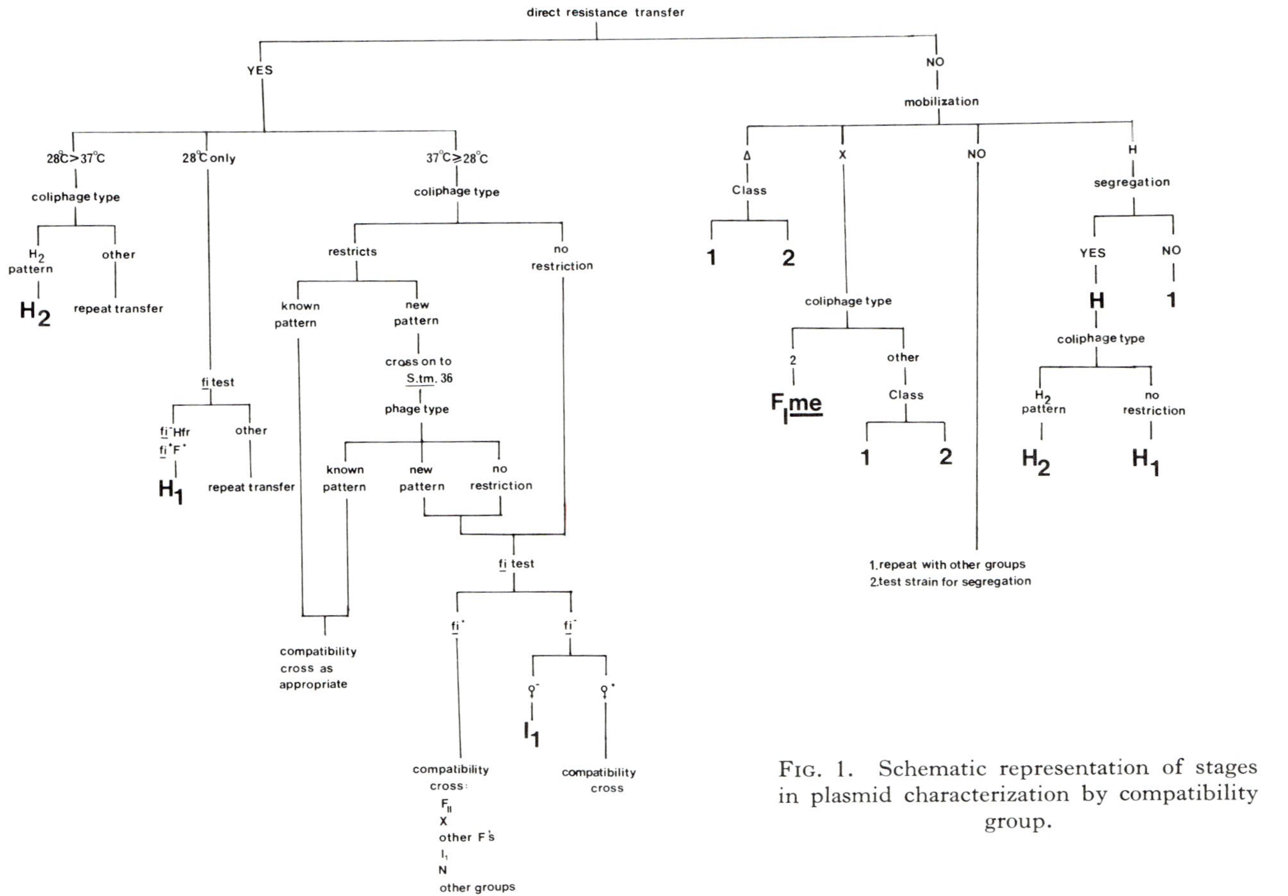

FIG. 1. Schematic representation of stages in plasmid characterization by compatibility group.

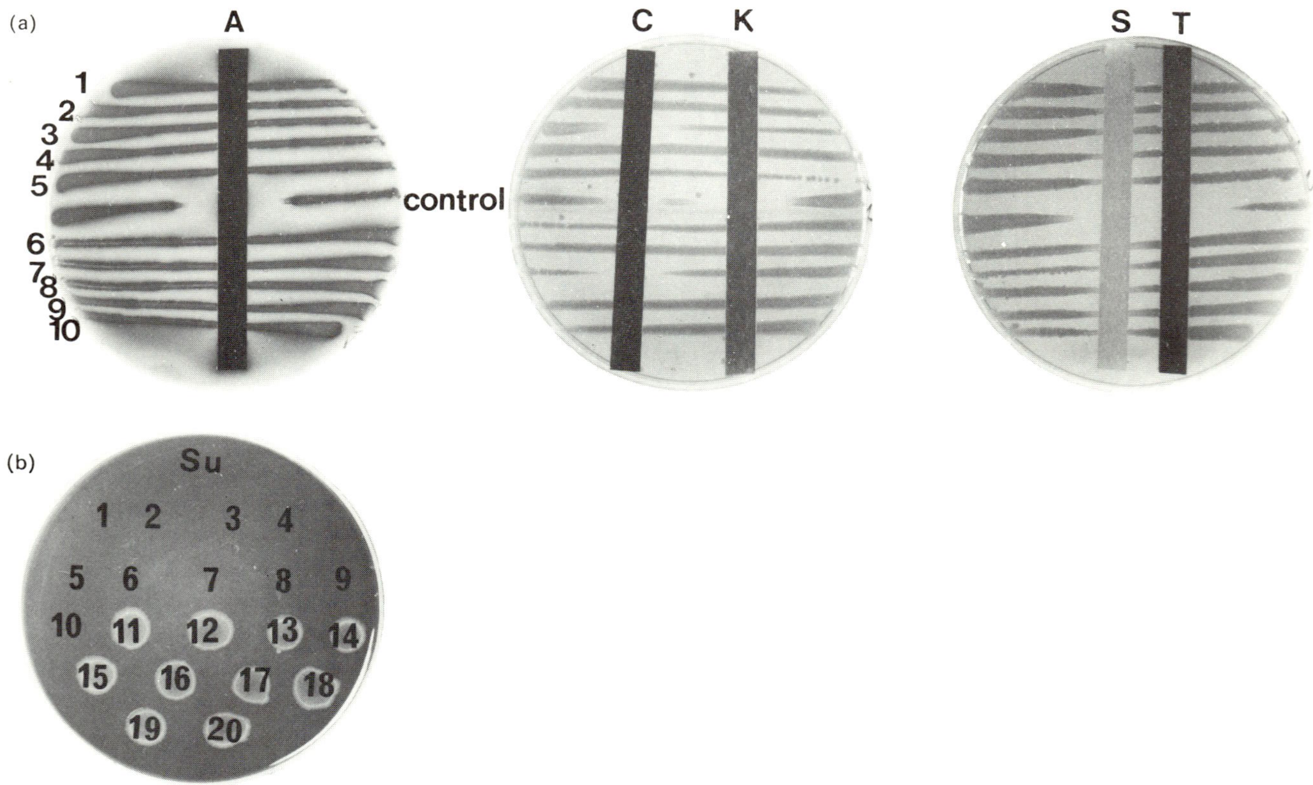

FIG. 2. Drug resistance tests—R-typing. (*a*) Example of R-typing against ampicillin (A), chloramphenicol (C), kanamycin (K), streptomycin (S) and tetracyclines (T). Picks 1, 2, 4, 5, 6, 7, 9 and 10 are resistant to ACKST. Picks 3 and 8 are resistant to AKST. (*b*) R-typing against sulphonamides (Su). Spots 1–10 are sensitive, spots 11–20 are Su resistant.

Testing for Drug Resistance

Resistance to most antibiotics is tested by a diffusion method on nutrient agar plates using blotting paper strips soaked with the respective drugs, then freeze-dried. Ten test cultures and one control are streaked across each plate and one or two strips laid at right angles to the cultures (Fig. 2*a*). Resistance to sulphonamides and trimethoprim is detected by spotting 0·01 ml drops of a 10^{-4} dilution of a late exponential culture onto a nutrient agar plate containing 5% v/v lysed horse blood and the appropriate drug. Resistance to spectinomycin, nalidixic acid and furazolidone is detected by spotting onto nutrient agar plus antibiotics. Up to 30 cultures can be tested on each plate plus positive and negative controls (Fig. 2*b*). The concentrations of antibiotics used in preparing strips and pouring plates are shown in Table 1.

TABLE 1

Antibiotic concentrations in strips and media

Code	Antibiotic	Concentration in plates (μg/ml)	Concentration in solution for preparing strips (μg/ml)
A	Ampicillin	100 or 50	1000
C	Chloramphenicol	20	300
G	Gentamicin	20	300
K	Kanamycin	20	5000
S	Streptomycin	20 or 40	2500
T	Tetracycline	5, 10 or 20	2500
Su	Sulphonamides	100*	Not applicable
Sp	Spectinomycin	100	Not applicable
Tm	Trimethoprim	0·5*	Not applicable
Fu	Furazolidone	20	Not applicable
Nx	Nalidixic acid	20	Not applicable

* Nutrient agar + 5% v/v lysed horse blood.

Colicinogeny Testing

This is performed by the method of Fredericq (1948). Broth cultures are stabbed with a straight wire onto nutrient agar plates. After overnight incubation at 37°C the colonies are killed by inverting the plates over watchglasses containing chloroform for 10–15 min, before drying for 30 min. Each plate is overlayered with 5 ml of 0·4% nutrient agar containing 0·3 ml of a broth culture of a sensitive indicator strain. The plates are incubated overnight and colicin production is detected as an inhibition zone

Table 2

Characterization of resistance plasmids in three multiresistant Salmonella typhimurium *strains*

Host strain		13M60 *Salm. typhimurium* phage type 193*	15M1030 *Salm. typhimurium* phage type 200†			18M3919 *Salm. typhimurium* phage type 122‡	
Direct transfer		AKT	ASSuT	K col Ib	CSSu		
	28°C	10^{-1}	10^{-3}	10^{-2}	10^{-1}	—	
	37°C	—	10^{-1}	10^{0}	10^{-3}	—	
Mobilization						SSu	ACKSSuSpTGTm
	I_1					10^{-1}	—
	F_{II}					—	10^{-2}
Fertility inhibition	F^+	+	—	—	—	—	+
	Hfr	—	—	—	—	—	+
Phage restriction	K12	—	9	3	16	—	2
	Stm 36	—	NC1	125	125	—	NC10
Compatibility group		H_1	N	I_1	H_2	2	$F_I me$
Molecular weight (daltons × 10^6)		>100	28	65	>100	6	90

* Isolated in England, 1973, from 5-year-old child; family outbreak of gastroenteritis (source unknown) resistant to AKT.
† Isolated in Belgium, 1975, from bovine source, resistant to ACKSSuT + col Ib.
‡ Isolated in India, 1978, from 40-year-old male with fatal septicaemia from nosocomial hospital infection, resistant to ACKSSuSpTGTm.

in the indicator lawn. The type of colicin can be identified by using standard indicator strains, each resistant to a known colicin.

Drug Resistance Transfer

Autotransferring plasmids

Ideally crosses are set up with one parent a lactose fermenter, the other *lac*⁻. Thus, by plating on MacConkey agar, the parents can easily be differentiated. The recipient strain carries chromosomal resistance to either nalidixic acid, rifamycin or streptomycin, depending on the sensitivity of the donor to these agents. If a suitable, chromosomally resistant strain is not available, then 0·3 ml of either colicin E_2 (titre 1 : 32) or salmonella phage 01 (Felix & Callow 1943) (titre > 10^{11}) is used to eliminate *Escherichia coli* and *Salm. typhimurium* respectively. These are spread over the selective plates immediately before inoculation.

Broth cultures of donor and recipient strains are grown with shaking at 37°C to exponential phase. The cultures are mixed in equal volumes, usually 1 ml, and incubated overnight. Crosses are set up at both 28 and 37°C because transfer frequencies vary between compatibility groups (see Fig. 1; Table 2).

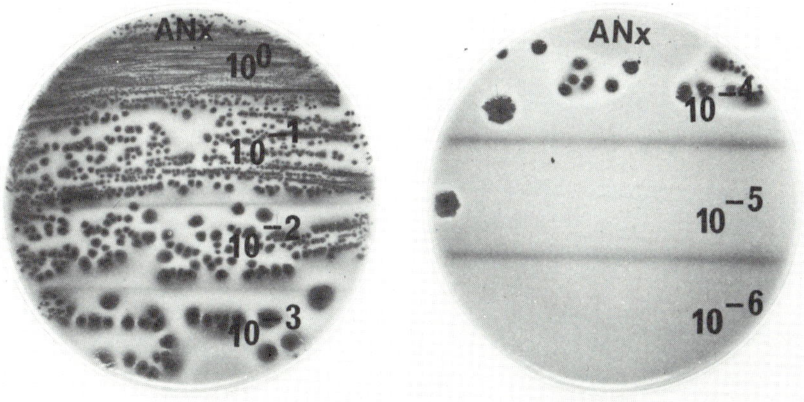

FIG. 3. Resistance transfer: 0·01 ml aliquots of mating mixture, dilutions 10^{0} to 10^{-6}, are plated on MacConkey agar containing an antibiotic (A) and nalidixic acid (Nx). Resistant recipients = 5×10^{6}/ml.

After incubation, serial decimal dilutions are prepared in phosphate buffer and 0·01 ml volumes plated on MacConkey agar with suitable selective agents, in duplicate (Fig. 3). The mating mixture dilutions are also plated on MacConkey agar without any selective agent to obtain colony counts for each parent. The plates are incubated overnight at 37°C and colonies counted. Transfer frequency is expressed as the proportion of resistant progeny per recipient cell. The transfer frequencies obtained with one of the representative strains are given in Table 3.

Ten colonies picked from each antibiotic plate are then R-typed against all the resistances present. Two colonies of each resistance pattern (= R-type) are retained for further study.

TABLE 3

Direct resistance transfer in overnight crosses from 15M1030—Salmonella typhimurium *200, ACKSSuT, to 14R525*—Escherichia coli *K12, F^-*lac$^+$ *Nal^r*

Incubation temperature	Selection		Transfer frequency	R-type 10 colonies	Plasmids present		
28°C	A	Nx	$2{\cdot}3 \times 10^{-3}$	ACKSSuT (10)	H_2	I_1	N
	C	Nx	$1{\cdot}3 \times 10^{-1}$	CSSu (10)	H_2		
	K	Nx	$2{\cdot}9 \times 10^{-2}$	CKSSu (8)	H_2	I_1	
				K (2)		I_1	
	S	Nx	$7{\cdot}0 \times 10^{-2}$	CSSu (10)	H_2		
	Su	Nx	$5{\cdot}2 \times 10^{-2}$	CSSu (10)	H_2		
	T	Nx	$4{\cdot}5 \times 10^{-4}$	ACKSSuT (8)	H_2	I_1	N
				ACSSuT (2)	H_2		N
37°C	A	Nx	$1{\cdot}1 \times 10^{-1}$	AKSSuT (9)		I_1	N
				ASSuT (1)			N
	C	Nx	$1{\cdot}8 \times 10^{-3}$	ACKSSuT (10)	H_2	I_1	N
	K	Nx	10^{0}	K (10)		I_1	
	S	Nx	$1{\cdot}4 \times 10^{-2}$	ACKSSuT (8)	H_2	I_1	N
				AKSSuT (2)		I_1	N
	Su	Nx	$1{\cdot}8 \times 10^{-2}$	ACKSSuT (10)	H_2	I_1	N
	T	Nx	$9{\cdot}8 \times 10^{-3}$	AKSSuT (10)		I_1	N

Resistance symbols: A, ampicillin; C, chloramphenicol; K, kanamycin; S, streptomycin; Su, sulphonamides; T, tetracyclines; Nx, nalidixic acid.

Mobilization of non-autotransferring plasmids

Where no direct transfer is detected, strains are examined for resistance mobilization in a triparental cross (Anderson 1965). Equal volumes of a late exponential culture of the donor strain, carrying a standard transfer factor, and the wild strain, are mixed and incubated at the appropriate temperature for at least 2 h. The plasmid-free recipient is then added and the mixture incubated overnight. The cross is plated on selective media with counter-selection against both the donor and wild strain. Resistant recipient colonies are then picked and R-typed as above.

Class of transfer system

At this stage it is important to establish how many plasmids are involved and whether the resistances transferred are linked to or independent of the transmissible plasmids. This distinction, between a Class 1 transfer system in which the resistance genes and transfer genes are covalently linked, and a Class 2 system where a transfer factor co-transfers a non-autotransferring resistance plasmid, must be made before compatibility crosses are attempted.

A Class 2 transfer system can usually be detected by interrupted crosses. Mating is interrupted at intervals from 15 min to 4 h and the cross plated in the usual manner. If the transfer and resistance genes are on different plasmids then some resistant progeny may only carry the one plasmid and be unable to transfer the resistance on to a subsequent cross. Progeny are therefore picked and R-typed and crosses set up to a further standard strain. If the transfer factor in a Class 2 system restricts coliphages, then this property can also be used to detect variations in the plasmid content of resistant progeny.

Initially each segregant of a different R-type from the wild strain is treated as though it carried a different plasmid. If, however, it seems that the wild strains carried two plasmids which are incompatible with each other they must, by definition, be segregants of the same plasmid. This can be confirmed by analysis of the plasmid DNA from appropriate strains.

Tests for Fertility Inhibition (*fi*)

Most F-like plasmids and some members of other compatibility groups inhibit the fertility of the sex factor F. This phenomenon can most easily be demonstrated as inhibition of visible lysis by the F-specific phage μ2.

The plasmid to be tested is transferred into both a K12 Hfr and a K12 F^+ strain as described above. Both strains are used because plasmids of some compatibility groups, notably H_1, displace the F factor from F^+ strains, but not Hfr. Phenotypically the plasmid therefore appears to be fi^+ in F^+ strains but fi^- in Hfr.

The progeny are R-typed and spotted onto nutrient agar using a platinum loop delivering 0·01 ml. The inoculum is then spread over an area of approximately 1 cm and allowed to dry for a few minutes. 0·01 ml of phage, approximate titre 10^{12} p.f.u./ml is spotted onto each culture and the plates incubated for 4 h at 37°C. Plates are prepared in duplicate and one of each pair spotted with phage μ2. The other plate is spotted with phage φ2, an *E. coli* specific phage which is restricted by certain group I_1 plasmids. Fertility inhibition is detected by loss of visible lysis by phage μ2 (Fig. 4).

Plasmid-determined Phage Restriction

Each plasmid is transferred into standard *E. coli* and salmonella strains and the progeny phage typed (Callow 1959; Ashley 1979).

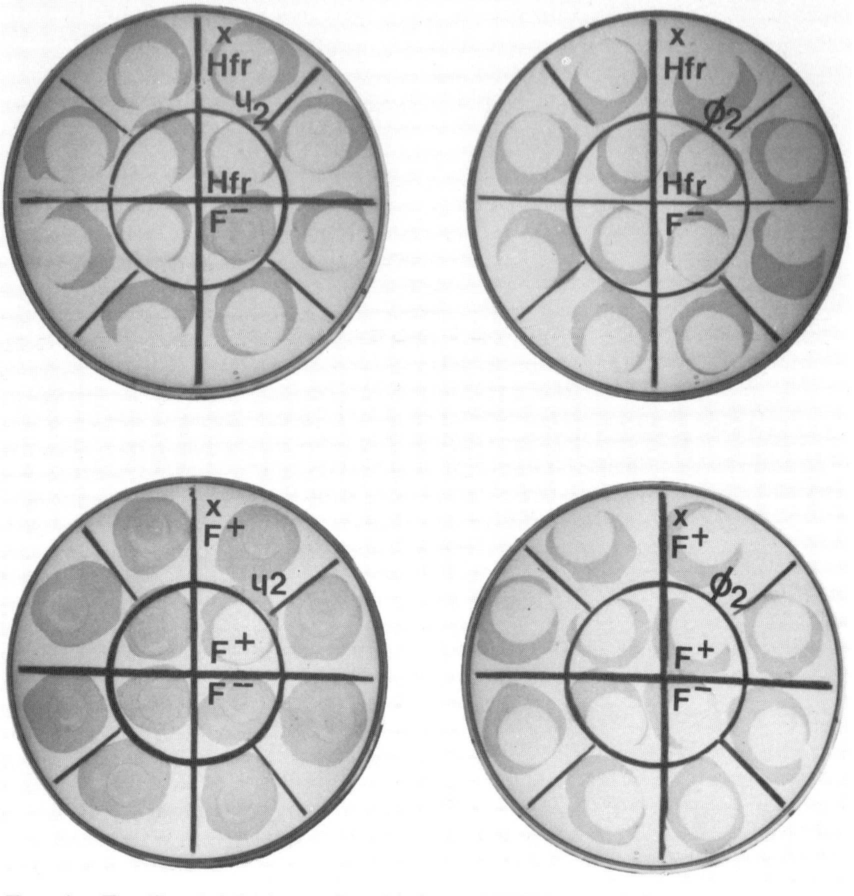

FIG. 4. Fertility inhibition: plasmid from 13M60 tested for inhibition of F fertility in Hfr and F^+; see text. Ten progeny plus Hfr or F^+ and F^- controls spotted with phages $\mu 2$ and $\varphi 2$.

Plasmids can be tested for coliphage restriction in the *E. coli* K12 host after direct transfer or mobilization. If the plasmid does not restrict, or gives an atypical restriction pattern, then the plasmid may be transferred on into *Salm. typhimurium* phage type 36 and phage typed in that organism. In many cases the resultant patterns in *E. coli* and *Salm. typhimurium* will indicate which compatibility crosses are necessary to confirm the plasmid's identity (Fig. 1). Although many plasmids restrict typing phages in *Salm. typhi*, transfer to this organism is only employed as a last resort because of the stringent safety precautions required. One advantage of the use of coliphage restriction is the ready availability of the phages employed to many laboratories. The coliphage restriction patterns determined by the plasmids described in Table 2 are shown in Table 4.

TABLE 4

Coliphage typing

Pick	R-type	Typing phages													Type
		1	2	3	4	5	6	7	8	9	10	11	12	13	
10R151 (13M60) A1	AKT	cl	< cl	cl	cl	cl	cl	< cl	cl	scl	cl	cl	cl	cl	1
10R151 (Δ/18M3919) S1	SSu	cl	+ +//scl	< cl	cl	< cl	±	< cl	< cl	+ + +	cl	scl	+ +	cl	6
10R151 (X/18M3919) A1	ACKSSuSpTGTm	–	scl	< cl	cl	cl	cl	scl	< scl	cl	cl	< cl	scl	cl	2
10R151 (15M1030) A14	ASSuT	+	< cl	cl	< cl	cl	cl	+ +	+ +	cl	+ + +	< cl	scl	+ + +	9
10R151 (15M1030) K3	K	< cl	< scl	cl	–	< cl	< cl	cl	cl	–	cl	< cl	< cl	cl	3
10R151 (15M1030) C1	CSSu	–	+ +	cl	+ +	< cl	< cl	+ + +	+ +	+ + +	+ + +	< cl	–	+ + +	16
10R151	sensitive	cl	< cl	cl	cl	cl	< cl	cl	scl	cl	cl	< cl	cl	cl	1 control

cl, confluent lysis; scl, semi-confluent lysis; + → + + +, increasing numbers of discrete plaques; –, no visible lysis.

Compatibility Tests

In most cases the results obtained with the above tests will give some indication of the compatibility group to which a plasmid belongs (Fig. 1). Compatibility crosses can be set up accordingly.

Compatibility between two plasmids is demonstrated by introducing one plasmid into a strain carrying the other and examining recipient colonies for stability of the two plasmids.

In general, if the plasmids belong to the same compatibility group, the resident plasmid will be displaced. Where both plasmids are present, the clones are tested for segregation after growth at 37°C for 6 and 24 h. The strains are then plated on nutrient agar and, the following day, replica-plated on selective media. Compatible plasmids will segregate at the same rate as their spontaneous loss from control strains carrying only one plasmid. If no segregation is observed the strains are tested for independent transfer of the two plasmids, since the resistance markers may have recombined or transposed onto the same plasmid.

Plasmids of the same compatibility group often exhibit a degree of entry exclusion (Novick 1969), the extent of which varies from group to group. Exclusion can be demonstrated by comparing the transfer frequency of a plasmid into a plasmid-free recipient with its frequency of transfer into a strain carrying a plasmid of the same compatibility group. In crosses with a high level of surface exclusion, it may be difficult to obtain transconjugants unless the cross is plated on media with selection for both plasmids.

Plasmid-specific Phage Propagation

A number of phages have been isolated whose attachment sites are on plasmid-determined pili. These phages can only infect cells carrying the appropriate plasmids and are usually specific for one, or a number of closely related, compatibility groups. Examples of such phages are given in Table 5.

Phage propagation can be demonstrated as described by Grindley & Anderson (1971). The phage and test strain are incubated together overnight; the bacteria are then removed by centrifugation and the supernatant titrated on a suitable plasmid-carrying indicator strain. Propagation is seen as an increase in titre in the presence of a suitable plasmid compared with a plasmid-free control.

This property is particularly useful in the identification of transfer factors in a Class 2 system where the resistance markers are on an independent plasmid and hence not displaced in a compatibility cross. It is also helpful in classifying plasmids with unusual compatibility properties.

TABLE 5

Plasmid-specific phages

Phage	Compatibility groups	Reference
μ2	$F_I - F_{IV}$	Dettori *et al.* (1961)
If1	I_1, I_2	Meynell & Lawn (1968)
IKe	N	Khatoon *et al.* (1972)
PRD1	N,P,W	Olsen *et al.* (1974)
C-1	C	Sirgel *et al.* (1981)

Methods for Preparation of Partially Purified Plasmid DNA

Many procedures are now published and some which differ in scale and principle are outlined below.

Small-scale method for rapid screening of plasmid-carrying strains

A technique of plasmid DNA preparation developed by Birnboim & Doly (1979) exploits the relative stability to denaturation by alkaline conditions of covalently closed circular plasmid DNA. The method is very rapid and reliable, and we have used it to detect plasmids in wild and laboratory strains of *E. coli*, in salmonellas, shigellas, yersinias and pseudomonads. A microcentrifuge capable of spinning samples at about 10,000 **g** is required. Cultures are grown in 2·5 ml volumes of nutrient broth without shaking for 18 h at 37°C; between 0·5 and 1·0 ml samples are harvested by centrifugation in 1·5 ml polypropylene tubes in an Eppendorf microcentrifuge. The cell pellet is resuspended in the same tubes by vortexing with 0·1 ml of a freshly prepared solution containing 2 mg/ml lysozyme, 10 mmol/l EDTA and 50 mmol/l glucose in 25 mmol/l Tris–HCl buffer pH 8·0. After 10–30 min on ice, the bacteria are lysed by adding 0·2 ml of 1% sodium dodecyl sulphate (SDS) in 0·2 N sodium hydroxide. Chromosomal DNA denatured under these conditions is then precipitated with 0·15 ml 3 mol/l sodium acetate pH 4·8 which is mixed with the cell lysate by several inversions of the tubes. After 60 min on ice, the heavy white precipitate is removed by a 5 min centrifugation and a 0·4 ml sample of the supernatant is transferred to a fresh microcentrifuge tube. Ice-cold ethanol (1 ml) is added to precipitate plasmid DNA and the tubes left at −30°C for 30 min. DNA is pelleted by centrifugation for 2 min, dissolved in 0·1 ml 100 mmol/l sodium acetate–50 mmol/l Tris–HCl pH 8·0 and re-precipitated with 2 vols of ethanol. The DNA is finally dissolved in 50 μl 10 mmol/l Tris–HCl pH 8·0 containing 1 mmol/l EDTA (TE) and this solution can be stored if necessary at −30°C before electrophoresis of the whole sample.

Larger scale procedures

These techniques are useful after initial screening of strains for plasmid content and provide samples that can be stored for comparison with future preparations. Plasmid-carrying organisms are harvested in late exponential phase from 20–100 ml volumes of nutrient broth. All subsequent steps are carried out at 0–4°C unless otherwise stated; volumes of reagents are those required for a 50 ml culture.

In one procedure (Clewell & Helinski 1969), bacteria are washed with 0·1 mol/l sodium phosphate buffer pH 7·0 and resuspended in 1·7 ml (25% w/v) sucrose in 50 mmol/l Tris–HCl pH 8·0 to which 0·35 ml lysozyme is added (5 mg/ml in 0·25 mol/l Tris–HCl pH 8·0). After 5 min, 0·7 ml of 0·25 mol/l EDTA pH 8·0 is added; 5 min later gentle lysis of the cells is achieved by the rapid addition of 2·7 ml of a mixture of 1% Brij 58, 0·4% sodium deoxycholate and 62·5 mmol/l EDTA in 0·05 mol/l Tris–HCl pH 8·0. Centrifugation in an angle rotor (MSE 10 × 10) at 48,000 **g** for 30 min removes more than 98% of chromosomal DNA to leave a cleared lysate which is treated as described below.

Another similar procedure uses SDS to lyse bacteria that have been treated with sucrose, lysozyme and EDTA as indicated above (Guerry *et al.* 1973). After lysis with 2·7 ml 2% SDS, chromosomal DNA and protein are precipitated with 1·4 ml 5 mol/l sodium chloride and the mixture kept at 4°C for 18 h. The dense white precipitate is removed by centrifugation at 17,000 **g** for 30 min to yield a cleared lysate.

Lysates obtained from these procedures are diluted with 0·5 vol. 30 mmol/l Tris–HCl pH 8·0 containing 50 mmol/l sodium chloride and 5 mmol/l EDTA (TES) and extracted with 1–2 vols of TES-saturated phenol at room temperature (Meyers *et al.* 1976). Phases are separated by centrifugation in a swinging bucket rotor of a bench centrifuge and phenol treatment is repeated until the upper aqueous phase is clear. This solution is transferred to a centrifuge tube and sodium acetate added to a final concentration of 0·3 mol/l. DNA is precipitated with 2 vols of ice-cold 95% ethanol and mixtures are kept at −10°C for 6 h or overnight. The precipitate obtained after centrifugation in a bench centrifuge for 5 min is dissolved in 150–200 μl of TE buffer and stored at −30°C.

Lysis with Brij is convenient and quick for *E. coli* and salmonella strains but significant loss of plasmids larger than 80 × 10^6 may occur. The SDS lysis method has been applied to a wide range of bacterial species and a modification of this technique has been devised specifically to isolate plasmids of mol. wt up to 300 × 10^6 (Hansen & Olsen 1978).

Agarose Gel Electrophoresis and Molecular Weight Determination

Plasmids of different molecular weights can be separated by electrophoresis on agarose gels. The method described here is that of Willshaw *et al.* (1979), in which electrophoresis is performed in vertical slab gels of approximate dimensions 16 × 15 × 0·4 cm. The gels contain agarose concentrations from 0·5 to 1·0% (w/v; Sigma, type II) depending on the molecular size of the plasmids to be separated. For most screening purposes, a 0·6% (w/v) gel is prepared in electrophoresis buffer pH 8·2 containing 89 mmol/l Tris, 2·5 mmol/l EDTA and 89 mmol/l boric acid. Samples of partially purified plasmid DNA (usually 15–60 μl) are mixed with a solution of 60% (w/v) sucrose and 0·25% (w/v) bromophenol blue in 10 mmol/l Tris–HCl pH 8·0 containing 1 mmol/l EDTA. The samples for electrophoresis contain 6–10% (w/v) sucrose and are loaded under electrophoresis buffer into 0·9 cm wide slots. Electrophoresis of DNA towards the anode is performed at 140 V, a voltage gradient of approximately 9 V/cm, for 2·5–4 h at room temperature.

Gels are soaked for 30 min in an aqueous solution of 0·5 μg/ml ethidium bromide and photographed by ultraviolet light on a short wavelength transilluminator (Ultra Violet Products, San Gabriel, California, USA). DNA bands, which fluoresce pinkish orange, are photographed on Polaroid type 52 Land film or Kodak Tri-X using a ×7 red filter. Plasmid bands containing covalently closed circular molecules appear sharp, in contrast to regions containing fragments of chromosomal DNA in which fluorescent bands are broader and diffuse. The presence of chromosomal DNA can obscure plasmid bands but these can be detected by alteration of gel strength to change the relative migration of chromosomal and plasmid DNA.

The distance migrated by a plasmid is inversely related to its molecular weight. The sizes of plasmids in DNA preparations under investigation can be determined relative to the mobility of reference plasmids, which range in size from 2·6 to 78 × 10^6 and are run as mixtures in two slots of the gel. Often a sample of one of these plasmids is mixed with the DNA under examination as an internal standard. The internal standard is chosen so that it does not co-migrate with, and therefore obscure, any plasmids present in the preparation and for this reason molecular sizes are generally determined after experimental plasmid preparations have been run on a preliminary gel. The mobilities of all plasmid bands are calculated relative to the migration of the internal standard. For the molecular weight standards, a graph of the logarithm of the relative mobility against logarithm of the molecular weight is approximately linear for plasmids from 4 to 80 × 10^6 run on 0·6% gels and this calibration can be used to determine the sizes of plasmids in the samples under investigation. We have compared the sizes of some plasmids measured by gel electrophoresis with those obtained by electron microscopy and found the values to be within 5% of each other. Detailed discussion of the factors affecting DNA migration and molecular weight determination on agarose gels can be found in Johnson & Grossman (1977) and Willshaw *et al.* (1979).

Applications of the Methods

The characterization of the resistance plasmids in three different *Salm. typhimurium* strains is summarized in Table 2. The first example, 13M60. belongs to phage type 193 and is resistant to ampicillin, kanamycin and tetracyclines. This strain was isolated in England in 1973 from a three-year-old child with gastroenteritis. The patient became infected during a family holiday and four other members of the family were also ill. Although the source of infection was not traced, organisms of this type carrying group H_1 plasmids have been isolated in the UK and are usually associated with infections originating in South East Asia.

Plasmids of group H_1 have two easily recognized characteristics. They transfer at a high frequency at 28°C but do not transfer at 37°C; they displace the F factor from an F^+ strain but not Hfr (see 'Fertility inhibition method'). The identity of a plasmid with these characteristics can be confirmed by testing for compatibility with a standard group H_1 plasmid.

Gel electrophoresis shows at least four bands that could correspond to different plasmid species in a DNA preparation from 13M60 (Fig. 5, track 1). These include a slowly migrating band, two species with mol. wt 60–70 $\times$ 10^6 and a band moving ahead of the chromosomal DNA region. The largest plasmid present in 13M60 has a mobility similar to that of a reference plasmid of mol. wt *ca.* 140 $\times$ 10^6 and is the only plasmid present in a K12 transconjugant of R-type AKT that carries the group H_1 plasmid from 13M60 (Fig. 5, track 2).

15M1030, a strain of *Salm. typhimurium*, phage type 200, R-type ACKSSuT, was isolated from a bovine outbreak in Belgium in 1975. This type was one of a number of phage types associated with bovine infections in North West Europe at that time.

Table 2 shows the transfer frequencies obtained by direct transfer from 15M1030 to *E. coli* K12. It is immediately apparent that there is more than one plasmid present since the frequencies vary, e.g. resistance to kanamycin is transferred at 10^0 at 37°C and 10^{-2} at 28°C, while chloramphenicol resistance is transferred at 10^{-1} at 28°C and 10^{-3} at 37°C, frequencies typically associated with group H_2. Coliphage typing of the different

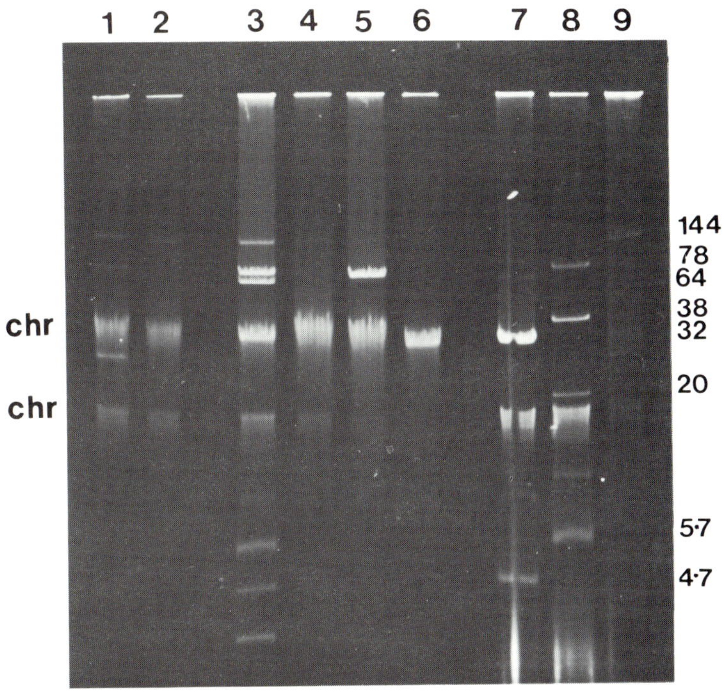

FIG. 5. Agarose gel electrophoresis of plasmids in *Salmonella typhimurium* strains and K12 transconjugants derived from them. Plasmid DNA run in tracks 1 to 6 and 9 was prepared by the alkaline SDS lysis method of Birnboim & Doly (1979). DNA of standard plasmids in tracks 7 and 8 was obtained by phenol treatment of cleared lysates prepared with Brij 58. Electrophoresis was on a 0·6% agarose gel run in Tris–borate buffer at 140 V for 3 h. The position of chromosomal DNA fragments (chr) are indicated, together with the sizes of the reference plasmids. The main region of chromosomal DNA in tracks 7 and 8 has migrated further than the principal chromosomal band in tracks 1 to 6. This difference is found consistently, and reflects the different DNA preparation methods employed. Migration towards the anode was downwards from the origin. The preparations run in tracks 1 to 9 are as follows. 1. *Salm. typhimurium* 13M60; 2. K12 carrying H_1 plasmid from 13M60; 3. *Salm. typhimurium* 15M1030; 4. K12 carrying H_2 plasmid from 15M1030; 5. K12 carrying KColI plasmid from 15M1030; 6. K12 carrying N group plasmid from 15M1030. Standard plasmids are of mol. wt 64×10^6, $31{\cdot}7 \times 10^6$, $4{\cdot}7 \times 10^6$ (track 7); $77{\cdot}6 \times 10^6$, 37·8, 20·2 and $5{\cdot}7 \times 10^6$ (track 8) and 144×10^6 (track 9). Faint bands running between the chromosomal DNA and the 4·7 and $5{\cdot}7 \times 10^6$ plasmids in tracks 7 and 8 are open circular forms of these plasmid molecules.

segregants obtained on R-typing identified a group H_2 plasmid coding for resistance to CSSu, a K-ColI, I_1 plasmid and an ASSuT group N plasmid. The compatibility grouping of these plasmids was confirmed by appropriate crosses. (Tables 2, 3, 4). These three types of plasmid are frequently encountered in both animal and human infections in North West Europe.

Gel electrophoresis of plasmid DNA from 15M1030 (Fig. 5, track 3) shows a very large plasmid, two plasmids in the size range 65–75 $\times$ 10^6 and one band visible within the chromosomal DNA region. Several fast-moving bands are also visible but detailed analysis would be required to determine whether each of these is an independent plasmid or if the bands represent open circular and linear forms of only one or two plasmids (see Johnson & Grossman 1977, and Willshaw *et al.* 1979 for discussion). Transconjugants in tracks 4 and 5 identify the plasmids from 15M1030 that belong to groups H_2 and I_1, and no other plasmids from the wild strain are present in these derivatives. The strain shown in track 6 carries the drug resistance markers of the group N plasmid and the DNA band corresponding to this is located within the chromosomal DNA region. The faint band well separated from that region may contain the open circular form of the group N plasmid.

The third example, 18M3919 is a *Salm. typhimurium* strain belonging to phage type 122, and resistant to ACKSSuSpTGTm. It was isolated in India in 1978. The patient, a 40-year-old male, developed fatal septicaemia as a result of cross-infection during a hospital outbreak of gastroenteritis. Outbreaks caused by this and related organisms have been reported from a number of hospitals throughout India (Rowe *et al.* 1980). Resistances in this strain were not directly transferable but could be mobilized by standard transfer factors (Table 2). Further study identified a non-autotransferring F_I*me* plasmid coding for the complete resistance spectrum and an SSu plasmid which could be mobilized with the standard I_1 transfer factor Δ.

The above examples illustrate how, by following the protocol in Fig. 1, the plasmid content of a strain can often be analysed relatively quickly.

In organisms such as *Salm. typhimurium* where a phage-typing scheme is available, the phage type may be altered by the presence of a plasmid. If the plasmids in such a strain are shown to restrict the typing phages in *Salm. typhimurium* type 36, which is sensitive to all the typing phages, then the possibility of its affecting the phage type of the host strains should be investigated. The restricting plasmid is displaced, either by spontaneous segregation or by transferring a non-restricting plasmid of the same compatibility group into the wild strain. The progeny are then phage typed. If a type change has occurred then the original type can be reconstructed by re-introducing the original plasmid. The value of this technique in the tracing of relationships between strains of different phage types is illustrated in the following chapter (pp. 285–297).

References

AKIBA, T., KOYAMA, K., ISHIKI, Y., KIMURA, K. & FUKUSHIMA, T. 1960 On the mechanism of development of multiple drug-resistant clones of *Shigella. Japanese Journal of Microbiology* **4,** 219–227.

ANDERSON, E. S. 1965 Origin of transferable drug resistance factors in the Enterobacteriaceae. *British Medical Journal* **2,** 1289–1291.

ANDERSON, E. S. 1968 The ecology of transferable drug resistance in the enterobacteria. *Annual Review of Microbiology* **22,** 131–179.

ANDERSON, E. S. 1975 The problems and implications of chloramphenicol resistance in the typhoid bacillus. *Journal of Hygiene, Cambridge* **74,** 289–299.

ANDERSON, E. S. 1977 The geographical predominance of resistance transfer systems of various compatibility groups in salmonellae. In *Topics in Infectious Diseases* Vol. 2. R-factors: Their Properties and Possible Control. ed. Drews, J. & Hogenauer, G. pp. 25–38. Wien, Springer-Verlag.

ANDERSON, E. S., THRELFALL, E. J. 1974 The characterisation of plasmids in the enterobacteria. *Journal of Hygiene, Cambridge* **72,** 471–487.

ASHLEY, A. 1979 *A study of the restriction of coliphages by enterobacterial resistance plasmids*. FIMLS Thesis, Institute of Medical Laboratory Sciences, London.

BIRNBOIM, H. C. & DOLY, J. 1979 A rapid alkaline extraction procedure for screening recombinant plasmid DNA. *Nucleic Acids Research* **7,** 1513–1523.

CALLOW, B. R. 1959 A new phage-typing scheme for *Salmonella typhimurium. Journal of Hygiene, Cambridge* **57,** 346–359.

CLEWELL, D. B. & HELINSKI, D. R. 1969 Supercoiled circular DNA-protein complex in *Escherichia coli*: purification and induced conversion to an open circular form. *Proceedings of the National Academy of Sciences of the United States of America* **62,** 1159–1166.

DATTA, N. 1962 Transmissible drug resistance in an epidemic strain of *Salmonella typhimurium. Journal of Hygiene, Cambridge* **60,** 301–310.

DETTORI, R., MACCACARO, G. A. & PICCININ, G. L. 1961 Sex-specific bacteriophages of *Escherichia coli* K12. *Giornale di Microbiologi* **9,** 141–150.

FELIX, A. & CALLOW, B. R. 1943 Typing of paratyphoid B bacilli by means of Vi bacteriophages. *British Medical Journal* **ii,** 127–130.

FREDERICQ, P. 1948 Actions antibiotiques réciproques chez les Entérobactériaceae. *Revue belge de Pathologie et de Médicine expérimentale* **19,** (Supplement IV), 1.

GANGAROSA, E. T., PERERA, D. R., MATA, L. J., MORRISON, C. M., GUZMAN, G. & RELLER, L. B. 1970 Epidemic shiga bacillus dysentery in Central America. II. Epidemiological studies in 1969. *Journal of Infectious Diseases* **122,** 181–190.

GRINDLEY, J. N. & ANDERSON, E. S. 1971 I-like resistance factors with the fi^+ characters. *Genetical Research* **17,** 267–271.

GRINDLEY, N. D. F., GRINDLEY, J. N. & ANDERSON, E. S. 1972 R factor compatibility groups. *Molecular and General Genetics* **119,** 287–297.

GRINDLEY, N. D. F., HUMPHREYS, G. O. & ANDERSON, E. S. 1973 Molecular studies of R factor compatibility groups. *Journal of Bacteriology* **115,** 387–398.

GUERRY, P., LEBLANC, D. J. & FALKOW, S. 1973 General method for the isolation of plasmid deoxyribonucleic acid. *Journal of Bacteriology* **116,** 1064–1066.

HANSEN, J. B. & OLSEN, R. H. 1978 Isolation of large bacterial plasmids and characterization of the P2 incompatibility group plasmids pMG1 and pMG5. *Journal of Bacteriology* **135,** 227–238.

JOHNSON, P. H. & GROSSMAN, L. I. 1977 Electrophoresis of DNA in agarose gels. Optimizing separations of conformational isomers of double- and single-stranded DNAs *Biochemistry* **16,** 4217–4224.

KHATOON, H., IYER, R. V. & IYER, V. N. 1972 A new filamentous bacteriophage with sex-factor specificity. *Virology* **48,** 145–155.

MEYERS, J. A., SANCHEZ, D., ELWELL, L. P & FALKOW, S. 1976 Simple gel electrophoretic method for the identification and characterization of plasmid deoxyribonucleic acid. *Journal of Bacteriology* **127,** 1529–1537.

MEYNELL, G. G. & LAWN, A. M. 1968 Filamentous phage specific for the I sex factor. *Nature, London* **217,** 1184–1186.

NOVICK, R. P. 1969 Extrachromosomal inheritance in Bacteria. *Bacteriological Reviews* **33,** 210–235.

OCHIAI, K., YAMANAKA, T., KIMURA, K. & SAWADA, O. 1959 Studies on the inheritance of drug resistance between shigella strains and *Escherichia coli* strains. *Nippon Iji Shimpo* **1835,** 38–42 (in Japanese).

OLSEN, R. H., SIAK, J. & GRAY, R. 1974 Characteristics of PRD1, a plasmid-dependent broad host range DNA bacteriophage. *Journal of Virology* **14,** 689–699.

ROWE, B., FROST, J. A., THRELFALL, E. J. & WARD, L. R. 1980 Spread of a multiresistant clone of *Salmonella typhimurium* phage type 66/122 in South East Asia and the Middle East. *Lancet* **ii,** 1070–1071.

SIRGEL, F. A., COETZEE, J. N., HEDGES, R. W. & LECATSAS, G. 1981 Phage C-1, an IncC Group Plasmid-specific Phage. *Journal of General Microbiology* **122,** 155–160.

WATANABE, T., NISHIDA, H., OGATA, C., ARAI, T. & SATO, S. 1964 Episome mediated transfer of drug resistance in Enterobacteriaceae. VII. Two types of naturally occurring R factors. *Journal of Bacteriology* **88,** 716–726.

WILLSHAW, G. A., SMITH, H. R. & ANDERSON, E. S. 1979 Application of agarose gel electrophoresis to the characterization of plasmid DNA in drug-resistant enterobacteria. *Journal of General Microbiology* **114,** 15–25.

The Use of Phage Typing and Plasmid Characterization in Studying the Epidemiology of Multiresistant *Salmonella typhimurium*

E. J. THRELFALL, LINDA R. WARD AND B. ROWE

Division of Enteric Pathogens, Central Public Health Laboratory, Colindale, London, UK

Phage Typing of *Salmonella typhimurium*

For the three years 1976–1978, salmonellas were responsible for about 75% (23,052 cases) of all food poisoning reported in England and Wales, which undoubtedly represents a severe under-estimate, as only a small proportion of salmonella cases are examined bacteriologically. *Salmonella typhimurium* is the commonest of all salmonellas isolated in Britain and during this period was responsible for 27% of cases (7410 infections) in England and Wales (Hepner 1980).

Salmonella typhimurium has many hosts and these include animals commonly used by man as food, such as chickens, calves and adult cattle, turkeys, pigs and ducks. Interhuman infection is considered to be relatively rare but may occur under special conditions, for example in closed institutions.

Because of the large number of cases involved, rapid and effective strain characterization is essential. The most useful method currently employed is bacteriophage typing. Over many years this has proved invaluable in epidemiological investigations; the technique is simple, and the reagents used are relatively inexpensive and easy to prepare and standardize. The emergence of new types is seen easily and further studies on new types can be initiated promptly.

At present over 200 distinct phage types are recognized by the scheme used in the Division of Enteric Pathogens (Anderson *et al.* 1977). The scheme used is that of Callow (1959), as extended by Anderson (1964), and is dependent on the patterns of lysis obtained when routine test dilutions (RTDs) of thirty bacteriophages are plated on strains of *Salm. typhimurium*.

ANTIBIOTICS
ISBN 0 12 604480 5

A supplementary scheme is under development for differentiating those strains which do not react with the phages of Callow (1959).

Changes of Phage Type

The pattern of lysis can be changed by the acquisition of both temperate phages and plasmids. To understand the relationships between strains, elucidation of the role of these extra-chromosomal elements in phage type determination may be necessary. Such studies are particularly important when studying the epidemiology of infections with multiresistant strains, in which antimicrobial drug resistance is encoded by one or more plasmids that may also change the phage type of carrier strains.

This is illustrated by an account of how the epizootic spread of multiresistant *Salm. typhimurium* in Britain was investigated, using a combination of phage typing, resistance typing and plasmid characterization. These strains were of phage types 204, 193, 204a and 204c. The methods used for the characterization of plasmids in the strains are those described in this volume pp. 265–284.

Accounts of the occurrence and spread of these strains and of their properties have been published elsewhere (Threlfall *et al.* 1978*a*, *b*; Rowe *et al.* 1979; Threlfall *et al.* 1980) and a detailed account of plasmid characterization is given by Willshaw *et al.* (1980).

Studies of Multiresistant *Salm. typhimurium* in Britain

Epidemiological aspects

The appearance dates of the strains and their phage type designations and drug resistance spectra are shown in Table 1.

(1) Type 204 of *Salm. typhimurium*, first identified in cattle in Britain in 1974, became the predominant phage type in bovine animals and humans in 1977. Until June 1977 the predominant R-type in type 204 was that of sulphonamides and tetracyclines.

(2) In June 1977, type 204 of R-type CSSuT (see Table 1 for meaning of symbols), was identified in calves. By September 1977 isolations of R-type CSSuT had exceeded those of R-type SuT. The first human infections of type 204 CSSuT occurred in August, 1977.

(3) In December 1977 *Salm. typhimurium* of R-type ACKSSuT were identified in cattle and humans. The strains did not react with the standard *Salm. typhimurium* typing phages and were assigned to phage type 193 on the basis of their reactions with a new scheme which is under development.

(4) In October 1978, type 204a of R-type SuT was recognized as a type distinct from 204. This phage type became common during 1979, particularly in Scotland, and has entered the food chain.
(5) In March 1979 *Salm. typhimurium* strains of R-type CSSuTTm were identified in calves. These strains were found to be related to type 204 and the phage type was designated type 204c. Human infections first occurred in May 1979.
(6) By December 1979 the predominant R-type in type 204c was that of ACKSSuTTm.
(7) In March 1978 strains of type 204a of R-type CKSSuT were identified in cattle and humans.

TABLE 1

Appearance of Salmonella typhimurium *phage type 204 and related strains*

Strain	R-type*	Date
Type 204	SuT	1974 January
	CSSuT	1977 June
Type 193	ACKSSuT	1977 December
Type 204a	SuT	1978 October
	CKSSuT	1980 March
Type 204c	CSSuTTm	1979 March
	ACKSSuTTm	1979 October

*Resistance (R) symbols: A, ampicillin; C, chloramphenicol; K, neomycin-kanamycin; S, streptomycin; Su, sulphonamides; T, tetracyclines; Tm, trimethoprim.

Infections in cattle

The proportions in cattle of *Salm. typhimurium* type 204 and the related types from 1977 to 1980 are shown in Table 2. Their distribution over this period is shown in Fig. 1.

In 1977 type 204 became the predominant phage type in cattle and isolations of this type comprised 34·1% of bovine *Salm. typhimurium.* Of this total, type 204 SuT comprised 20% and type 204 CSSuT 14·1%. In subsequent years type 204 and related types have comprised 43·6%, 54·2% and 54·0% of bovine *Salm. typhimurium.*

The clone of type 204 CSSuT became the predominant strain in cattle in Britain by late 1977 but has subsequently disappeared. Type 193 peaked in 1978/79 but the frequency of isolation of this clone was greatly reduced in 1980. Type 204c, which appeared in 1979, became the predominant multiresistant clone in cattle during 1980.

TABLE 2

Isolations of Salmonella typhimurium *types 204, 193, 204a and 204c from cattle, 1977–1980*

Year	Number referred	Type 204 (%)		Type 193 (%)	Type 204a (%)		Type 204c (%)	Type 204 and related types as % of number referred
		SuT	CSSuT	ACKSSuT	SuT	CKSSuT	CSSuTTm and ACKSSuTTm	
1977	1194	20·0	14·1	0·6	0	0	0	34·7
1978	1790	12·8	13·6	15·8	1·4	0	0	43·6
1979	1732	13·2	2·3	16·4	13·6	0	8·7	54·2
1980	1585	10·0	0	3·4	18·8	0·9	20·9	54·0

Source: strains referred to the Division of Enteric Pathogens.

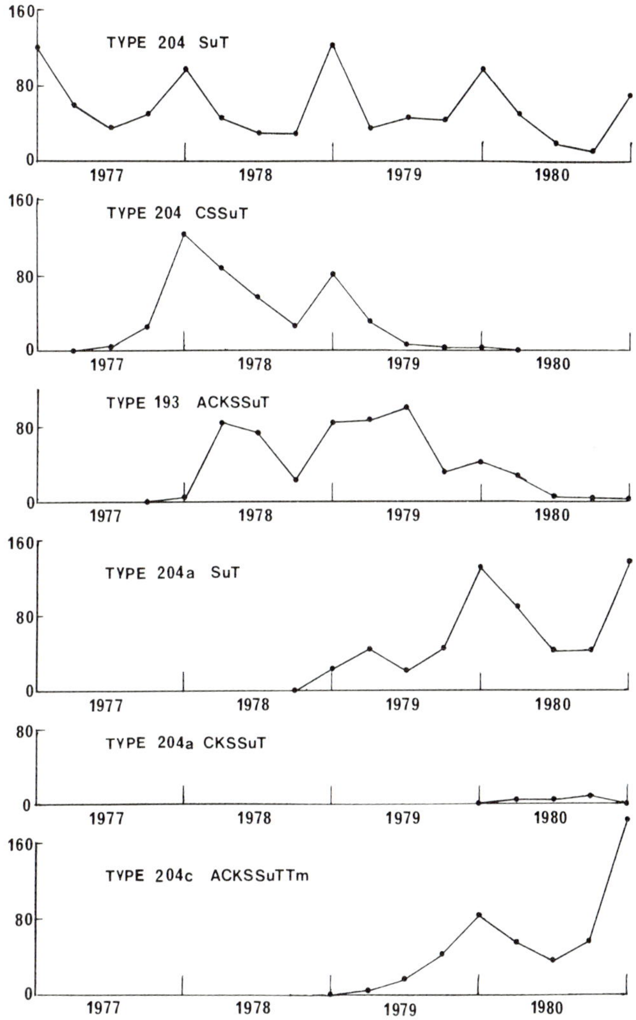

Fig. 1. Numbers of drug-resistant *Salmonella typhimurium* type 204 and related strains in cattle 1977–1980.

The frequency of isolations of type 204a SuT has increased each year since this type was recognized in 1978. Type 204a CKSSuT has come into prominence in 1980. Type 204 SuT has been isolated regularly during the four-year period 1977–1980, but the proportion of infection with this strain was reduced in 1980. Up to 50% mortality has been reported in infected herds and economic losses have been severe.

TABLE 3

Human infections with Salmonella typhimurium *types 204, 193, 204a and 204c, 1977–1980*

	Type 204		Type 193	Type 204a		Type 204c		
Year	SuT	CSSuT	ACKSSuT	SuT	CKSSuT	CSSuTTm or ACKSSuTTm	SSuTTm	Total
1977	203	37	4	0	0	0	0	
1978	103	51	89	7	0	0	0	
1979	153	15	94	83	0	20	0	
1980	164	0	29	363	48	102	16	
	623	103	216	453	48	122	16	1581

Source: strains referred to the Division of Enteric Pathogens.

TABLE 4

Phage typing reactions

Type designation	Typing phages in routine test dilution																	
	2	3	7	8	12	14	15	16	17	20	21	26	27	28	29	32	35	S1*
49	+++	++	SCL	+++	CL	CL	+	CL	SCL	CL	CL	+	OL	+	CL	+++	CL	SCL
204	+	–	–	+	–	SCL	–	++	+	+	+	–	++	–	SCL	–	SCL	SCL
204c	+	+	–	+	–	SCL	–	+	–	+	+	+	SCL	+	++	–	SCL	SCL
204a	–	–	–	–	–	++	–	–	–	–	–	–	+	–	+	–	–	SCL
193	–	–	–	–	–	–	–	+	–	–	–	–	–	–	–	–	–	SCL
36	CL	CL	CL	CL	CL	CL	CL	CL	CL	CL	CL	CL	CL	CL	CL	CL	CL	SCL
NC1	+	–	–	+	–	SCL	–	+++	+	+	+	+	SCL	SCL	SCL	+	CL	SCL
125	CL	CL	CL	CL	–	CL	CL	CL	CL	CL	CL	CL	CL	CL	CL	CL	CL	SCL
NC9	+	++	–	SCL	–	SCL	SCL	SCL	+	++	++	–	++	OL	++	+	OL	SCL

CL, confluent lysis; OL, opaque lysis; SCL, semi-confluent lysis. –, +, ++, +++, increasing numbers of discrete plaques.
* S1, phage of supplementary typing scheme.

Infections in humans

One thousand five hundred and eighty-one human infections with strains of phage type 204 and the related types have been recognized since 1977.

Of these, 441 infections were caused by multiresistant strains of types 204, 193 and 204c. In addition, a further 16 people were infected with a type 204c variant of R-type SSuTTm which appeared in 1980; 48 patients have been infected with type 204a CKSSuT (Table 3).

Enteritis was reported as the cause of the death of two patients infected with the multiresistant strains, and there was extra-intestinal spread in a further 10 patients. One child died with a septicaemic illness following infection with type 193 ACKSSuT and one patient has died of salmonella meningitis following infection with a strain of type 204c (Ellis *et al.* 1981).

Phage typing and plasmid characterization

Phage typing

The reactions of types 49, 204, 204a and 204c with seventeen of the *Salm. typhimurium* typing phages of Callow and with one phage of the supplementary typing scheme are shown in Table 4. Also included in Table 4 are the reactions of phage type 36 and of type 36 into which resistance plasmids from the various strains have been transferred. The phages selected were chosen because their reactions demonstrate the differences between the types and show the patterns of restriction produced by the drug resistance plasmids carried.

Plasmid characterization

The genetic properties of the plasmids identified are summarized in Table 5.

Phage types

Type 204 SuT

Sulphonamides and tetracycline resistance in type 204 SuT were non-autotransferring but could be mobilized independently by autotransferring plasmids (see pp. 265–284). Tetracycline resistance was specified by a plasmid of mol. wt 63 $\times$ 10^6. This plasmid was compatible with representative plasmids of defined compatibility groups and was not assigned to a compatibility group. The tetracycline resistance plasmid also specified resistance to lysis by 24 of the *Salm. typhimurium* typing phages and when introduced into a strain of type 36, which is sensitive to lysis by all 30 of the typing phages, the resultant pattern corresponded to the type designated

Table 5

Properties of plasmids in type 204 and related strains

Resistance	Cryptic*	Su	T	CSSuT†	AKS	AK	CKSSuT
Transferability	−	−	−	+	+	+	+
Mobilization	nt	+	+	·	·	·	·
Compatibility group	nt	nt	nc	H_2	I_1	X	H_1
Mol. wt ($\times 10^6$)	5·3	4·2	63	> 100	76	40	> 100
Phage restriction:							
in type 36	nt	NR	NC1	125	NC9	125	NR
in type 49	NR	NR	204	NR	NC	NR	NR
in type 204	NR	NR	NR	NR	193	NR	NR
in type 204a	NR	NR	NR	NR	193	NR	NR
in type 204c	NR	NR	‡	NR	193	NR	NR
Type 49, Su	———	———					
Types 204 and 204a, SuT	———	———	———				
Types 204 and 204c, CSSuT	———	———	———	———			
Type 193, ACKSSuT	———	———	———	———	———		
Type 204c, ACKSSuTTm	———	———	———	———		———	
Type 204a, CKSSuT	———	———	———				———

nt, not tested; NC, does not conform to a designated type; NR, non-restricting; nc, not classified.
* Does not specify drug resistance.
† CSSuTTm in type 204c.
‡ Loss of property of phage restriction from T plasmid.

NC (= non-conforming) 1. If spontaneously lost from a strain of phage type 204, the resultant strain had enhanced sensitivity to the typing phages and the reactions corresponded to those of type 49 (Table 4). These results indicated that the probable progenitor of type 204 was a strain of phage type 49.

In contrast, the sulphonamide resistance plasmid was of mol. wt $4{\cdot}2 \times 10^6$ and did not have a phage type-determining role.

Type 204 strains also carried a third plasmid, mol. wt $5{\cdot}3 \times 10^6$, detected by agarose gel electrophoresis. This plasmid did not code for antibiotic resistance and is of unknown function.

Type 204 CSSuT

Plasmid characterization demonstrated that type 204 CSSuT had been derived from a strain of type 204 SuT following the acquisition of a single autotransferring resistance plasmid of compatibility group H_2. This plasmid coded for the complete resistance spectrum (CSSuT), and abolished lysis of type 36 by two of the typing phages, thereby converting type 36 to type 125. However, restriction of these phages was also specified by the tetracycline resistance plasmid described above. Consequently, acquisition of the H_2 plasmid by phage type 204 SuT changed the R-type to that of CSSuT but there was no alteration in phage type.

Type 193 ACKSSuT

Plasmid characterization and displacement studies showed that type 193 ACKSSuT had been derived from type 204 CSSuT as a result of the acquisition of an autotransferring group I_1 plasmid. This plasmid encoded resistance to ampicillin, kanamycin and streptomycin (AKS), and also determined restriction of 15 of the *Salm. typhimurium* phages, thereby converting type 36 to a type designated NC9 and type 204 to type 193 (Table 4). When displaced from type 193 ACKSSuT the resultant strain was of type 204 R-type CSSuT.

Type 204a SuT

Genetic examination of type 204a isolations of R-type SuT showed that their plasmid content was indistinguishable from that of type 204 SuT but that an additional temperate bacteriophage was present. This phage had the ability to restrict lysis of carrier strains by the typing phages and when plated on type 204 strains, abolished lysis by seven of the ten phages with which type 204 reacted. The resultant typing phage pattern was that designated type 204a (Table 4).

Type 204a CKSSuT

Strains of this R-type had been derived from a strain of type 204a SuT following the acquisition of a plasmid of compatibility group H_1 which encoded the complete resistance spectrum, CKSSuT. This H_1 resistance factor did not specify restriction of the typing phages.

Type 204c CSSuTTm

Because their pattern of reactions with the typing phages did not conform to a designated type, *Salm. typhimurium* of R-type CSSuTTm were originally designated as RDNC (reacts but does not conform). The type was subsequently designated type 204c after characterization of plasmids and carried phages had demonstrated its derivation from type 204 CSSuT by the following series of events.

(i) Loss of the typing phage restriction property from the tetracycline resistance plasmid present in all strains of type 204. This resulted in the conversion of type 204 to type 49 without plasmid loss.
(ii) Acquisition of a trimethoprim resistance transposon by the CSSuT group H_2 resistance plasmid.
(iii) Acquisition of a small-plaque temperate bacteriophage, the presence of which changed the phage typing reactions of type 49 to those of the new type, subsequently designated type 204c.

Type 204c ACKSSuTTm

Isolations with this resistance spectrum had been derived from type 204c CSSuTTm by the acquisition of an R factor of compatibility group X which coded for ampicillin and kanamycin resistance (AK) and specified restriction of two of the typing phages. However, strains of type 204c did not react with the phages restricted by the group X plasmid. Thus, in this instance, plasmid acquisition did not result in change of phage type.

The stages in development of the strains are shown in Fig. 2.

The plasmid characterization studies have demonstrated that:

(1) All strains of types 204, 204a, 204c and 193 have a common plasmid content. This consists of a cryptic plasmid, a sulphonamide resistance plasmid and a plasmid which conferred resistance to tetracyclines (Table 5).
(2) The probable progenitor strain was of phage type 49.
(3) The appearance of the different phage types and R-types has followed the sequential acquisition of resistance plasmids and temperate bacteriophages. Some resistance plasmids also specified restriction of lysis by the typing phages.
(4) The epidemiological study of infections with multiresistant strains of types 204, 193, 204a and 204c is an extension of that of type 204 SuT. However, the influence of the increasing spectrum of antimicrobial drug resistance on the spread of the various types is an important factor.

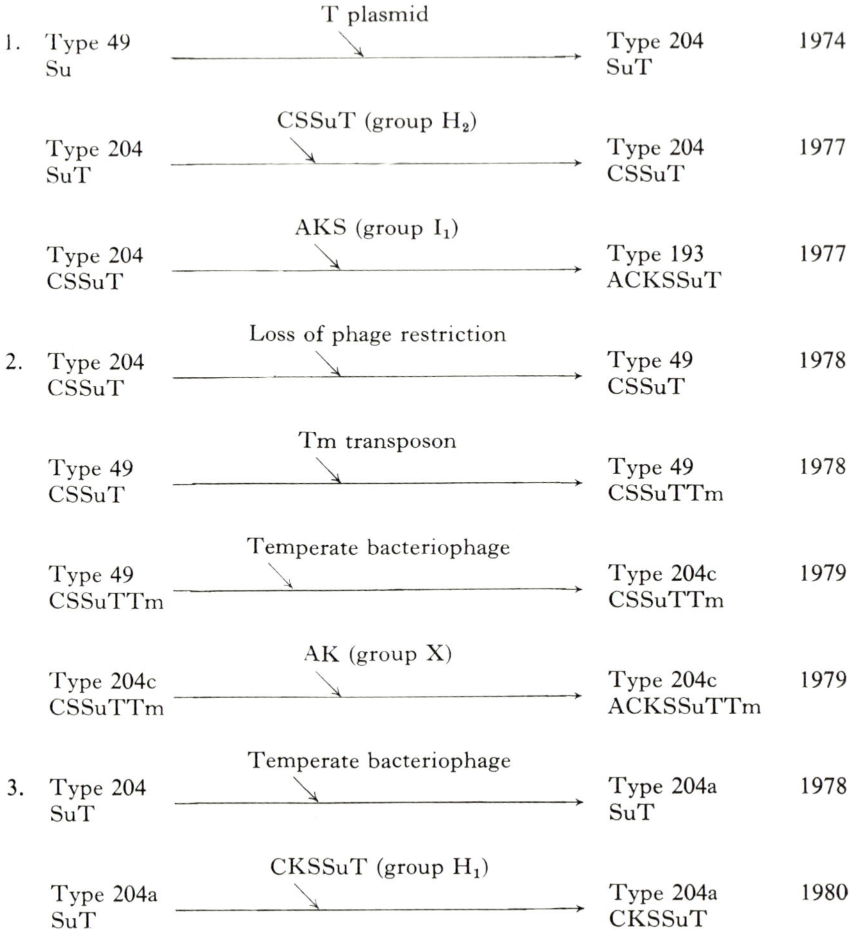

FIG. 2. The development of multiresistant strains of *Salmonella typhimurium* types 204, 193, 204c and 204a.

Conclusions

This study illustrates:

(1) The use of phage typing for the initial discrimination of strains of *Salm. typhimurium*.

(2) The use of resistance typing as a secondary genetic marker, enabling strains of different resistance spectra within a phage type to be recognized.

(3) The use of plasmid characterization in understanding: (a) Change of resistance spectra within a phage type; (b) Change of phage type; (c) The relationships between strains with different phenotypes; (d) The evolutionary development of multiresistant strains.

The combined use of phage typing and plasmid characterization may be widely applicable in epidemiological investigations of enterobacterial infections with *Salm. typhimurium* and other salmonella serotypes.

References

Anderson, E. S. 1964 The phage typing of salmonellae other than *S. typhi*. In *The World Problem of Salmonellosis* ed. Van Oye, E. pp. 89–110. The Hague: Dr. W. Junk.

Anderson, E. S., Ward, L. R., DeSaxe, M. J. & DeSa, J. D. H. 1977 Bacteriophage-typing designations of *Salmonella typhimurium*. *Journal of Hygiene* **78,** 297–300.

Callow, B. R. 1959 A new phage-typing scheme for *Salmonella typhimurium*. *Journal of Hygiene* **57,** 346–359.

Ellis, M. E., Smith, C. C., Reid, T. M. S. & Porter, I. A. 1981 Chloramphenicol-resistant *Salmonella typhimurium* meningitis in an adult. *British Medical Journal* **283,** 273.

Hepner, E. 1980 Food poisoning and salmonella infections in England and Wales, 1976–1978. *Public Health, London* **94,** 337–349.

Rowe, B., Threlfall, E. J., Ward, L. R. & Ashley, A. S. 1979 International spread of multiresistant strains of *Salmonella typhimurium* phage types 204 and 193 from Britain to Europe. *Veterinary Record* **105,** 468–469.

Threlfall, E. J., Ward, L. R. & Rowe, B. 1978*a* Spread of multiresistant strains of *Salmonella typhimurium* phage types 204 and 193 in Britain. *British Medical Journal* **ii,** 997.

Threlfall, E. J., Ward, L. R. & Rowe, B. 1978*b* Epidemic spread of a chloramphenicol-resistant strain of *Salmonella typhimurium* phage type 204 in bovine animals in Britain. *Veterinary Record* **103,** 438–440.

Threlfall, E. J., Ward, L. R., Ashley, A. S. & Rowe, B. 1980 Plasmid-encoded trimethoprim resistance in multiresistant epidemic *Salmonella typhimurium* phage types 204 and 193 in Britain. *British Medical Journal* **280,** 1210–1211.

Willshaw, G. A., Threlfall, E. J., Ward, L. R., Ashley, A. S. & Rowe, B. 1980 Plasmid studies of drug-resistant epidemic strains of *Salmonella typhimurium* belonging to phage types 204 and 193. *Journal of Antimicrobial Chemotherapy* **6,** 763–773.

Measurement of Combined Antibiotic Action

ANGELA S. BEALE AND R. SUTHERLAND

Beecham Pharmaceuticals Research Division,
Chemotherapeutic Research Centre,
Brockham Park, Betchworth, Surrey, UK

Combined antibacterial therapy is very common, and the most frequent reason for its use is to provide broad-spectrum antibiotic cover in seriously ill patients, often before the identity of the infecting organism is known. In theory, combined therapy would be replaced by appropriate monotherapy based upon the laboratory findings, but in practice combined treatment is often continued if the patient shows signs of improvement. A particular situation where combined therapy is preferred to monotherapy, even when the antibiotic sensitivity of the causal organism is known, is that of febrile patients being treated with immunosuppressive therapy. In such cases, a regimen which is likely to be synergistic *in vitro* is often selected as first choice, e.g. an aminoglycoside antibiotic with a broad-spectrum penicillin such as carbenicillin or ticarcillin, or combined with a cephalosporin. Less frequently, a combination of antibiotics may be chosen specifically on the basis of laboratory tests showing synergy against the patient's infecting organism. An outstanding example is the use of combined penicillin/aminoglycoside therapy to provide enhanced bactericidal activity in the treatment of enterococcal endocarditis.

Although much emphasis is placed on the demonstration of synergistic effects it is also important to ensure that antagonism is not likely to ensue as a result of combining two or more antibiotics, and this aspect has received renewed attention. It is important therefore that a laboratory is competent to measure the results of interaction of two or more antibacterial agents and to define the types of effect produced, namely (1) *synergistic*, when the effect produced by the agents in combination is greater than the sum of individual effects of either drug alone, (2) *antagonistic*, when the activity of one drug is reduced by the presence of another,

ANTIBIOTICS
ISBN 0 12 604480 5

and (3) *indifferent* or *additive*, when the combined action is no greater than that to be predicted from the activities of the individual drugs.

Antibacterial agents may interact with each other by a number of different mechanisms and consequently no one single test method is likely to be suitable for the measurement of the effects produced by combinations of all or most of the available agents. Accordingly, a variety of different methods has been employed to demonstrate synergism (or antagonism) between antibacterial drugs, but in many instances the relevance of the *in vitro* testing procedures to the *in vivo* situation is uncertain. For instance, the production of a synergistic effect at antibiotic concentrations much above those attainable *in vivo* is unlikely to be of clinical value. Experimental infection studies in animals may provide a better indication of the likely clinical effects of combined therapy but such *in vivo* studies are not within the province of the usual clinical laboratory.

It is the purpose of this brief review to provide an outline of the methods used most frequently *in vitro* to measure the interaction of antibiotic combinations and to comment upon the advantages or disadvantages of the various techniques. No attempt is made to provide a detailed account of the methodology of combined antibiotic interaction, for which the reader is referred to the excellent reviews by Krogstad & Moellering (1980) and Waterworth (1978, 1981).

Chessboard Method

The most common method used in *in vitro* studies to measure combined antibacterial activity is the chessboard (or checkerboard) titration technique. In this test, the organisms are exposed to serial dilutions of two drugs so that all possible combinations of drug concentrations (within the range of dilutions used) are tested. The resulting pattern of growth produces the so-called 'chessboard' effect responsible for the name of the technique.

The test consists of preparing a range of six or more dilutions of each drug starting from just above the expected minimum inhibitory concentration (MIC). Tubes or Petri dishes are placed in the form of a square, which consists of columns containing the same amount of one drug, diluted along the horizontal axis, and rows which contain the same amounts of the other drug diluted along the vertical axis. The test may be carried out in agar, which is relatively cumbersome, and many workers prefer tests using broth, particularly the use of microdilution plates which may or may not be part of an automated system (Fig. 1).

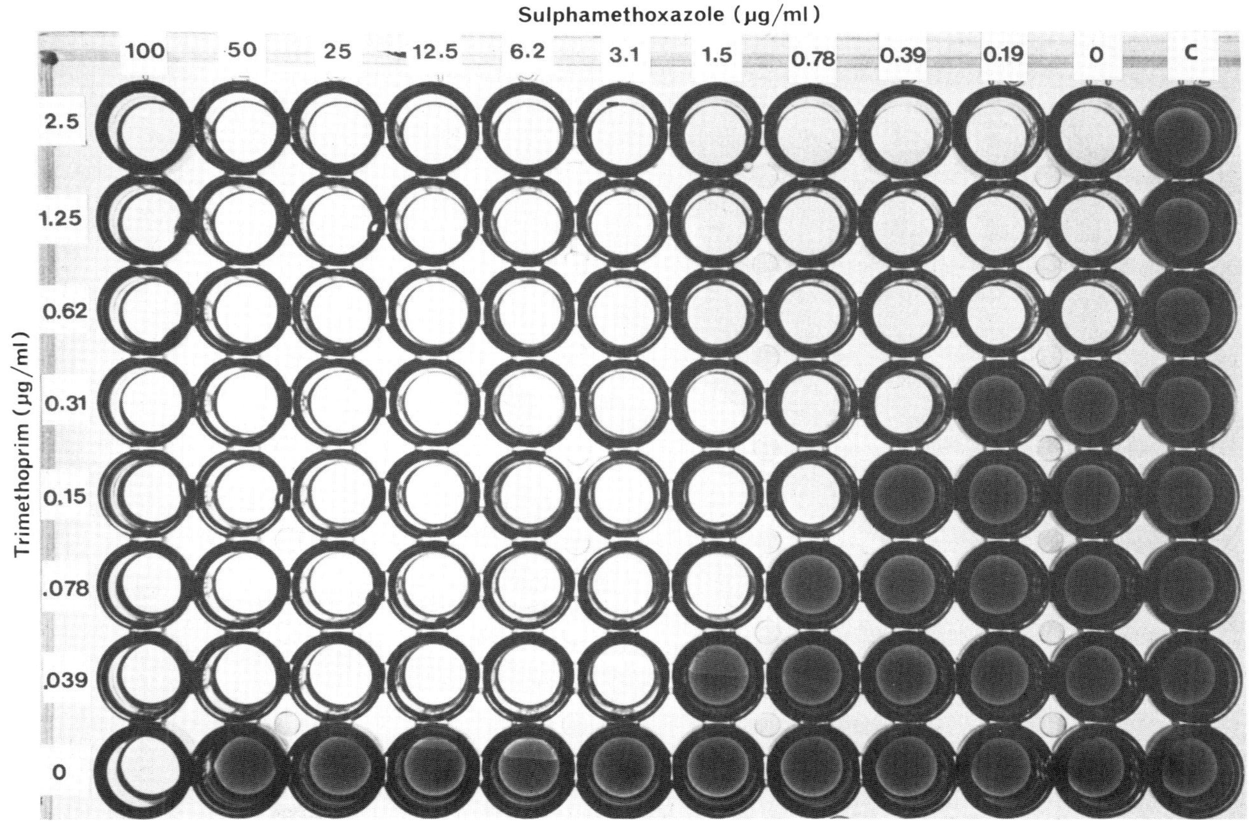

FIG. 1. Microtitre chessboard titration of sulphamethoxazole and trimethoprim against *Escherichia coli* showing bacteristatic synergy, i.e. MIC of sulphamethoxazole = 100 μg/ml, MIC of trimethoprim = 0·62 μg/ml. In the presence of 0·078 μg/ml trimethoprim, the MIC of sulphamethoxazole is reduced to 1·5 μg/ml. C = drug-free control.

The end-point is usually defined as the MIC after overnight incubation and the results are conveniently interpreted as follows (Andriole 1971):

(1) synergistic: $\frac{1}{4}$ MIC of drug A + $\frac{1}{4}$ MIC of drug B inhibits growth;

(2) partially synergistic: $\frac{1}{4}$ MIC of drug A + $\frac{1}{2}$ MIC of drug B inhibits growth;

(3) additive: $\frac{1}{2}$ MIC of drug A + $\frac{1}{2}$ MIC of drug B or higher concentrations are needed to inhibit growth.

The test may be adapted to measure bactericidal activity, in which case the results are expressed in terms of minimum bactericidal concentration (MBC) (Krogstad & Moellering 1980; Waterworth 1981).

The results may also be interpreted graphically by plotting the isobol (line connecting points of equivalent biological effect) between the MIC values for each drug in combination and alone. Several isobols may be presented in a single isobologram: a concave isobol represents synergy and a convex isobol indicates antagonism (Fig. 2*a*). Isobols of MBC or FIC values (see below) may also be plotted (Fig. 2*b*).

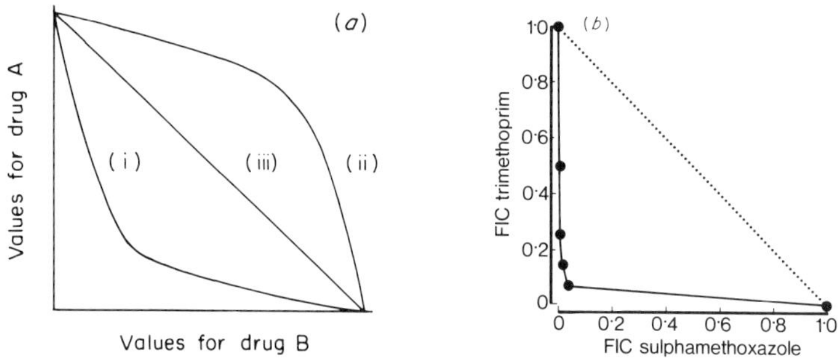

FIG. 2. (*a*) Isobologram with three isobols representing possible results of drug A and B acting together. The concave isobol (i) represents synergy, the convex isobol (ii) antagonism and the isobol (iii) indicates no effect of either drug on the other (indifference). (*b*) Isobologram of FICs for trimethoprim and sulphamethoxazole derived from data in the chessboard titration shown in Fig. 1.

An alternative interpretation involves calculation of the fractional inhibitory concentration (FIC) index (Elion *et al.* 1954). The FIC of each drug in each row is calculated as the minimum concentration of the drug in combination causing inhibition divided by the MIC of the drug alone, and the FIC index is the sum of the FIC values in the most effective combination.

$$\text{i.e.}\quad \frac{\text{MIC of A in combination}}{\text{MIC of A alone}} + \frac{\text{MIC of B in combination}}{\text{MIC of B alone}}$$

$$= \text{FIC A} + \text{FIC B} = \Sigma\text{FIC}.$$

The reciprocal of the FIC index has been called 'the factor of synergy'.

When the FIC index is $\leqslant 0{\cdot}5$, the combination is synergistic, and when it is $\geqslant 2{\cdot}0$ the combination is antagonistic. If the two drug effects are unchanged the FIC index should be 1·0 (Krogstad & Moellering 1980). Other authors conclude the combination is synergistic if the isobol is concave and the ΣFIC at the point of maximum synergy is $\leqslant 0{\cdot}7$; antagonistic if the ΣFIC at any point on the isobol is $\geqslant 1{\cdot}3$, and additive if the FICs do not vary by more than $\pm$ 0·3 around the 'central line' (connecting MIC of A alone and MIC of B alone) at any point (Kerry *et al.* 1975).

Half chessboard

In cases in the clinical laboratory where it is considered necessary to test the interaction of a number of drugs, most often to find a bactericidal combination, a modified chessboard involving the use of a single concentration of each drug may be preferred. The choice of concentration of each drug is important, and is usually based on a level which is readily attainable in the blood (Waterworth 1978).

TABLE 1

Results of a half-chessboard test to determine the bactericidal effects of antibiotic combinations against a penicillin-resistant strain of Staphylococcus aureus

	μg/ml	Penicillin G	Methicillin	Gentamicin	Erythromycin	Lincomycin	Fusidic acid	Rifampicin	Vancomycin
Penicillin G	10	++	(+)	−	+	+	+	−	−
Methicillin	10		−	−	++	++	++	−	−
Gentamicin	5			+	−	−	−	−	−
Erythromycin	2·5				+	+	+	−	+
Lincomycin	10					(+)	(+)	−	+
Fusidic acid	5						−	−	+
Rifampicin	5							−	−
Vancomycin	10								+

Results of subcultures: ++ growth similar to original inoculum (static effect only); + some reduction in the number of colonies; (+) < 10 colonies; − no growth (complete cidal effect).

The containers (usually tubes) are placed in a square rack in the form of a half chessboard, and are filled with antibiotic-containing broth to produce the desired antibiotic combinations as is illustrated by the example shown in Table 1. After incubation, usually overnight, but occasionally for 6 h, the tubes are examined for growth and a subculture is taken from all cultures showing no growth onto drug-free agar. Results are read after 18–24 h incubation, and the killing effects of the various combinations of antibiotics are compared with those produced by the individual compounds.

Viable Count Tests

Another widely used method is the quantitative measurement of bactericidal activity in viable count studies. The organism is incubated in broth medium containing selected concentrations (usually clinically achievable concentrations) of the antimicrobial agents, alone and in combination. Samples are taken at suitable intervals of time during the course of the test and are plated on drug-free agar. It is desirable that the agar should contain a neutralizing agent to prevent inhibition of growth as a result of 'carry-over' of the antibacterial agent. Examples of such agents include a β-lactamase for β-lactam antibiotics, thymidine for trimethoprim and *p*-aminobenzoic acid for sulphonamides. After incubation, colonies are counted and the viable bacterial counts of the cultures are calculated. The effects of interaction are assessed by comparison of the kill-curves obtained, alone and in combination, as is illustrated by the results in Fig. 3, which show the synergistic interaction of ticarcillin and tobramycin against *Pseudomonas aeruginosa*.

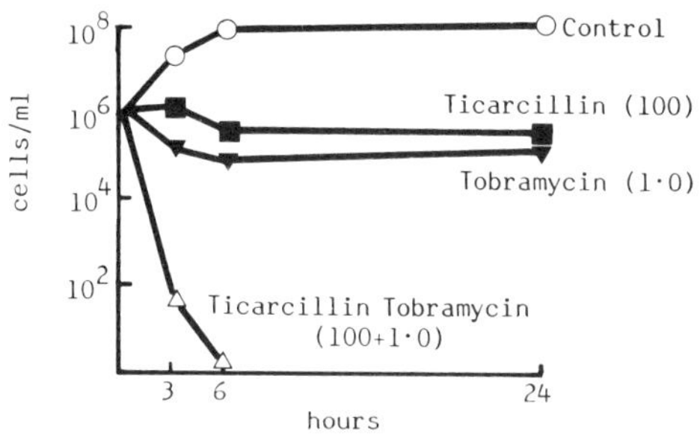

FIG. 3. Kill-curves by ticarcillin and tobramycin, alone and in combination, against logarithmically growing *Pseudomonas aeruginosa* showing bactericidal synergy. Figures in parentheses are concentrations of antibiotics (μg/ml).

Various workers have used different criteria to define bactericidal synergy from the results of viable count tests. For example, Jawetz, who was the first worker to conduct systematic investigations of antibiotic interactions, originally defined synergy as a large increase in the rate of bactericidal action (Jawetz & Gunnison 1952). Subsequently, the definition was modified to embrace both early bactericidal activity and total bactericidal kill (Jawetz 1968). A more recent and more widely used definition proposes bactericidal synergy as being a hundred-fold or greater increase in bactericidal killing at 24 h with both drugs, compared with either alone (Moellering *et al.* 1971).

The quantitative measurement of bactericidal activity in viable count tests is undoubtedly the best method for the assessment of bactericidal interaction, but the techniques to measure killing are relatively laborious and limit the number of antibiotic combinations that can be studied.

Turbidimetric Studies

The interaction of antibiotics may be assessed conveniently by continuous turbidimetric monitoring of the growth curves of bacteria exposed to the individual drugs and in combination. Synergy can be assessed on the basis of the minimum antibacterial concentration (MAC) (Lorian 1975); in this system, this is the minimum concentration required to produce a deviation in the growth curve from that obtained with the organism in the absence of the antibiotic. According to Greenwood (1979) the method has the advantage that the measurement of synergy is not affected by the emergence of resistant mutants as may occur in tests involving overnight incubation.

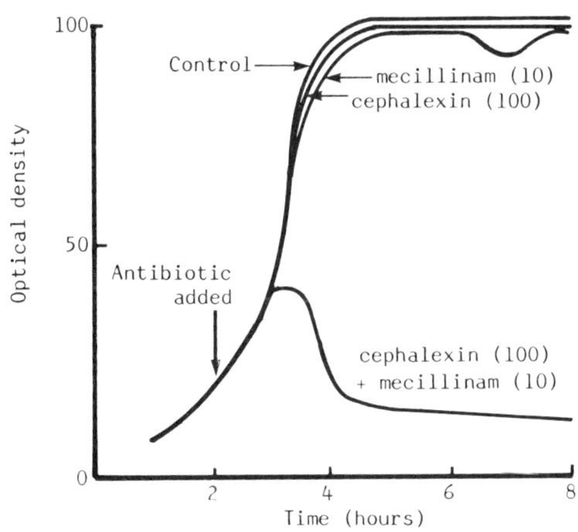

FIG. 4. Bacteriolytic activities of cephalexin and mecillinam against *Escherichia coli* alone and in combination, showing the synergistic effects of the combination of drugs. Figures in parentheses are concentrations of antibiotics (μg/ml).

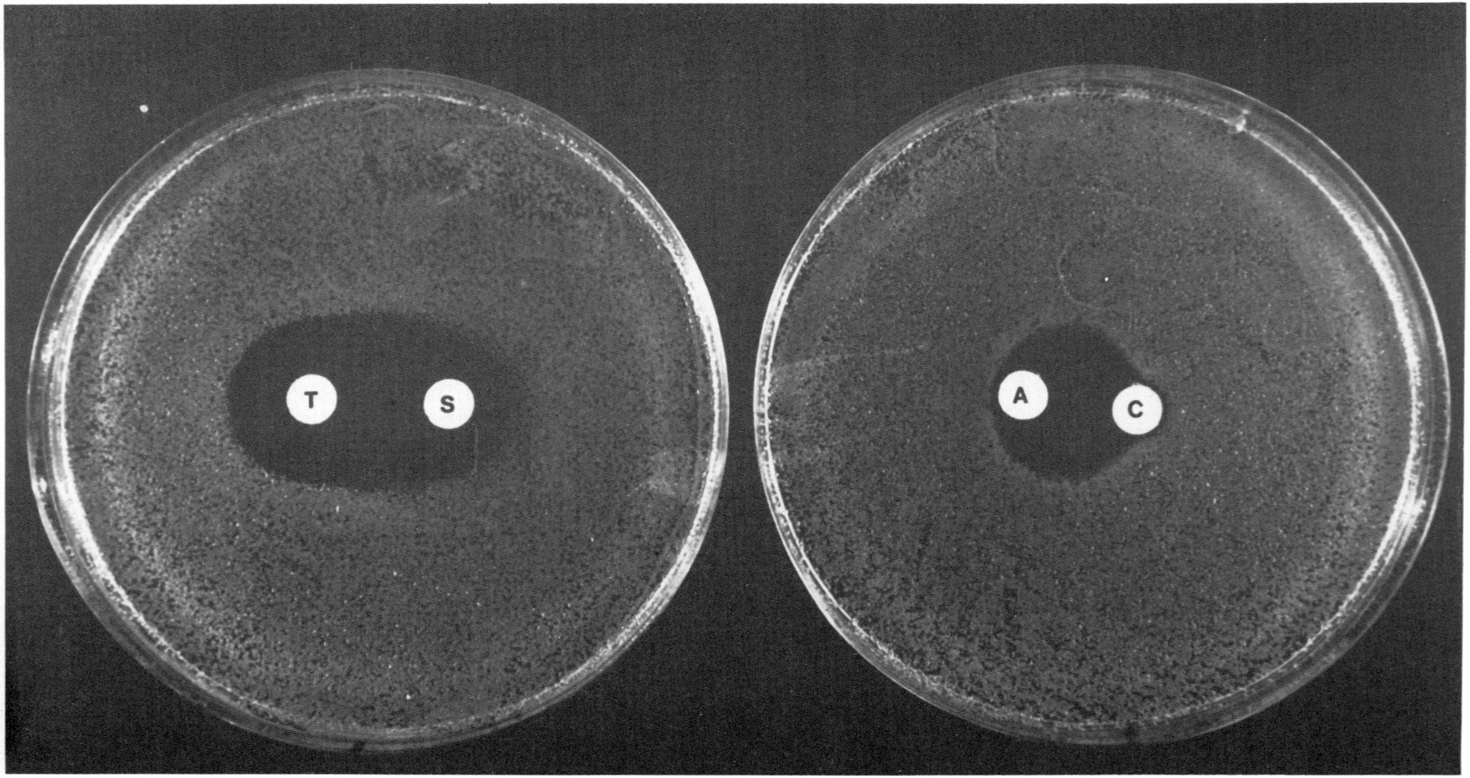

FIG. 5. Disc tests showing synergy between trimethoprim (T) and sulphamethoxazole (S) (on the left) and amoxycillin (A) and clavulanic acid (C) (on the right) against *Escherichia coli*.

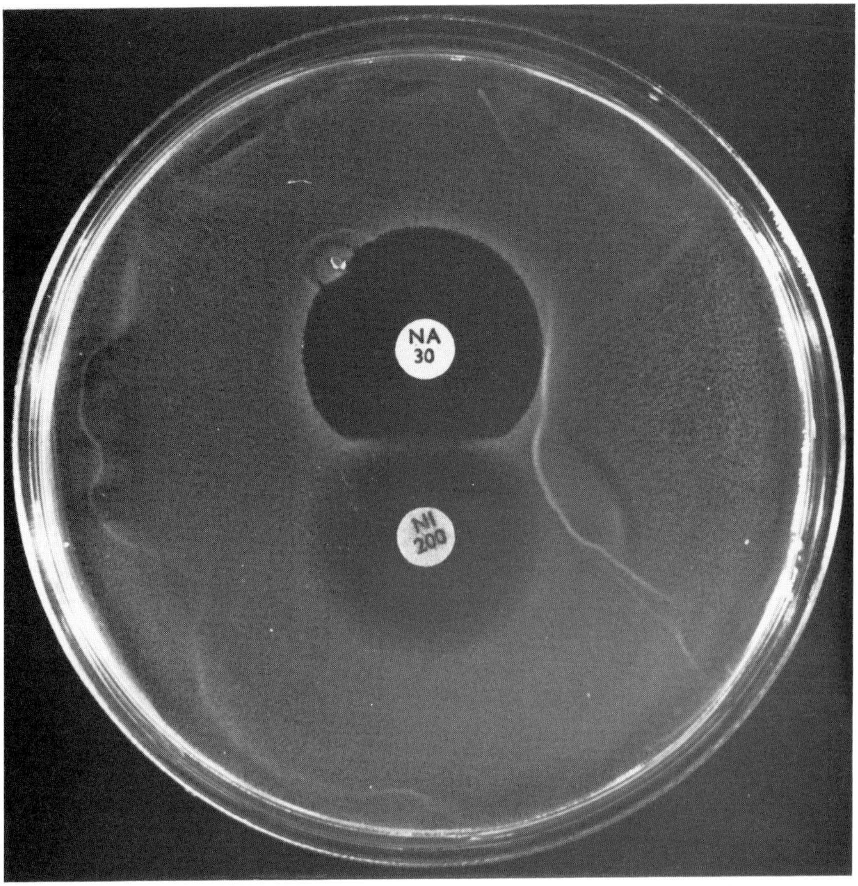

FIG. 6. Disc test showing antagonism between nitrofurantoin (NI) and nalidixic acid (NA) against *Klebsiella aerogenes*.

An outstanding example of synergy demonstrated by turbidimetric measurement was that demonstrated by Greenwood & O'Grady (1973) in studies with two β-lactam antibiotics, mecillinam and cephalexin. Mecillinam is unusual among the β-lactam antibiotics in that exposure of bacteria to the compound causes the formation of osmotically stable spherical cells, as a result of preferential binding to penicillin-binding protein 2 (PBP 2) (Spratt 1975). In contrast, cephalexin binds to PBP 3 causing the production of filamentous cells which lyse only slowly. When the antibiotics are combined, a rapid lytic effect is obtained (Fig. 4) and morphological observation shows that the presence of the spheroplast forms are responsible for the rapid lytic effects associated with β-lactam antibiotics. The interaction between the two β-lactam compounds binding to different PBPs was defined by Greenwood (1979) as complementation, a form of double blockade resulting from the action of the drugs at different, but related sites.

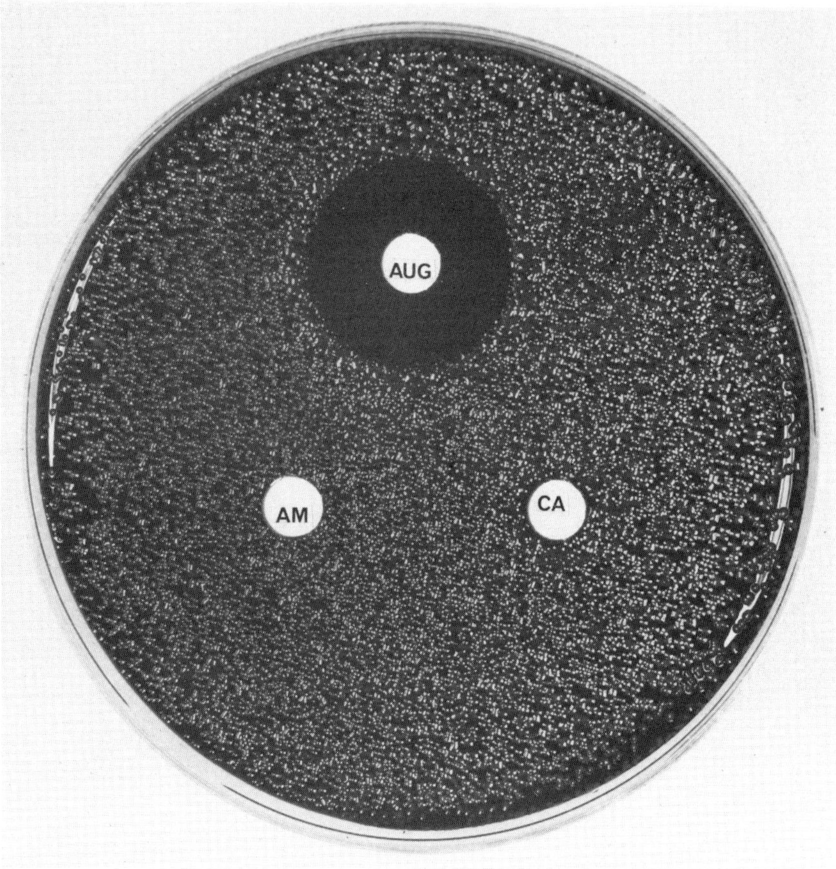

FIG. 7. Synergism between amoxycillin (AM) and clavulanic acid (CA) against *Escherichia coli* when combined in a single disc (AUG).

Diffusion Tests

Serial dilution tests to determine MIC, MBC or MAC values, or the determination of kill-curves by viable count studies, are relatively laborious and time-consuming, and simple diffusion methods are often preferred, despite yielding qualitative results which may be difficult to interpret. Apart from the relative ease of performance of diffusion tests, an additional advantage is that commercially available antibiotic sensitivity discs may often be employed.

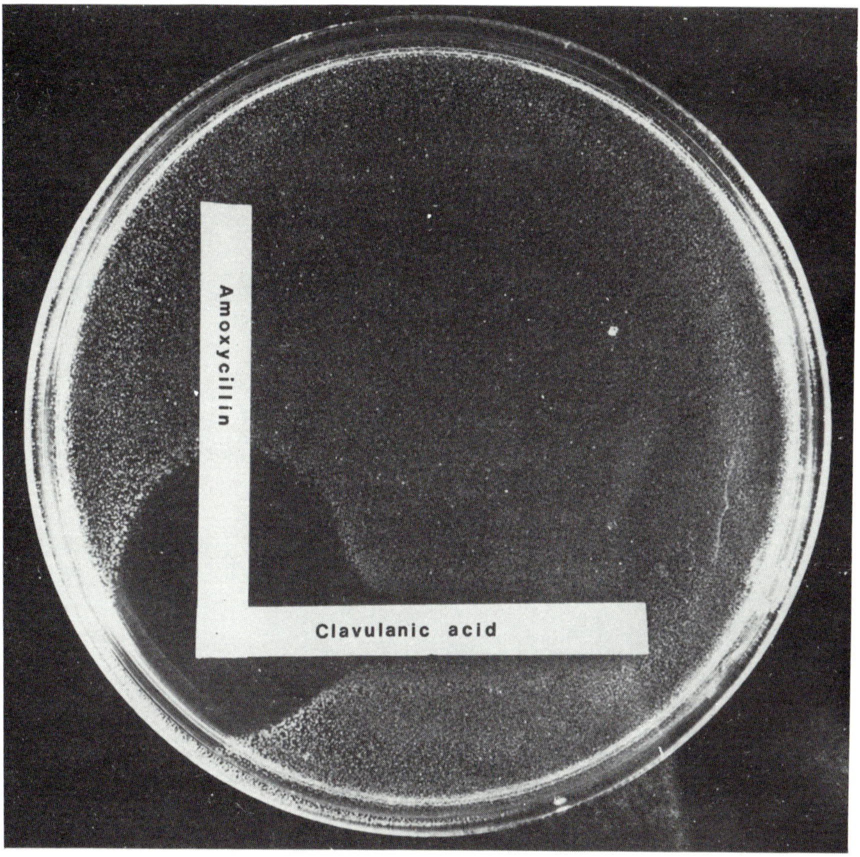

FIG. 8. Paper strip test showing synergy between amoxycillin and clavulanic acid against a β-lactamase-producing strain of *Escherichia coli*.

In the simplest method, paper discs containing each of the two antibiotics are placed at a suitable distance from one another on an agar plate seeded with the test organism. The size and appearance of the inhibition zones may be greatly influenced by the density of the inoculum used, and for best results it is recommended that the inoculum should be such as to produce 'dense but not confluent growth' (Waterworth 1981). After overnight incubation the interaction between the compounds is assessed from the appearance of the zones of inhibition (Möller & Holmgren 1969;

Quesnel & Handley 1974). Synergy may be reported when the inhibition zones are enlarged or when there is bridging between the discs (Fig. 5); antagonism is reported when there is a reduction or 'flattening' of the zones (Fig. 6) and indifference is associated with two independent circular zones. Alternatively, the performance of a single disc containing both antibiotics may also be compared with single discs containing the individual compounds (Fig. 7), but in some cases there may be greater difficulty in the interpretation of results.

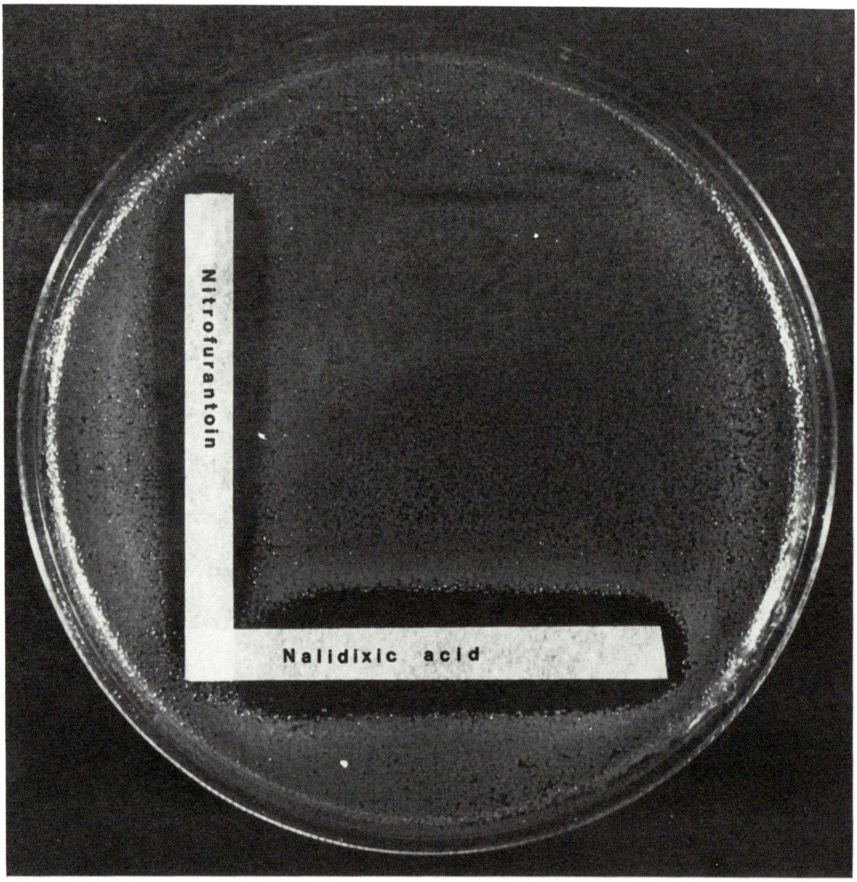

FIG. 9. Paper strip test showing antagonism between nitrofurantoin and nalidixic acid against *Proteus morganii*.

In place of paper discs, two antibiotic-impregnated paper strips placed at right angles to each other may yield inhibition patterns signifying synergy (Fig. 8) (enhancement of inhibition at the junction of the strips), antagonism (reduction of inhibition areas) (Fig. 9) and indifference (no obvious effect). A modification involves placing a paper strip impregnated with one agent on the surface of agar containing a subinhibitory concentration of another drug. Several test organisms may be streaked to the edge of the strip (Waterworth & Emmerson 1979).

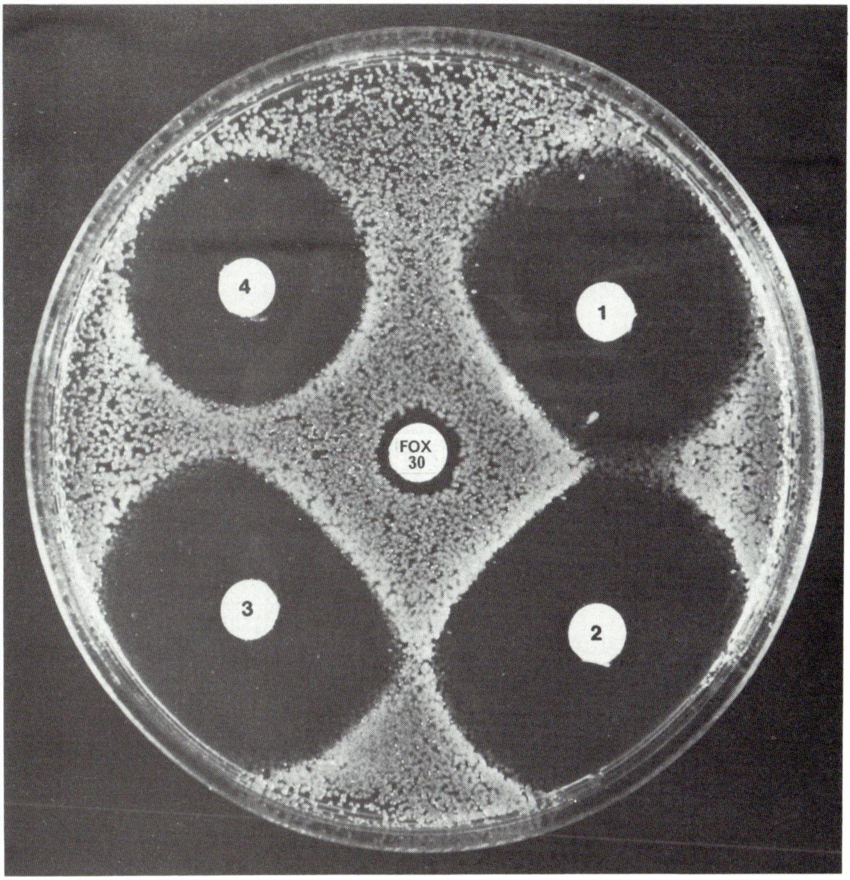

FIG. 10. Antagonism as a result of β-lactamase induction by cefoxitin (centre). Inhibition zones of moxalactam (1), cefotaxime (2) and ceftazidime (3) are flattened but no antagonism is seen with temocillin (4) which is stable to the β-lactamase produced by the test strain of *Enterobacter cloacae*.

The development in recent years of potent broad-spectrum penicillins and cephalosporins has led to an interest in the use of combinations of β-lactam antibiotics for the treatment of serious infections. Unexpectedly, antagonism has been demonstrated *in vitro* with some combinations of penicillins or cephalosporins in tests against certain Gram negative bacilli such as *Enterobacter* spp., *Serratia marcescens*, indole-positive *Proteus* spp., *Ps. aeruginosa* etc. (Waterworth & Emmerson 1979; Sanders & Sanders 1979; Kuck *et al.* 1981) (Fig. 10). The antagonism probably occurs as a result of the induction of bacterial β-lactamases resulting in the inactivation of one or both of the β-lactam compounds. The clinical relevance of the phenomenon is uncertain but it has resulted in renewed interest in antibiotic interactions.

The simple diffusion tests described above suffer from the disadvantage of measuring inhibition of growth only, and modified methods are employed

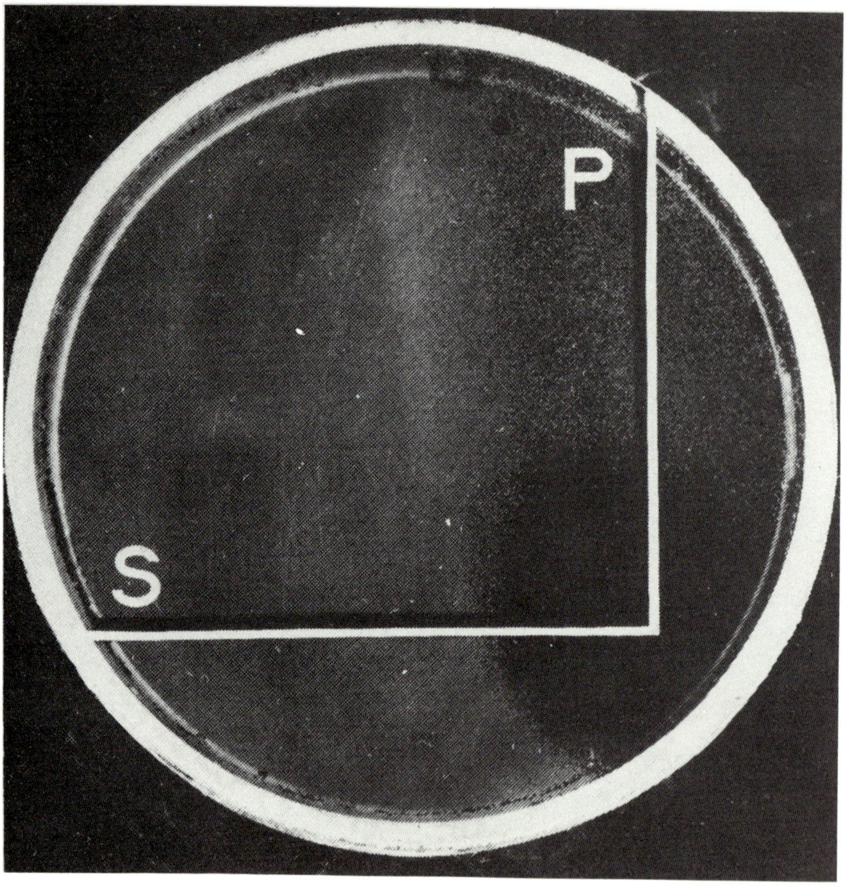

FIG. 11. The cellophane transfer method used on a strain of *Streptococcus faecalis*. The transfer shows bactericidal synergy between penicillin and streptomycin after incubation on antibiotic-free medium (from Waterworth 1981).

to detect bactericidal interactions. In the cellophane transfer technique first described by Chabbert (1957), a cellophane tambour is inoculated on the inside with the test organism and placed on an agar plate in which antibiotics have been allowed to diffuse from paper strips placed at a right angle (Waterworth 1978). After incubation, the cellophane is removed from the plate and transferred to antibiotic-free agar. The bactericidal effects of each drug and of the combination can be observed after incubation, from the zones at the ends of the strips in comparison with the zones seen at the junction of the strips (Fig. 11). Care must be taken in the choice of antibiotic concentrations used in the strips, otherwise if the concentration is too high sufficient antibiotic will be carried over to cause inhibition of growth after transfer (Chabbert & Waterworth 1965). In a modification of the method, a membrane filter is used as the transferable material in place of the cellophane (Lorian & Fodor 1974).

In tests involving β-lactam antibiotics the transfer method has largely been replaced by a simple technique involving the use of β-lactamase to inactivate the β-lactam component of the combination (Lee & Komarmy 1975; Anand & Paull 1976). The most common method is to spray the plate with a solution of β-lactamase after the first incubation period, and to examine the plate after further incubation for the presence of organisms which may have been inhibited by the combination but which were able to grow after inhibition of the β-lactam compound. In the triple layer modification of the technique, a layer of agar incorporating the β-lactamase is overlaid on the discs or strips after the initial incubation period (Yourassowsky *et al.* 1976).

Conclusions

Although it is often considered that combinations of antibiotics are used too frequently without good cause, nevertheless there are numerous clinical situations which justify combined therapy. It is important therefore that the routine laboratory is familiar with the techniques most suited for measuring combined antibiotic effects, and of interpreting the data obtained. In addition, as new compounds are discovered and introduced into clinical practice it is essential that the interaction with existing agents is monitored, even although the mechanism of action of the new drug may be well known. The demonstration of synergistic effects may hold the greatest interest but awareness of potential antagonism arising from combined therapy is equally important.

We wish to thank Mr S. Lomax and Mr C. Blackmore for their skilled assistance in the preparation of the figures and photographs.

References

ANAND, C. M. & PAULL, A. 1976 A modified technique for the detection of antibiotic synergism. *Journal of Clinical Pathology* **29,** 1130–1131.

ANDRIOLE, V. T. 1971 Synergy of carbenicillin and gentamicin in experimental infection with *Pseudomonas*. *Journal of Infectious Diseases* **124** (Supplement), S46–S55.

CHABBERT, Y. A. 1957 Une technique nouvelle d'étude de l'action bactericide des associations d'antibiotiques: le transfert sur cellophane. *Annales de l'Institut Pasteur* **93,** 289–299.

CHABBERT, Y. A. & WATERWORTH, P. M. 1965 Studies on the "carry-over" of antibiotics using the cellophane transfer technique. *Journal of Clinical Pathology* **18,** 314–316.

ELION, G. B., SINGER, S. & HITCHINGS, G. H. 1954 Antagonists of nucleic acid derivatives. VIII: Synergism in combinations of biochemically related antimetabolites. *Journal of Biological Chemistry* **208,** 477–488.

GREENWOOD, D. 1979 Laboratory methods for the evaluation of synergy. In *Antibiotic Interactions* ed. Williams, J. D. pp. 53–67. London & New York: Academic Press.

GREENWOOD, D. & O'GRADY, F. 1973 The two sites of penicillin action in *Escherichia coli*. *Journal of Infectious Diseases* **128,** 791–794.

JAWETZ, E. 1968 Combined antibiotic action: some definitions and correlations between laboratory and clinical results. In *Antimicrobial Agents and Chemotherapy* 1967 ed. Hobby, G. L. pp. 203–209, Washington: American Society for Microbiology.

JAWETZ, E. & GUNNISON, J. B. 1952 An experimental basis of combined antibiotic action. *Journal of the American Medical Association* **150,** 693–695.

KERRY, D. W., HAMILTON-MILLER, J. M. T. & BRUMFITT, W. 1975 Trimethoprim and rifampicin: *in vitro* activities separately and in combination. *Journal of Antimicrobial Chemotherapy* **1,** 417–427.

KROGSTAD, D. J. & MOELLERING, R. C. 1980 Combinations of antibiotics, mechanisms of interaction against bacteria. In *Antibiotics in Laboratory Medicine* ed. Lorian, V. Ch. 11, pp. 298–341, Baltimore & London: Williams & Wilkins.

KUCK, N. A., TESTA, R. Y. & FORBES, M. 1981 *In vitro* and *in vivo* antibacterial effects of combinations of beta-lactam antibiotics. *Antimicrobial Agents and Chemotherapy* **19,** 634–638.

LEE, W. S. & KOMARMY, L. 1975 Simple technique for the assay of antibiotic synergism against enterococci. *Antimicrobial Agents and Chemotherapy* **7,** 82–84.

LORIAN, V. 1975 Some effects of sub-inhibitory concentrations on bacteria. *Bulletin of the New York Academy of Medicine* **9,** 1046–1055.

LORIAN, V. & FODOR, G. 1974 Technique for determining the bactericidal effect of drug combinations. *Antimicrobial Agents and Chemotherapy* **5,** 630–633.

MOELLERING, R. C. JR., WENNERSTEN, C. B. G. & WEINBERG, A. N. 1971 Synergy of penicillin and gentamicin against enterococci. *Journal of Infectious Diseases* **124** (Supplement), S207–S209.

MÖLLER, O. & HOLMGREN, J. 1969 A paper disc technique for studying antibacterial synergism. *Acta pathologica et microbiologica Scandinavica* **76,** 141–143.

QUESNEL, L. B. & HANDLEY, P. S. 1974 Synergism between polymyxins, polysorbate and antimetabolites of folic acid synthesis, and a paper disc technique for routine testing for synergism. *Microbios* **10,** 199–210.

SANDERS, C. C. & SANDERS, W. E. 1979 Emergence of resistance to cefamandole: possible role of cefoxitin-inducible beta-lactamases. *Antimicrobial Agents and Chemotherapy* **15,** 792–797.

SPRATT, B. G. 1975 Distinct penicillin-binding proteins involved in the division, elongation and shape of *Escherichia coli* K12. *Proceedings of the National Academy of Sciences, USA* **72,** 2999–3003.

WATERWORTH, P. M. 1978 Tests of combined antibacterial action. In *Laboratory Methods in Antimicrobial Chemotherapy* ed. Reeves, D. S., Phillips, I., Williams, J. D. & Wise, R. Ch. 4, pp. 41–49. Edinburgh: Churchill Livingstone.

WATERWORTH, P. M. 1981 Laboratory control. In *Antibiotic and Chemotherapy* 5th edn, ed. Garrod, L. P., Lambert, H. P. and O'Grady, F. Ch. 27, pp. 464–504, Edinburgh: Churchill Livingstone.

WATERWORTH, P. M. & EMMERSON, A. M. 1979 Dissociated resistance among cephalosporins. *Antimicrobial Agents and Chemotherapy* **15,** 497–503.

YOURASSOWSKY, E., VANDERLINDEN, M. P. & SCHOUTENS, E. 1976 A rapid simple method for demonstrating synergy of amikacin and penicillin against various microorganisms. *Journal of Infectious Diseases* **134** (Supplement), S275–S279.

A Novel Multi-channel Biophotometer and its Use in Determining Antibiotic Effects

K. COLEMAN, PAMELA A. HUNTER AND P. RIDGWAY WATT

Beecham Pharmaceuticals Research Division,
Brockham Park, Betchworth, Surrey, UK

The value of turbidimetric monitoring of bacterial growth is well established, but the equipment currently available for the average research laboratory is limited either by cost, as for example, with the Autobac (General Diagnostics, Warner Lambert Co., Morris Plains, NJ, USA) and the MS-2 (Abbot Laboratories Ltd, Basingstoke, Hants., UK), or by the small number of channels, as for example, with the Bonet-Maury biophotometer (Jobin Yvon, Longjumeau, France). Some laboratories have designed their own equipment (see Mackintosh *et al.* 1973; Marcelis *et al.* 1980), but this has often been rather large and cumbersome. We have designed a simple automatic instrument (Fig. 1) with 24 channels, which can be built at little cost and which can be interfaced to a low-cost microcomputer.

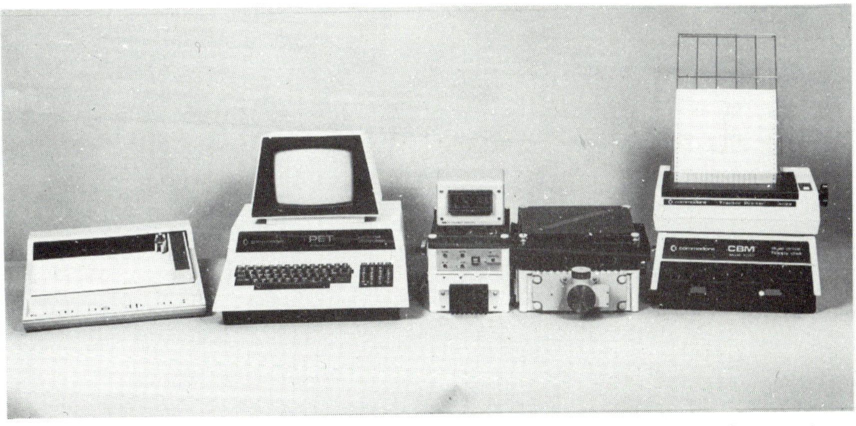

FIG. 1. General view of the equipment. Left to right: X-Y plotter, Commodore PET microcomputer, biophotometer and interface box, disc drive and printer.

ANTIBIOTICS
ISBN 0 12 604480 5

Biophotometer: General Principles

The biophotometer measures bacterial concentrations by optical means: a beam of light is passed through the bacterial suspension, and its transmission is monitored at intervals. The measured transmission is used to estimate the amount of bacterial growth, and the growth curves for a series of cultures are recorded automatically under microprocessor control for subsequent analysis. A system of this type (Fig. 2) requires the provision of a sample carrier, a light source and detector, a housing, and appropriate electronics; these are discussed below.

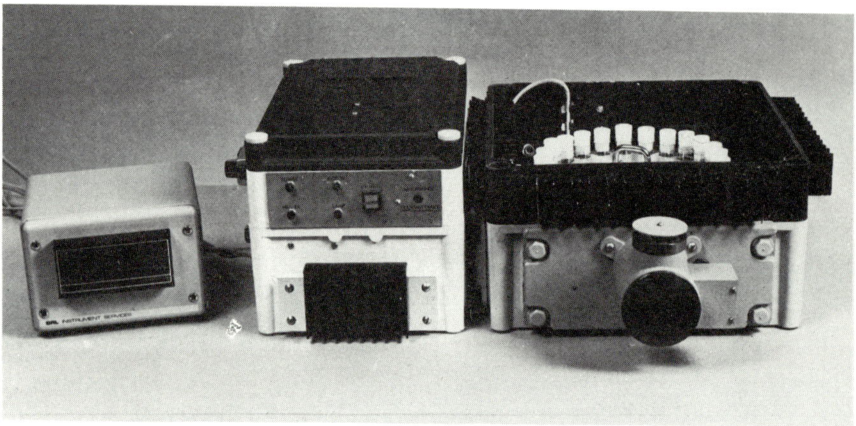

FIG. 2. The biophotometer showing the sample carrier in place.

Sample carrier

It is important to ensure that conditions for growth are as uniform as possible if growth rates are to be compared from culture to culture. In order to reduce the influence of local temperature variations within the housing, it was decided to use a rotating sample carrier which would expose all cultures equally to any such variations. The carrier is in the form of a removable turntable, with twenty-four evenly spaced sample positions whose centres lie on a circle of 6·5 inches diam. The turntable is arranged to fit over a drive unit, which centres and rotates it. In order to simplify the positioning of the turntable on the drive unit, the centre section has been constructed from transparent polycarbonate sheet. Experience with a commercial photometer, which employed glass cuvettes to hold bacterial cultures, had shown that the glass surfaces developed grey, uneven areas after a few sets of measurements. It was therefore decided that disposable plastic cuvettes (Fig. 3) would be preferable to re-usable glass ones: the turntable was provided with square, punched holes which would accept 1·0 cm stoppered cuvettes (W. Sarstedt, Leicester, UK).

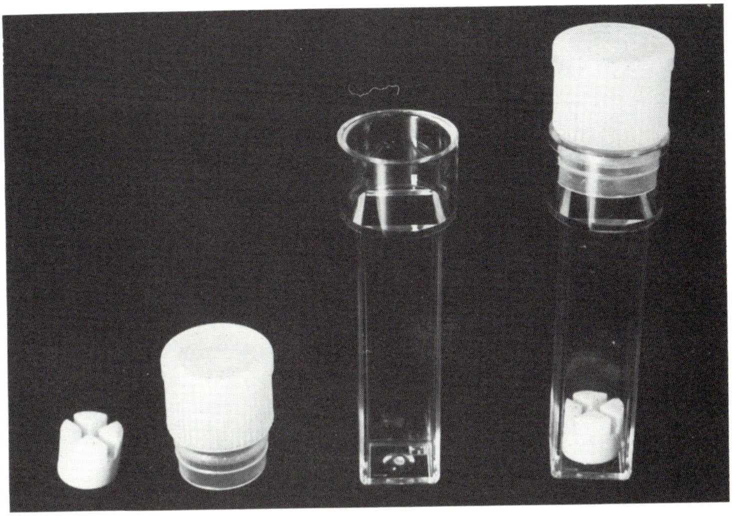

FIG. 3. Cuvette, magnetic stirrer and cap assembly.

Drive unit

Motive power to the turntable is provided by a small geared electric motor, which turns the input shaft of a commercial worm-drive gear box.

Light source

A quartz-iodine, A1/220, projector lamp is used as a light source. The lamp is contained in an external housing and is provided with a heat filter and a glass lens so that a narrow light beam may be projected through the cuvette being measured. In order to reduce the heating effect of the lamp on the system, intermittent operation is used. The lamp is run at full brightness only for the few seconds that are needed for measurement; at other times the filament is merely kept warm by a small current.

The light-scattering effect resulting from bacterial growth is most conveniently measured at the blue end of the spectrum. Normal silicon photodiodes, however, have a maximum sensitivity at the red end, around 800 nm. In practice, a reasonable compromise has been achieved by the use of a blue–green filter, fitted permanently into the optical path.

Detector

The transmitted light is detected by means of a PIN photodiode (IPL 33) and associated circuitry. Standard neutral density filters are used from time to time, to check the accuracy of the system. Additionally, a cuvette has been adapted to receive a rectangle of neutral density Perspex, to provide a further check on the measuring system; this may be incorporated with the samples in the turntable as required.

Stirring

It is desirable that the contents of each cuvette should be stirred at intervals. This is accomplished by the use of magnetic stirrers (Fig. 3): each cuvette contains a Teflon-encapsulated follower magnet (Bel-Art 'Cell Spinbar'; R. B. Radley), and there are three equally spaced driver magnets rotating at 500–600 r/min under the path of the turntable.

Housing

The biophotometer turntable, stirrers and optical components are housed in a sealable fibreglass container so that they may, if necessary, be operated in a controlled atmosphere. The housing also contains a small fan and heater so that it can be maintained at constant temperature.

Hardware

The system is designed to operate in association with a microcomputer. In this instance a 32 Kbyte PET (Commodore Business Machines, CBM, Slough, UK) is used with a disc-drive (3040 CBM), a tractor feed printer (4022 CBM) and an X-Y plotter (7225A Hewlett-Packard, Winnersh, Bucks, UK). This is a relatively low-cost arrangement which provides a control system for the biophotometer and also allows the host laboratory to use the PET for other work between experiments.

Software

A suite of programs has been written to handle all data and to control the biophotometer turntable. All programs can be loaded from a common 'menu' (Fig. 4) which resides in the PET throughout a run. The initialization program allows the user to vary the speed of rotation of the turntable which holds the cuvettes. In practice, the speed that has been found suitable for most experiments is 4 r/h.

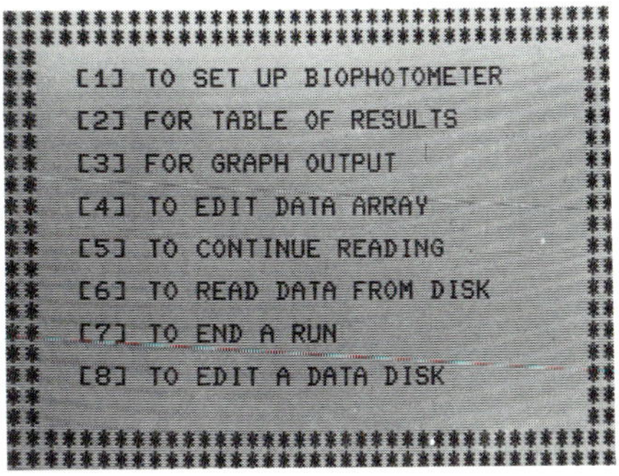
[1] TO SET UP BIOPHOTOMETER
[2] FOR TABLE OF RESULTS
[3] FOR GRAPH OUTPUT
[4] TO EDIT DATA ARRAY
[5] TO CONTINUE READING
[6] TO READ DATA FROM DISK
[7] TO END A RUN
[8] TO EDIT A DATA DISK

FIG. 4. Available programs listed on screen of the PET.

The data collection program sends a pulse to the biophotometer to move the next cuvette into the light path. The biophotometer waits for the previously selected interval, checks that the lamp is on, and then takes a series of transmission readings from the interface. The average transmission reading is stored in memory and on disc, along with the time of the reading, the cuvette number and the revolution number. If the event marker is detected, the program checks that there were 24 readings taken on the previous revolution, updates the revolution counter, and resets the cuvette counter to 'one'. Throughout the read cycle, the last reading obtained for each cuvette is displayed on the screen in the form of a bar chart (Fig. 5). This program may be interrupted at any time to obtain a numeric and/or graphic display of the data, with options to resume reading, or to end the experiment without taking further readings.

At the end of an experiment, the disc file is closed. A print-out of all transmission readings taken at pre-selected times during the period of the experiment may then be obtained, providing a hard copy record of the entire experiment. The results from any number of the 24 cuvettes can be plotted graphically, either during, or more usually at the end of, an experiment. Since the data are stored on magnetic disc, further graphs may be obtained at a later date, if desired.

Further programs allow for: (a) data for one or more cuvettes to be displayed graphically to the screen (Fig. 6) or to an X-Y plotter (Fig. 7) for hard copy; (b) various editing options such as conversion of transmission values to optical density; (c) data from a previous experiment to be re-loaded from the magnetic disc for further processing; (d) erasure of old data files which are no longer required.

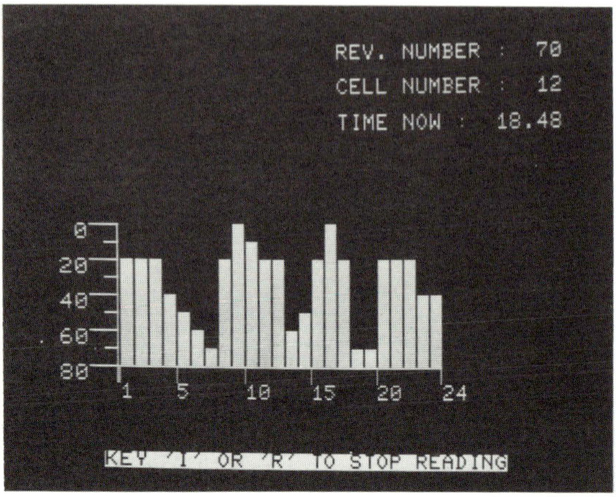

FIG. 5. An example of a screen display on the PET during an experiment, showing the transmission of each cuvette. The reading for cuvette no. 12 has just been entered; it is the 70th revolution and 18·48 h have elapsed from the start of the experiment.

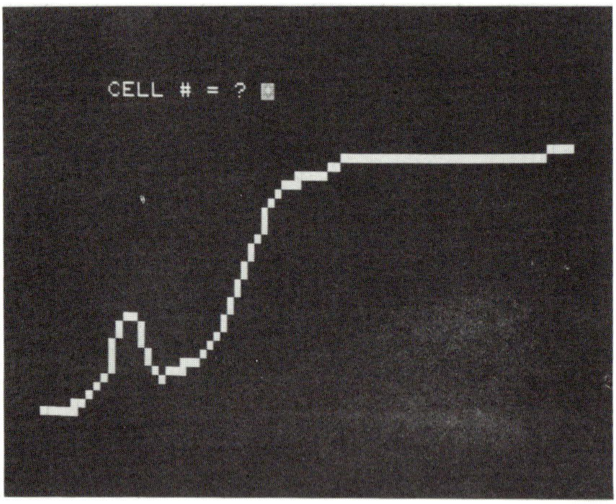

FIG. 6. An example of a screen display of the transmission readings of a cuvette. This display may be obtained at any time during the experiment to check the progress of one or more cuvettes. The display may also be used to select which data are suitable for printing by the X-Y plotter.

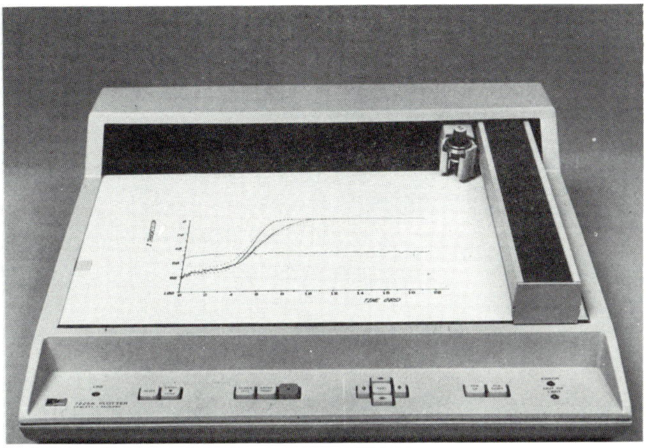

FIG. 7. The X-Y plotter with a completed graph *in situ*.

Use of the Biophotometer

The magnetic stirrers are placed in a suitable container and sterilized by autoclaving. A stirrer is placed in each cuvette and the cuvette closed with a cap (Fig. 3). The disposable cuvettes and caps are 'clean packed', and provided they are handled and stored carefully, no problems with contamination should be encountered.

At the end of an experiment the magnetic stirrers are removed from the cuvettes, sterilized, cleaned, and can then be used again.

Bacterial cultures are grown in suitable broth media, mixed thoroughly, diluted in warm broth and 3·5 ml placed in each cuvette. Tryptone Soy broth (Lab M) has been used for the majority of Gram negative organisms and Brain Heart Infusion Broth (Lab M) for staphylococci. The machine is switched on approximately 30 min prior to the start of the experiment to allow the chamber to warm up and equilibrate before loading the cuvette carrier. Most of our experiments have used log-phase cultures, the organisms being allowed to grow for 1–3 h in the biophotometer before the addition of antibiotics.

The machine has produced good results with a range of organisms including Enterobacteriaceae, staphylococci and *Haemophilus influenzae*. Results with *Pseudomonas* species have been less successful, some strains clumping and producing pellicles. The addition of nitrate to the broth reduced clumping, allowing more strains to be used successfully, but there were still a significant number of strains which did not grow satisfactorily.

It is hoped that modifications to the method of stirring will allow more strains to be used.

Inoculum Effects

The biophotometer is a convenient instrument for determining the effect of the size of inoculum on antibiotic activity, since it reveals that many antibiotics exert a considerable effect on the growth of bacteria at concentrations below their minimum inhibitory concentration (MIC). Using a biophotometer, Greenwood (1976) has described the activity of several different types of antibiotics against a strain of *Escherichia coli*. Such studies are particularly convenient to carry out in the instrument we are describing, since the large number of channels, the ease with which additions of antibiotic can be made, and the constant visual display of the growth in each cuvette, allow greater variety of experimental design.

Part of an experiment investigating the activity of Augmentin (Beecham Pharmaceuticals) against a β-lactamase-producing strain of *E. coli* is illustrated in Fig. 8. Augmentin is the co-formulation of the β-lactam antibiotic amoxycillin and the β-lactamase inhibitor clavulanic acid

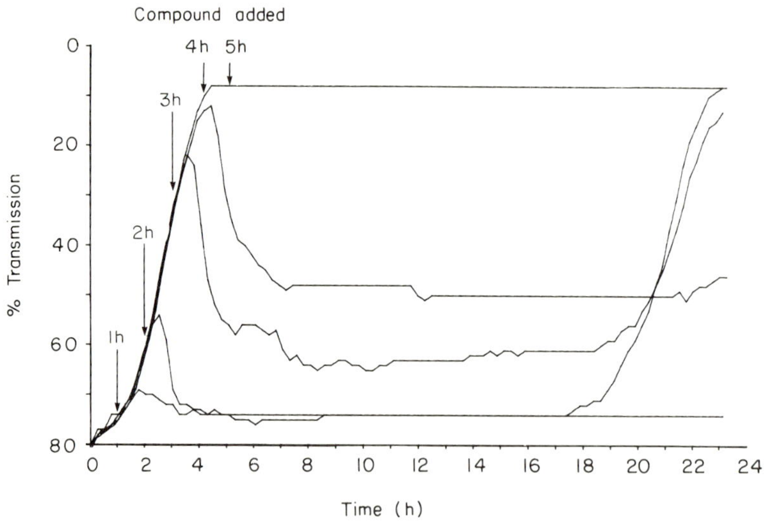

FIG. 8. Turbidimetric response of *Escherichia coli* cultures to which Augmentin (10 μg amoxycillin/ml + 5 μg clavulanic acid/ml) has been added after varying periods of incubation. Output from the X-Y plotter.

(Comber *et al.* 1980). Amoxycillin has poor stability to the plasmid-mediated β-lactamase produced by this strain of *E. coli* and consequently its addition to the culture does not affect the rate at which turbidity develops. Clavulanic acid is a potent inhibitor of this type of β-lactamase (Reading & Cole 1977) and is able to protect amoxycillin from enzymic degradation, so that a synergistic effect is seen when it is used in conjunction with amoxycillin (Hunter *et al.* 1980). In the example illustrated in Fig. 8, 10 μg of amoxycillin/ml and 5 μg of clavulanic acid/ml were used, additions being made to the growing culture after 1, 2, 3, 4 and 5 h incubation. When the compounds were added after 1 h to the culture which contained 10^6 c.f.u./ml, the development of turbidity was prevented for 24 h, whereas addition at 5 h, when the culture contained 8×10^8 c.f.u./ml, had no effect. Additions at 2, 3 and 4 h all produced a rapid lytic effect characteristic of the mode of action of amoxycillin (Rolinson *et al.* 1977) but as would be expected from the increased numbers of organisms present at 3 and 4 h, the reduction in turbidity was incomplete. (The viable count of the culture was 7×10^6 at 2 h, 7×10^7 at 3h and 2×10^8 c.f.u./ml at 4 h.)

Correlation of Turbidimetric Readings with Viability

In any study of the activity of antibiotics against bacterial cultures, it is desirable to determine the numbers of viable organisms remaining after exposure to the antibiotic for varying periods of time. However, techniques for determining viability are time-consuming, even with equipment such as the spiral plater and laser counter (Don Whitley Scientific, Shipley, UK). Generally, counts are only performed during the working day and the following morning; if a fall in numbers is followed by regrowth, the time at which this regrowth occurs is not always known. A biophotometer of the type we are describing has the advantage of requiring very little effort to set up and allows monitoring of the growth in cuvettes without the operator being present. The major disadvantage to turbidimetric monitoring is that no drop in bacterial numbers below *ca.* 5×10^6 c.f.u./ml can be detected, only an increase. Nevertheless, the use of a multi-channel biophotometer can provide valuable information on a larger number of antibiotic/bacterial inter-reactions than the average laboratory could cope with using viability determinations. However, for the best use of such an instrument, an understanding of the correlation between the viability of a culture and the turbidimetric readings is necessary.

We have followed the viability of cultures in various experiments performed in the biophotometer, and in most instances have found a good correlation between viable counts and turbidimetric readings. Examples are quoted here of experiments in which a Gram positive coccus and a Gram negative bacillus were exposed to β-lactam antibiotics.

Using a plasmid-carrying strain of *E. coli* which produced large quantities of β-lactamase, the addition after 2·75 h incubation of Augmentin (10 μg amoxycillin/ml + 5 μg clavulanic acid/ml) or 10 μg cefazolin/ml (Kefzol, Eli Lilly) resulted in a rapid fall in the turbidity of the culture. The onset of this fall occurred 1–1·5 h after the addition of the compounds. Neither compound was able to maintain this reduction in turbidity, and after 6–7 h exposure to the antibiotics, the turbidity of the cultures increased rapidly at a rate similar to that seen earlier in the control cuvette (antibiotic absent). A rapid fall in bacterial numbers was apparent when the first viable count was performed at 45 min after the addition of the compounds. Both antibiotics reduced the viable count from 7×10^7 to 10^5 c.f.u./ml in 3 h, but subsequently were unable to maintain this rate of kill; numbers then increased rapidly (Fig. 9).

In this experiment a slight change in turbidity was seen at 1·5 h, at which point the viable count was 3×10^6 c.f.u./ml, which corresponds to the approximate lower limit of detection with the biophotometer. If numbers fall below this figure and subsequently increase, as occurred in the experiment described above, there will be a delay in the detection of this increase by the biophotometer, since the turbidity of the culture will only increase when numbers exceed 1 to 5×10^6/ml. In the experiment illustrated in Fig. 9, the numbers of organisms fell initially following antibiotic treatment, and then, at 6 h after the start of the experiment, started to increase. The turbidity of these cultures, although falling initially, did not show an increase until the numbers of organisms had reached 3 to 6×10^6 c.f.u./ml. Apart from these minor differences, the two methods produce remarkably similar results.

Figure 10 illustrates the effect of adding 0·1 μg cefazolin/ml or 0·1 μg benzylpenicillin/ml (Beecham Pharmaceuticals) to a culture of *Staphylococcus aureus* after 2 h incubation. As noted above, the correlation between viable count and turbidity for the control culture (antibiotic absent) was excellent; the biophotometer recordings show an initial lag-phase of 1·5 h, followed by a phase of rapid growth which ceased at 6–7 h. The addition of benzylpenicillin at 2 h initially reduced the rate of increase in numbers, followed by a slow, steady fall in numbers, which was maintained at 24 h. The turbidity of these cultures also increased at a slower rate than that of the control cultures initially, and then decreased slowly, remaining constant after *ca.* 8–9 h.

The addition of cefazolin produced a far slower bactericidal effect; numbers continued to increase at a reduced rate for 3 h after the addition of

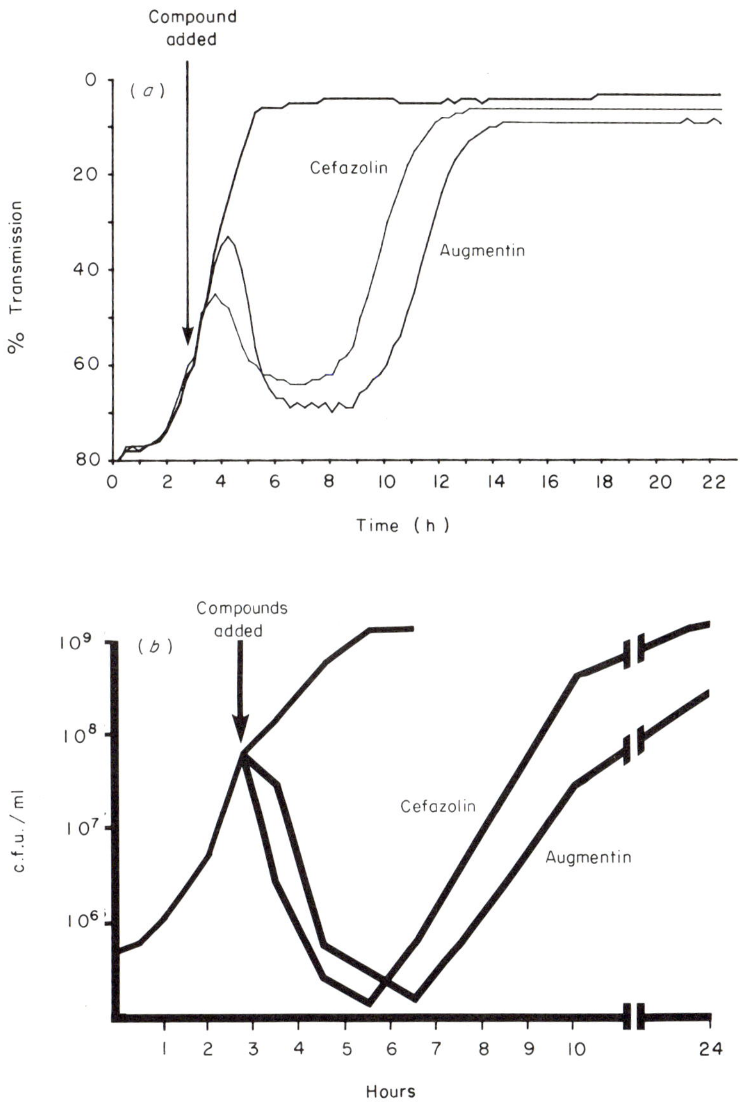

FIG. 9. Effects of augmentin and cefazolin on an *Escherichia coli* culture. (*a*) Biophotometric response (output from X-Y plotter). (*b*) Viable count.

antibiotic, and then fell slowly, so that after a further 4 h there were still 10^7 c.f.u./ml present. This pattern was reflected in the readings from the biophotometer, but whereas the viable count continued to fall to a low figure overnight, the biophotometer output did not change significantly after 10 h. We have previously observed such a discrepancy between the viable count and the turbidity of antibiotic-treated cultures, and it has been associated with the addition of suboptimal levels of antibiotic to a large inoculum of bacteria. In the example illustrated here, the numbers of bacteria in the cefazolin-treated culture reached 10^8 c.f.u./ml before any killing effect was evident; the subsequent rate of kill was then slow.

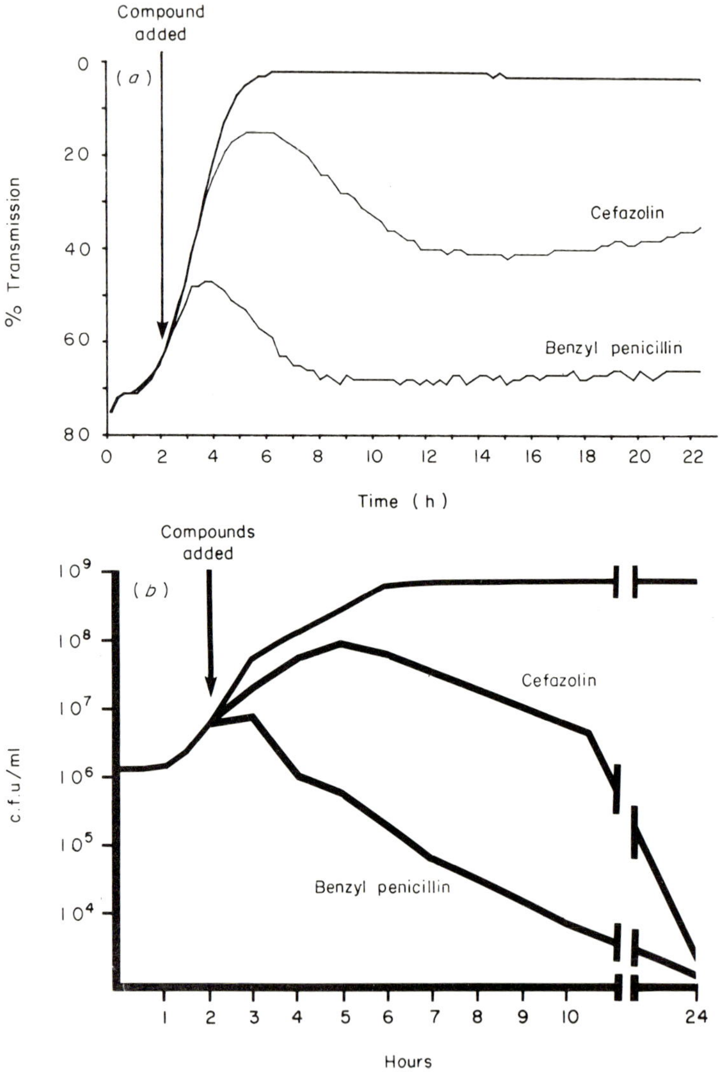

FIG. 10. Effects of benzylpenicillin and cefazolin on a *Staphylococcus aureus* culture. (*a*) Biophotometric response (output from X-Y plotter). (*b*) Viable count.

Our experience has been that even lytic β-lactam antibiotics may not always produce complete clearing of the broth when dense populations are exposed to suboptimal levels. A slow and incomplete fall in turbidity is particularly marked when β-lactam antibiotics which are pronounced filament-producers are used, e.g. cefotaxime and moxalactam (Greenwood *et al.* 1981; Hunter & Coleman, unpublished results). Antibiotics which do not affect the cell wall, generally do not produce a marked fall in turbidity (Greenwood 1976). Ideally, microscopic examination of the contents of the cuvettes should be carried out at intervals, but this is not always practicable. In our laboratory the machine is frequently used to give an indication of the relative activity of compounds prior to the performance of more detailed studies. When this is the case, and in order that data from the biophotometer should not be misinterpreted, the contents of all cuvettes are sampled at the end of an experiment to determine the numbers of organisms present. This routine also serves to check the purity of the cultures. Whenever possible, samples from any cuvettes showing a slow fall in turbidity are also examined microscopically.

The experiments described here serve to illustrate the value of this biophotometer in determing the effects of antibiotics against bacterial cultures. Correlation between turbidity and viability is particularly good when antibiotic effects are rapid. Some discrepancy can occur when antibiotics are added to large inocula of bacteria and produce a slow rate of kill, the biophotometer occasionally underestimating the effect of the antibiotic. However, provided that cuvette contents are sampled at the end of an experiment, any such discrepancy should not lead to misinterpretation of the data, since the initial fall in numbers is accurately reflected. As with many techniques, the value of biophotometry depends on a proper understanding of the shortcomings, as well as the advantages, of the equipment.

Summary

The novel instrument described has been developed for the routine measurement of bacterial growth in stirred culture broths. The instrument monitors growth by measuring light transmission through the broth samples in disposable plastic cuvettes, and is capable of handling up to 24 samples. The cuvettes are held in a turntable, which is contained within a temperature-controlled, sealable casing; movement of the turntable is under microprocessor control, and can be varied to suit the particular requirements of the procedure. The microprocessor itself is a low-cost, commerically available unit which controls the biophotometer and various peripherals including a disc drive, a printer and an X-Y plotter. Experimental data are stored on a disc file: under the direction of a specialized program they may then be presented in graphical or numerical form, on a screen display or as hard copy. The use of the instrument to determine the effect of the size of inoculum on antibiotic activity is described. Further examples of antibiotic effects are given, in which light-transmission readings have been correlated with viable counts. A useful feature of the system is that the microprocessor may be applied to general calculation and the running of other programs when the biophotometer is not in use.

References

COMBER, K. R., HORTON, R., MIZEN, L., WHITE, A. R. & SUTHERLAND, R. 1980 Activity of amoxycillin/clavulanic acid (2:1) (BRL 25000, Augmentin), *in vitro* and *in vivo*. *Current Chemotherapy and Infectious Diseases* **1,** 343–344.

GREENWOOD, D. 1976 Differentiation of mechanisms responsible for inoculum effects in the response of *E. coli* to a variety of antibiotics. *Journal of Antimicrobial Chemotherapy* **2,** 87–95.

GREENWOOD, D., ELEY, A., PEARSON, N. & O'GRADY, F. 1981 *In vitro* activity of the novel oxa-β-lactam antibiotic, moxalactam (LY 127935) against dense populations of selected Gram-negative bacteria. *Journal of Antimicrobial Chemotherapy* **7,** 353–362.

HUNTER, P. A., COLEMAN, K., FISHER, J. & TAYLOR, D. 1980 *In vitro* synergistic properties of clavulanic acid with ampicillin, amoxycillin and ticarcillin. *Journal of Antimicrobial Chemotherapy* **6,** 455–470.

MACKINTOSH, I. P., O'GRADY, F., GREENWOOD, D., WATSON, B. W., CRICHTON, T. C., PIPER, R. & FERRER, A. 1973 A 12-channel bacterial growth monitoring system. *Biomedical Engineering* **8,** 514–515, 526.

MARCELIS, J. H., VERSTEEG, H., MANSVELT-BECK, H. J. & VINKE, D. 1980 Semi-electronic turbidimeter for automated monitoring of bacterial growth in test tubes. *Applied and Environmental Microbiology* **39,** 281–284.

READING, C. & COLE, M. 1977 Clavulanic acid: a β-lactamase-inhibiting β-lactam from *Streptomyces clavuligerus*. *Antimicrobial Agents and Chemotherapy* **11,** 852–857.

ROLINSON, G. N., MACDONALD, A. C. & WILSON, D. A. 1977 Bactericidal action of β-lactam antibiotics on *Escherichia coli* with particular reference to ampicillin and amoxycillin. *Journal of Antimicrobial Chemotherapy* **3,** 541–553.

Identification of Antibiotics by High Voltage Electrophoresis

A. F. LOTT AND D. R. VAUGHAN

Laboratory of the Government Chemist, Department of Industry, Cornwall House, Stamford Street, London, UK

It is not uncommon to encounter antimicrobial activity in foods and in animal feeding stuffs. Inhibitory substances may occur naturally or may be added deliberately, for example as preservatives in food and as growth-promoting antibiotic additives in feeds, and such additions may be legitimate or otherwise. Inadvertent contamination during manufacture or the residues persisting from veterinary treatment are other obvious sources. A method for identifying antibiotics and other antibacterial substances similarly employed in human and veterinary medicine is therefore a valuable tool in the analytical laboratory.

Foods

Most methods for detecting antibiotic residues in foods discussed elsewhere in this volume (Corry *et al.*, pp. 349–373) are based simply on the demonstration of an antibacterial effect. Screening tests for meat, for example the proposed four plate test (FPT) of the European Community (Bogaerts & Wolf 1980), must be kept very simple to enable the anticipated large numbers of samples to be handled. A positive response in the FPT is not invariably due to a recognizable antibiotic residue (Smither 1978). In a series of 5442 UK-produced meat samples reported by Smither *et al.* (1980) 34 initially failed the FPT. Electrophoresis demonstrated that only two failures were due to recognizable antibiotics. Of the remainder, 20 passed the FPT upon re-testing and 12 were recognized as containing naturally produced inhibitors.

ANTIBIOTICS
ISBN 0 12 604480 5

Feeding Stuffs

Official methods for determining antibiotics added to animal feeding stuffs (Anon. 1976) assume that the additive declared on the feed label is solely responsible for the measured antibacterial response. The presence of undeclared inhibitory substances may lead to erroneous results which may not be obvious even to an experienced analyst. From eight official referee samples of feeding stuffs examined in the Laboratory of the Government Chemist (LGC) four were found to contain an undeclared antibiotic. These results should not be regarded as representative of feeding stuffs generally; the operation of the referee system ensures that it is the unusual 'problem' samples which reach the Laboratory. Another 21 feeding stuff samples were examined for suspected contamination with lincomycin, an antibiotic which may be added to pig feed on veterinary direction but which is known to produce adverse reactions in dairy cattle. The results are shown in Table 1. Recently the feeding stuff industry has adopted a code of practice which is designed to end the problem of cross-contamination with medicated feeds.

Electrophoresis was also used to confirm the presence of various unlicensed antibiotics in three samples of imported calf feed which had been intercepted by the authorities.

Electrophoresis

Electrophoresis is a separation technique in which charged molecular species are caused to migrate in a buffered gel by the application of a potential difference. In an agar gel most antibiotics migrate towards the cathode, some towards the anode. Migration distances vary according to the size and shape of the molecules and their net charge. The positions taken up are visualized by bio-autography using a sensitive bacterial culture. Early descriptions of the technique (Marten 1964; Lightbown & de Rossi 1965) have been followed by numerous other workers who have evolved their own variations on the general theme. Published methods include those of Bozzi & Valdebouze (1973), Grynne (1973), Reeves & Holt (1975), Billon & Tao (1979), Horng *et al.* (1979) and Stadhouders *et al.* (1981).

LGC electrophoresis system

A full description of the LGC electrophoresis system has already been published by Smither & Vaughan (1978) whose paper includes a table describing the results obtained with 50 named antibacterial substances (see Table 2). These data should be used as a general guide followed by 'runs' alongside selected standards.

TABLE 1

Cattle feeds suspected of lincomycin contamination

Source	Estimated lincomycin content (μg/g)	Other contaminating antibiotics
A	0·15	Furazolidone or nitrofurazone
	0·25	—*
	0·05	Tylosin
	Nf†	Penicillin; virginiamycin or chloramphenicol (trace)
	0·5	—
	1·0	—
	Nf	—
	1·0	—
	1·0	—
	1·0	—
	Nf	—
	Nf	Tylosin
B	Nf	Penicillin; chlortetracycline
	Nf	—
	2·0	Penicillin
	2·0	Tylosin; penicillin
C	Nf	Tylosin
D	Nf	Tylosin
E	3·0	Penicillin
F	Nf	Tylosin; dimetridazole‡
	Nf	Tylosin; dimetridazole‡

* None detected.
† Nf, not found.
‡ Identified by GLC.

The method features the use of low ionic-strength buffer systems to restrict current flow and therefore to reduce unwanted electrolytic and heating effects. Electrophoresis is carried out at pH 6 and 8 in both agar and agarose gels. Differences in the electro-endosmotic characteristics of agar and agarose lead to substantial changes in migration distances which enables additional information to be obtained from the plates. The original paper should be consulted for full details of the experimental technique which may be summarized as follows:

Extractant for feeding stuffs and powdered freeze-dried meat samples. Acetonitrile–distilled water (9 : 1, by vol.). Extracts may be applied directly to the plate or be concentrated by evaporation in a fume cupboard depending upon the anticipated antibiotic concentration.

Standard antibiotic solutions. Prepared in acetonitrile–distilled water (1 : 1, by vol.) and diluted in buffer solution.

TABLE 2

Sensitivity and migration profiles

Antibiotic: Family	Antibiotic: Substance	Antibiotic: Source	Minimum amount, pH 6·0: *Bacillus cereus*	Minimum amount, pH 6·0: *Micrococcus luteus*
Aminoglycoside	Dihydrostreptomycin SO_4	Sigma	1	1
	Gentamicin SO_4	Sigma	5	20
	Hygromycin B	IBS	10	10
	Kanamycin SO_4	Sigma	5	10
	Neomycin SO_4	Sigma	20–50†	> 100
	Paromomycin SO_4	IRP	10	20
	Streptomycin SO_4	Sigma	1	1
β-Lactam	Ampicillin trihydrate	BRL	5	0·002
	Amoxycillin trihydrate	BRL	5	0·002
	Benzylpenicillin Na	Sigma	10–20	0·002–0·005
	Cloxacillin Na	BRL	100	0·1–0·2
	Flucloxacillin	BRL	50–100	0·05–0·2
	Methicillin Na	BRL	1–100	0·05–0·1
	Phenethicillin K	BRL	20 50	0·005–0·02
	Phenoxymethylpenicillin K	Sigma	20	0·002–0·01
	Propicillin K	BRL	20–100	0·005–0·01
	Cephalexin	BPAS	2–10	0·05
	Cephaloridine hydrate	Glaxo	1–2	0·02–0·05
	Cephalothin	Glaxo	20–50	0·05–0·2
	Cephradine	Squibb	1–2	0·01
Macrolide	Erythromycin	Sigma	0·2–0·5†	0·05
	Oleandomycin PO_4	Sigma	0·5	0·2
	Spiramycin base	MB	10	0·4–1
	Spiramycin embonate	R-P	20	1–2
	Tylosin base	EL	1	0·1
Polypeptide	Bacitracin Zn	Dumex	4	0·05–0·2†
	Viomycin SO_4	Pfizer	20	50–100
	Virginiamycin	SKF	0·4	0·01
Tetracycline	Chlortetracycline HCl	Sigma	0·004	0·02
	Clomocycline	Pharmax	0·01	0·05
	Demethylchortetracycline	Pfizer	0·01	0·05
	Oxytetracycline dihydrate	Sigma	0·04	0·1
	Tetracycline HCl	Sigma	0·02	0·1
Sulphonamide	Sulphadiazine	Sigma	> 100	10
	Sulphadimidine	BPAS	> 100	50
	Sulphamethoxazole	BW	100	5–10
	Sulfaquinoxaline	MSD	50	15
	Sulphathiazole	Sigma	> 100	20
Other	Avoparcin SO_4	Cyanamid	0·1	0·1–0·2
	Chloramphenicol	Sigma	2	0·5
	Flavomycin	Hoechst	0·1	5–10
	Furazolidone	SKF	0·1	100
	Lincomycin HCl	Upjohn	20	0·2–0·5
	Monensin Na	Dista	0·5	0·5
	Nalidixic acid	Sigma	1	20
	Nitrovin	Cyanamid	0·05	> 100
	Novobiocin Na	Upjohn	0·05	0·01
	Rifamycin SV	Sigma	0·05	0·002–0·004†
	Spectinomycin HCl	Upjohn	20	10
	Trimethoprim	BW	> 100	10

* Where sensitivity is given as a range, e.g. benzylpenicillin 0·002–0·005 μg at pH 6·0 with *Micrococcus luteus*, the first figure represents the sensitivity in agarose, whilst the second figure represents the sensitivity in agar.

† Here the first figure represents the sensitivity in agar.

‡ Conditions in which antibiotics normally streak. (Figure given for neomycin (pH 6·0, agar) represents total length of streak, which originates from the well.)

§ Conditions in which antibiotics only streak when overloaded (flavomycin streaked with *Bacillus cereus* only).

of 50 antibacterial substances

detected (μg)*		Migration distance (mm)			
pH 8·0		pH 6·0		pH 8·0	
Bacillus cereus	*Micrococcus luteus*	Agar	Agarose	Agar	Agarose
0·2	0·1	31(A)	234	14	206
0·5	0·5–1†	71(A)§	240‡	77(A)§	177‡
10	2–4	11(A)	260	174	201
0·5	1	66(A)	253	66	185
2	1	66(A)‡	190‡	84(A)§	112‡
0·5–1†	2	71(A)§	234‡	60(A)§	170‡
0·2	0·2–0·4	32(A)	237	4	200
10	0·002–0·005	135	23	12	111(A)
5	0·002–0·005	138	28	23	95(A)
10–20	0·005	30(A)	149(A)	20(A)	138(A)
> 100	0·1–0·2	22(A)	131(A)	13(A)	123(A)
> 100	0·1–0·2	21(A)	93(A), *129(A)*‖	12(A)	123(A)
50–> 100	0·05–0·1	17(A)	127(A)	13(A)	124(A)
50–100	0·01–0·02	20(A)	134(A)	19(A)	131(A)
20	0·005	32(A)	148(A)	21(A)	138(A)
50–100	0·01–0·02	23(A)	131(A)	13(A)	126(A)
5–20†	0·05	134	21	12	108(A)
2	0·02	154	40	156	40
50	0·1–0·2	19(A)	132(A)	13(A)	131(A)
2–5†	0·02	146	31	36	85(A)
0·05	0·005	250	151	237	134
0·2	0·02	250	154	236	135
1	0·02–0·1†	238	204	226	125
2	0·05–0·2†	239	203	225	123
0·5	0·05	232	128	181	64
20	0·4–1†	193§	87§	123§	5(A)§
10	10–20	14	258	6	227
4	0·05	157	41	73, *164*‖	*42*, 43(A)‖
0·04	0·2–0·4	150	34	87	21(A)
0·1	0·5	147	30	88	22(A)
0·1	0·4	146	30	112	2
0·4	0·5	150	34	98	14(A)
0·2	0·5	149	35	123	5
> 100	50	101	18(A)	37(A)	161(A)
> 100	15	168	41	42	88(A)
100	5	20	96(A)	53(A)	167(A)
50	5	33	85(A)	31(A)	149(A)
100	2–5	155	32	32(A)	145(A)
0·2	0·2	*107*, 135‖	83, *120*‖	123, *151*‖	*34*, 65‖
2	0·5	167	43	157	40
0·04	5	17, *33(A)*§‖	97(A), *147(A)*§‖	17, *27(A)*§‖	100(A), *152(A)*§‖
0·1	50	162	40	152	37
5	0·05	266	180	219	105
2	4	58	64(A)	52	74(A)
4	100	76	52(A)	11	140(A)
0·01	> 100	215§	163§	168§	62§
0·25	0·02–0·05†	44	76(A)	39	81(A)
0·05	0·002	167	61	77	50(A)
20	5–10	242	257	250	179
> 100	3	290	208	190	68

‖ Antibiotic produced two zones of inhibition; those in italic represent the more potent of the two components.
(A) Migration towards anode.
IBS, International Biological Standard; IRP, International Reference Preparation; BRL, Beecham Research Laboratories; BPAS, BP Authentic Specimen; MB, May & Baker; R-P, Rhône-Poulenc, Paris; EL, Eli Lilly; SKF, Smith, Kline & French; BW, Burroughs Wellcome; MSD, Merck, Sharpe & Dohme.

TABLE 3

Sensitivity and migration profiles of additional antibacterial substances

Antibacterial substance		Minimum amount detected (μg)						Migration distance (mm)			
		pH 6·0			pH 8·0			pH 6·0		pH 8·0	
		B. cereus	*M. luteus*	*B. subtilis* BGA	*B. cereus*	*M. luteus*	*B. subtilis* BGA	*Agar*	*Agarose*	*Agar*	*Agarose*
Clindamycin		1·0	0·1–0·2*	1·0	0·05	0·02	0·03	255	178	196	95
Mocimycin		0·05	0·1–0·2†	0·2–0·5†	0·5	1·0	2·0	69	34(A)	60	46(A)
Lasalocid		0·05	0·15–0·25†	0·1	0·5	2·0	0·6	27	77(A)	34	73(A)
Olaquindox		12·5–25	100	20	10–15	100	15	142	42	147	44
Nosiheptide‡											
Robenidine		200	200	200	100	50	100	14(A)	112(A)	9(A)	70(A)
Acinitrazole		2·0	50	0·5	2·0	50	1·0–1·5	156	44	7	100(A)
Ronidazole		25	25	5·0	50	25	10	155	45	142	42
Tiamutin		25	0·5	20	10	0·1	5	242	172	—	—
Carbadox	(1)	10	100	5	25	50	10	159	44	135	36
	(2)	—	—	10	—	—	20	0	3	—	2
2-Amino-5-nitro	(1)	50	50	50	—	—	50	147	41	5	104(A)
-thiazole	(2)	—	—	100	—	—	—	128	25	—	—
Diaveridine	(1)	50	10	10	50	10	10	265	197	155	65
	(2)	—	—	—	—	—	100	—	—	—	3
Halquinol	(1)	—	—	2·0	—	—	0·5	152	44	132	36(A)
	(2)	—	—	2·0	—	—	0·5	0	0	66	76(A)
	(3)	—	—	—	—	—	0·5	—	—	2	1
	(4)	—	—	—	—	—	0·5	—	—	—	21
Nifursol	(1)	—	—	10	—	—	50–100	157	40	143	37
	(2)	—	—	50	—	—	—	—	0	—	—
Apramycin		—	—	1·0–2·0	—	—	0·2–0·4	100(A)	256	85	170
Narasin		0·2	0·2	0·1	1·0	2·0	2·0	43	60(A)	48	55(A)
Salinomycin		0·5	0·5	0·2	10	10	10	42	60(A)	45	60(A)

* Where sensitivity is given as a range, e.g. clindamycin 0·1–0·2 μg at pH 6·0 with *Micrococcus luteus*, the first figure represents the sensitivity in agarose and the second the sensitivity in agar.
† Here, the first figure represents the sensitivity in agar.
‡ Nosiheptide tends to give somewhat erratic/unreproducible zones.
(A) Migration towards anode.
Substances with numbers in parentheses: these yielded multiple 'spots'.

Plates. 60 × 40 cm, divided in half longitudinally. Operating temperature 17–18°C. Potential difference 1200 V; current approx 140 mA; duration 1·5 h.
Electrolytes. Tris 1·82 g, succinic acid 0·98 g, water to 1000 ml; pH 6. Tris 3·03 g, succinic acid 0·85 g, water to 1000 ml; pH 8.
Support gels. 1·6 mm deep, 1% (w/v) Bacto-agar (Difco) and 1% (w/v) agarose (Miles Laboratories) in the appropriate electrolyte.
Bio-autography. Antibiotic Medium No. 1 (Difco).
Micro-organisms. Micrococcus luteus ATCC 9341 (NCTC 8340) and *Bacillus cereus* var. *mycoides* ATCC 11778 (Difco Spore Suspension); incubation 18–24 h at 30°C.

Slight variations in such conditions as the make and batch of agar and agarose, the ambient temperature and humidity and the precise configuration of the electrolytic cell itself may considerably affect migration distances obtained. Results should therefore be confirmed by running appropriate control antibiotic solutions alongside sample extracts.

Certain antibiotics, when applied in excessive quantities, have been found to yield additional subsidiary zones of inhibition. For example, an overload of tylosin may produce an extra zone in a position normally taken up by lincomycin. Care must be taken therefore to apply antibiotic solutions which are adequately diluted. The interpretation of results when one antibiotic is present at a very much greater concentration than another may be difficult.

A certain amount of trial and error must be anticipated with totally 'unknown' samples. Conversely, many feeding stuff samples arrive already accompanied by information which renders it unnecessary to work through the method to its fullest extent.

As new antibiotics and other antibacterial agents come into use it is necessary to determine their behaviour in the system (Table 3). The majority prove to have characteristic patterns of migration but there are exceptions and limitations. With the newer feeding stuff antibiotics, narasin cannot be distinguished from another similar polyether antibiotic salinomycin while nosiheptide does not migrate satisfactorily presumably due to its restricted solubility.

The authors thank the Editors of the *Journal of Applied Bacteriology* for permission to reproduce Table 2 from the paper by Smither & Vaughan (1978).

References

ANON. 1976 *The Medicines (Animal Feeding Stuffs) (Enforcement) Regulations* 1976. London: Her Majesty's Stationery Office.

BILLON, J. & TAO, S. H. 1979 Détection des antibiotiques dans le lait. Identification et dosage par la méthode électrophorétique. *Le Lait* **59**, 361–375.

BOGAERTS, R. & WOLF, F. 1980 A standardized method for the detection of residues of anti-bacterial substances in fresh meat. *Fleischwirtschaft* **60**, 672–673.

BOZZI, F. & VALDEBOUZE, P. 1973 Méthode d'identification des antibiotiques dans les aliments des animaux par électrophorèse sur gélose. *Journal of Chromatography* **87**, 305–310.

GRYNNE, B. 1973 Identification of small amounts of antibiotics by electrophoresis and bioautography. *Acta pathologica et microbiologica scandinavica*, Section B **81**, 583–588.

HORNG, C. B., HSIEH, J. T., KO, H. C., JAN, R. H. & LI, J. R. 1979 Systematic analysis of antibiotics via agar gel electrophoresis and antimicrobial spectrum—Candidacy for detecting residual antibiotics in foods. *Proceedings of the National Science Council, Republic of China*, **3**, 382–387.

LIGHTBOWN, J. W. & DE ROSSI, P. 1965 The identification and assay of mixtures of antibiotics by electrophoresis in agar gel. *Analyst* **90**, 89–98.

MARTEN, G. 1964 Die mikrobiologische Antibioticabestimmung in Futtermitteln. *Landwirtschaftliche Forschung* **17**, 277–280.

REEVES, D. S. & HOLT, H. A. 1975 Resolution of antibiotic mixtures in serum samples by high-voltage electrophoresis. *Journal of Clinical Pathology* **28**, 435–442.

SMITHER, R. 1978 Bacterial inhibitors formed during the adventitious growth of micro-organisms in chicken liver and pig kidney. *Journal of Applied Bacteriology* **45**, 267–277.

SMITHER, R. & VAUGHAN, D. R. 1978 An improved electrophoretic method for identifying antibiotics with special reference to animal feeding stuffs. *Journal of Applied Bacteriology* **44**, 421–429.

SMITHER, R., LOTT, A. F., DALZIEL, R. W. & OSTLER, D. C. 1980 Antibiotic residues in meat in the United Kingdom; an assessment of specific tests to detect and identify antibiotic residues. *Journal of Hygiene, Cambridge* **85**, 359–369.

STADHOUDERS, J., HASSING, F. & GALESLOOT, T. E. 1981 An electrophoretic method for the identification of antibiotic residues in small volumes of milk. *Netherlands Milk and Dairy Journal* **5**, 23–33.

Actual and Potential Methods of Testing Antibiotics for Sterility

A. S. Breeze and Ann M. Simpson

Microbiology Laboratory, Department of Pharmacy, Heriot-Watt University, Edinburgh, UK

Sterile pharmaceutical preparations must be examined for the presence of microbial contaminants whether they have been manufactured aseptically or have been subjected to a sterilization process as the final stage in their manufacture. The procedures for sterility testing are contained in the various statutory pharmacopoeias (e.g. European Pharmacopoeia 1980). The limitations of sterility tests and the philosophy behind them have been discussed elsewhere (Knudsen 1949; Bryce 1956; Kelsey 1972) and are beyond the scope of this article.

There are two main methods for the detection of bacterial or fungal contaminants of pharmaceutical preparations: (i) direct inoculation into suitable nutrient media which will allow the growth of aerobes, anaerobes and fungi; (ii) membrane filtration to collect organisms on the surface of a membrane which is then brought into contact with media as in (i) above.

The direct inoculation of antibiotic-containing products into nutrient media is unlikely to be successful in diluting the activity of the antibiotic to a sufficiently low level unless impossibly large volumes of media are used. In some cases the activity of the drug can be neutralized by the addition of an antagonistic metabolite, e.g. *p*-aminobenzoic acid (PABA; 3-aminobenzoic acid) for sulphonamides, thymidine for trimethoprim. In others the antibiotic can be enzymically inactivated, e.g. penicillin by an appropriate β-lactamase (penicillinase), chloramphenicol by chloramphenicol acetyltransferase.

However, very many antibiotics are not, as yet, subject to such inactivation mechanisms and for them the prescribed method is membrane filtration. Indeed most pharmacopoeias recommend this technique for all antibiotic sterility testing. There are several disadvantages associated with

ANTIBIOTICS
ISBN 0 12 604480 5

this method, however, and it is interesting to note the way in which manufacturers have responded to the challenge by designing increasingly more sophisticated, and hence expensive, filtration systems to overcome these problems.

The method requires a high level of aseptic skill to ensure accurate and reliable results, particularly with regard to the problem of 'false positives' caused by accidental contamination. There is also the possibility of adsorption of antibiotic onto the filter and its subsequent release into the nutrient medium; this can be partly overcome by extensive rinsing of the membrane, but at the risk of further contamination.

Membrane Filtration

The simplest form of apparatus for membrane filtration is shown in Fig. 1. The whole apparatus, less the collecting flask, can be autoclaved

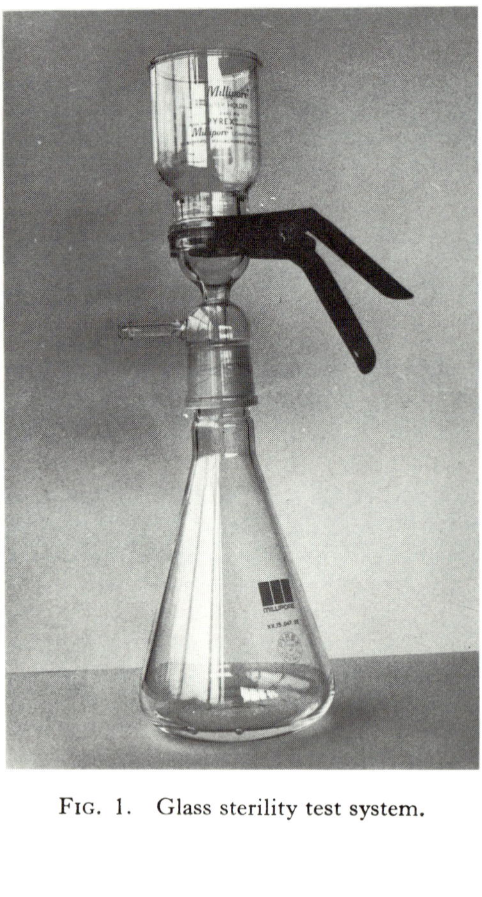

FIG. 1. Glass sterility test system.

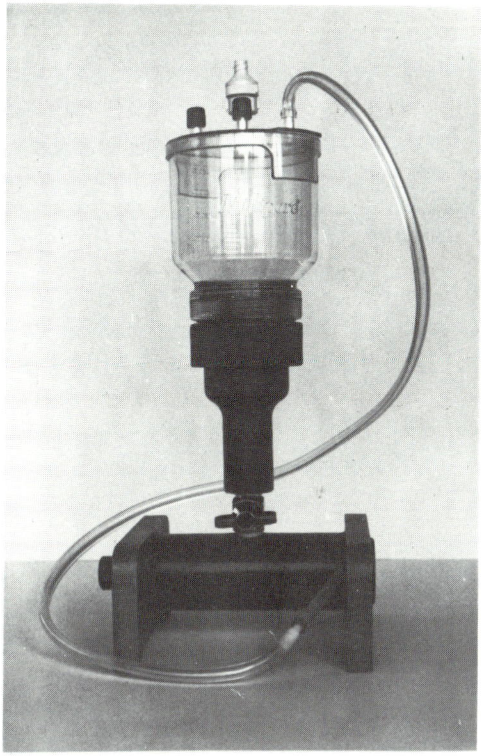

FIG. 2. Sterifil system attached to vacuum manifold.

with the membrane *in situ* by wrapping in Kraft paper. The inherent disadvantages of this apparatus for sterility testing are obvious: the top is open to contamination and the edge of the membrane may also be exposed. Less obvious is the occlusion of the circumference of the membrane by the ground glass surfaces of the funnel and the filter holder. Antibiotic may diffuse into this outer portion of the membrane and resist removal by rinsing. This can be overcome by the use of a filter with a hydrophobic edge which prevents this diffusion. With very great care and under ideal aseptic conditions, i.e. totally enclosed or laminar flow cabinets, this system can yield reliable results. An improved form of this apparatus is the "Sterifil" system (Millipore (UK) Ltd) shown in Fig. 2. This is manufactured in polycarbonate, can also be autoclaved with the filter(s) in position and has the advantages that the membrane is enclosed and the apparatus has a tight fitting lid. The lid has several ports to which sterile tubing can be attached for filling, and a filter may be attached to allow venting of the apparatus with sterile air. Unused ports are capped with rubber seals through which needles may be passed to introduce small samples. Vacuum is applied via a manifold, as shown, or by attaching the filter holder to a collecting vessel with a suitable vacuum outlet. Before use the apparatus is assembled with a 47 mm 0·45 μm pore size membrane with a hydrophobic edge (e.g. Millipore HAEP 047 OW), wrapped in Kraft paper and autoclaved.

Samples for testing are introduced by lifting the lid slightly, by gravity feed via sterile tubing attached to one of the ports, or by injection through one of the rubber caps. The membrane is rinsed 3 times with 200 ml of a sterile diluent such as 0·1% Peptone Water (Oxoid). The membrane must then be removed aseptically, divided into two equal parts, each part being put into a suitable nutrient medium, e.g. Tryptone Soya Broth (Oxoid) for aerobic bacteria and fungi; and Thioglycollate Medium USP (Oxoid) for anaerobes.

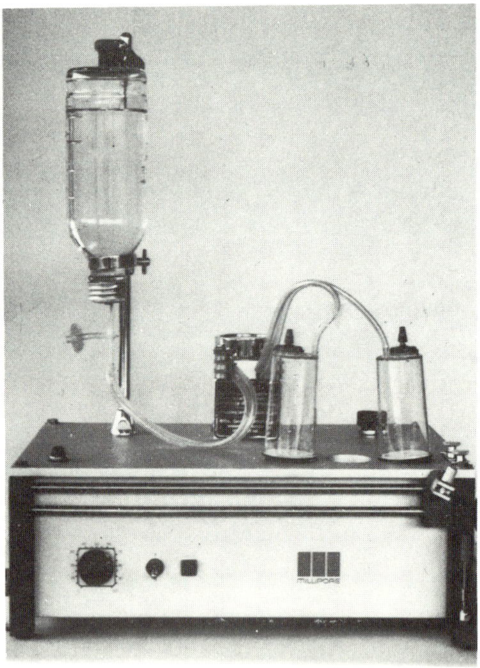

FIG. 3. Steritest apparatus shown with two filtration units during rinsing with diluent from inverted container.

This method, in common with the previous one, requires the aseptic removal of the filter and its division into two parts. This is rather a delicate operation even though there is a plethora of instruments available for cutting and folding the membrane for its easy insertion into culture vessels.

Figure 3 illustrates the third stage in the development of membrane filtration. This, the 'Steritest' system (Millipore (UK) Ltd), is a completely enclosed system which minimizes further the occurrence of external contamination. The membrane filter (0·45 μm pore size, hydrophobic edge) forms the base of a transparent incubation vessel to which is attached plastic tubing engaged in a peristaltic pump and terminating in a sampling needle which is introduced aseptically into the sample container. After filtration of the sample, the same needle is used to penetrate firstly the rinsing diluent container and secondly the containers of nutrient media. When the incubation chambers have been filled with nutrient medium they are suitably plugged before incubation.

Because the units are necessarily disposable after a single use, and because the system is quite sophisticated, this method is much more expensive than those previously described yet still requires a high degree of aseptic skill. The manufacturers recommend its use under laminar air flow conditions. It does of course avoid any possibility of contamination during manipulation of the membranes which is arguably the most hazardous stage of previous methods. The cost may be discounted because of its greater convenience and reliability. There remains, however, a potentially serious disadvantage with this apparatus: the peristaltic mechanism ensures the thorough oxygenation of anaerobic media—as seen by the reappearance of the green colouration if Brewer's thioglycollate medium is used. This may mean that a contaminant which is a strict anaerobe may fail to grow. Preliminary results from this laboratory show that this may be true for the test organism *Clostridium sporogenes* NCTC 532: 50% of containers filled with Brewer's medium via the peristaltic pump and challenged with 100 cells of *Cl. sporogenes* failed to show any growth after 14 days incubation. There does not appear to be any simple method for deoxygenating the medium without affecting the survival of contaminants or compromising the sterility of the system.

Enzymic Inactivation

Penicillins and cephalosporins

Many of the penicillins and cephalosporins are subject to attack by β-lactamases and thus should, if possible, be inactivated prior to being tested for sterility. Several preparations of β-lactamase are available from different species of bacteria: one, for example, from *Bacillus cereus* will inactivate several penicillins including cloxacillin; another, from *Enterobacter cloacae* will inactivate many cephalosporins. The preparation available from Wellcome Reagents Ltd will serve as an illustration of the method. It is supplied as a sterile filtrate of a broth culture of *B. cereus* such that 1 ml of solution will inactivate 100,000 units of penicillin per hour at 35°C. Because the preparation contains 0·25% w/v phenol as preservative it is necessary to ensure that the final dilution of the penicillinase solution is at least 1 : 50. The calculated amount of penicillinase is added to an appropriate sample of penicillin and incubated at 35°C for 1 h. The inactivated penicillin is then distributed to the containers of nutrient medium for incubation. This method achieves the highest enzyme to substrate ratio and avoids the possibility of contaminants being affected by the penicillin before inactivation is complete.

Chloramphenicol

The acetylation of chloramphenicol by chloramphenicol-acetyltransferase (CAT) renders it biologically inactive (Shaw 1967). This has been used in the inactivation of the antibiotic prior to sterility testing (Breeze & Macadam 1974). A reaction mixture containing 100 mmol/l Tris-HCl, pH 7·8; 1 mmol/l acetyl CoA; 2·5 mg crude CAT in a total volume of 10 ml inactivated 1·6 mg chloramphenicol in 30 min at 37°C.

Aminoglycoside antibiotics

Aminoglycoside antibiotics may be inactivated by a variety of enzyme mechanisms (Haas & Dowding 1975). Using a 3-*N*-acetyltransferase (AAC-3) with wide substrate specificity we have inactivated gentamicin, neomycin, kanamycin and tobramycin prior to testing them for sterility (Simpson & Breeze 1981). Using a reaction mixture containing 100 mmol/l Tris–HCl, pH 7·8; 1 mmol/l acetyl CoA; 1·5 mg AAC-3 in a total volume of 1 ml, 495 μg gentamicin, 290 μg kanamycin, 430 μg neomycin and 390 μg tobramycin were inactivated individually during 1 h incubation at 37°C. These amounts of antibiotics inactivated are, of course, at least 100-fold less than would be required to be inactivated for a full-scale sterility test, but there appears to be no reason why the reaction mixture should not be scaled up to this level, apart, that is, from the cost of the acetyl CoA needed. This is the major disadvantage of this method, and of that for chloramphenicol, but a later development of the method (Breeze & Simpson 1982) uses a recycling system for acetyl CoA which reduces dramatically the overall cost of each test. A reaction mixture containing

0·26 mmol/l CoA; 8 mmol/l acetyl phosphate; 1·9 μg phosphotransacetylase; 1·5 mg AAC-3 and 100 mmol/l Tris–HCl, pH 7·8 in a total volume of 2 ml inactivated 4 mg gentamicin in 1 h at 26°C.

Inactivation by Metabolites

The biologically active portion of the sulphonamide molecule is a structural analogue of PABA. Hence the addition of PABA to nutrient media overcomes the antibacterial activity of this group of drugs and this forms the basis of a sterility test for them (Sykes 1956). Ten mg of PABA in 100 ml nutrient medium is sufficient to neutralize the contents of a 1 g ampoule of, for example, sulphadiazine.

Trimethoprim

Trimethoprim is an inhibitor of dihydrofolate reductase, a critical enzyme in the synthesis of thymidylic acid. Exogenously supplied thymidine will reverse the effect of trimethoprim and will also antagonize sulphonamides. Thus this appears to be a candidate for use as an inactivating agent in testing these antibiotics for sterility, especially as trimethoprim is frequently administered in combination with sulphamethoxazole as cotrimoxazole. It has been reported that there is an upper limit to the amount of trimethoprim which can be antagonized in this way (Koch & Burchall 1971) but in practice this does not seem to be important in a sterility test. We have obtained good results using Brain Heart Infusion broth (Difco) which contains reasonable levels of thymidine (Koch & Burchall 1971) and gives copious growth of test organisms compared to nutrient broth, even when the latter is supplemented with 20 μg/ml of thymidine. Fifty mg trimethoprim is effectively neutralized in 100 ml Brain Heart Infusion broth although this can be supplemented by the addition of, say, 1 mg thymidine.

Discussion

The limitations of sterility testing are irrelevant in the context of this article. Nevertheless, it is important that every effort is made to improve the methods of testing that are available. Such improvement is a continuous process and it would be erroneous to suggest that further progress cannot be made.

The technique of membrane filtration has achieved a high level of sophistication and many of the problems have been eliminated. There remains, however, the problem of antibiotic binding to organisms or to the filter, which may not be removed by rinsing. This may be overcome in the examples cited above by the use of metabolite or enzymic inactivation on the filter. Reliance upon the physical removal of contaminants from the sphere of influence of the antibiotic is unlikely, given current techniques, to be completely satisfactory.

The methods of enzymic inactivation presented do have the appeal of elegant simplicity, and the aseptic manipulations involved are probably rather more familiar and thus less likely to be performed incorrectly. We envisage the production of reaction mixtures lyophilized in ampoules, the contents needing to be reconstituted with sterile water and added to the vial containing the antibiotic or vice versa. There is of course no expensive equipment involved but it is difficult to predict the cost of preparing the necessary ingredients on a large scale.

There is, however, a potentially serious disadvantage. It has been tacitly assumed that because the antibiotics have been inactivated with respect to the test organisms, other potential contaminants are also insusceptible to them, e.g. acetylated gentamicin. Preliminary experiments in this laboratory (H. E. D'Arcy, unpublished results) have indicated that this is true for a rather limited range of organisms but further work is needed to establish this. Similar considerations might also apply to neutralization of sulphonamides by PABA: the inhibition of some organisms might not be overcome in this way.

Sources of Materials

1. β-Lactamase

Wellcome penicillinase (MR 79): 1 ml inactivates 100,000 units of penicillin in 1 h at 35°C. British Drug Houses penicillinase. Miles Laboratories cephalosporinase.

2. Chloramphenicol acetyltransferase

Prepared from *Escherichia coli* K12 (RI). 2·5 mg inactivates 1·6 mg chloramphenicol in 30 min at 37°C in the presence of 1 mmol/l acetyl CoA (Breeze & Macadam 1974).

3. Aminoglycoside acetyltransferase (AAC-3)

Prepared from *E. coli* JR225. 1·5 mg inactivates 495 μg gentamicin in 1 h at 37°C in the presence of 1 mmol/l acetyl CoA (Simpson & Breeze 1981).

4. *Phosphotransacetylase*

Prepared from *E. coli* NCTC 10537. 1·9 μg regenerates sufficient acetyl CoA for the inactivation of 4 mg gentamicin by 1·5 mg AAC-3 in 1 h at 26°C. Reaction mixture also contains 0·26 mmol/l CoA; 8 mmol/l acetyl phosphate; 100 mmol/l Tris–HCl pH 7·8 in a total volume of 2 ml (Breeze & Simpson 1982).

5. *Filtration apparatus*

Glass filtration system, 'Sterifil' and 'Steritest' all by Millipore. Membrane filters with hydrophobic edges, 47 mm, 0·45 μm pore size (Millipore, HAEP 047 OW).

6. *Sulphonamide neutralization*

10 mg *p*-aminobenzoic acid in 100 ml nutrient broth effectively neutralizes 1 g of sulphadiazine.

7. *Trimethoprim neutralization*

100 ml Brain Heart Infusion broth (Difco) contains sufficient thymidine to neutralize 50 mg trimethoprim, but may be supplemented by the addition of 1 mg thymidine.

8. *Media*

For aerobic bacteria and fungi, Tryptone Soya Broth (Oxoid); for anaerobic bacteria, Thioglycollate Medium USP (Oxoid).

We gratefully acknowledge the co-operation of Millipore (UK) Ltd in lending some of the equipment shown at the original demonstration. We thank Mr I. J. Lamont for the photographs.

References

Breeze, A. S. & Macadam, G. A. 1974 A novel sterility test for chloramphenicol. *Journal of Pharmacy and Pharmacology* **26,** 122p.

Breeze, A. S. & Simpson, A. M. 1982 An improved method using acetyl-coenzyme A regeneration for the enzymic inactivation of aminoglycosides prior to sterility testing. *Journal of Applied Bacteriology* **53,** 277–284.

Bryce, D. M. 1956 The design and interpretation of sterility tests. *Journal of Pharmacy and Pharmacology* **8,** 561–572.

EUROPEAN PHARMACOPOEIA 1980 2nd Edn Part I Saint Ruffine, France: Maisonneuve S.A.

HAAS, M. J. & DOWDING, J. E. 1975 Aminoglycoside-modifying enzymes. *Methods in Enzymology* **43,** 611–628.

KELSEY, J. C. 1972 The myth of surgical sterility *Lancet* **ii,** 1301–1303.

KNUDSEN, L. F. 1949 Sample size of parenteral solutions for sterility testing. *Journal of the American Pharmaceutical Association* **38,** 332–337.

KOCH, A. E. & BURCHALL, J. J. 1971 Reversal of the antimicrobial activity of trimethoprim by thymidine in commercially prepared media. *Applied Microbiology* **22,** 812–817.

SIMPSON, A. M. & BREEZE, A. S. 1981 The sterility testing of aminoglycosides: a new approach using enzymic inactivation. *Journal of Applied Bacteriology* **50,** 469–474.

SHAW, W. V. 1967 The enzymatic acetylation of chloramphenicol by extracts of R-factor resistant *Escherichia coli*. *Journal of Biological Chemistry* **242,** 687–693.

SYKES, G. 1956 The technique of sterility testing. *Journal of Pharmacy and Pharmacology* **8,** 573–588.

Detection of Antibiotic Residues in Milk and Animal Tissues

JANET E. L. CORRY AND M. R. SHARMA

Ministry of Agriculture, Fisheries and Food (MAFF), Food Science Division, Romney Street, London, UK

M. L. BATES

MAFF, Food Science Division, Colney Lane, Norwich, UK

Antibiotics were used for veterinary purposes almost as soon as they had been developed for human medicine. They have been an extremely important aid during the development of intensive methods of animal husbandry and are almost indispensable for treatment of infection. They also serve a useful function when added to feed for growth promotion purposes.

The presence of residues of antibiotics in milk quickly became a problem because they inhibited dairy starter organisms used for making cheese and yoghurt. Fermentation failure due to residues can cause enormous economic losses. There was ample incentive, therefore, for screening methods to be developed to exclude contaminated milk; some of these will be discussed below.

Later, in the late 1950s and early 1960s, attention was drawn to the toxic and allergic hazards posed by antibiotic residues. Concern was further stimulated by the discovery of plasmid-mediated transferable antibiotic-resistance in strains of Enterobacteriaceae, and later in other groups of bacteria. In the UK the Swann Report (Report 1969) recommended measures to restrict antibiotic use, particularly to ban the use of certain antibiotics (chlortetracycline, oxytetracycline and penicillin) important in human medicine from use as growth-promoters in animals. Further recommendations included monitoring other animal products, as well as milk, for antibiotic residues and their degradation products.

ANTIBIOTICS
ISBN 0 12 604480 5

Hazards of Antibiotic Residues

There are four hazards that could be posed by antibiotic residues in foods: (i) inhibition of fermentation; (ii) allergic reactions; (iii) toxic effects; (iv) selection of resistant micro-organisms. There is no doubt that residues do inhibit fermentation in milk (Marth & Ellickson 1959). Acid production by starters has been estimated to be reduced by 0·01–0·02 u penicillin/ml and completely inhibited by 0·03–0·05 u/ml (Tramer 1974), although some authors have reported that lactic starters are becoming more resistant to antibiotics, presumably because of selective pressure (Jacquet *et al.* 1959; Jacquet & Auxpaules 1978). Allergic reactions have occasionally been attributed to the consumption of food containing antibiotics, especially penicillin in milk (Vickers 1964; Gounelle & Szakvary 1966). Other antibiotics which have been implicated include tetracyclines, oleandomycin and chloramphenicol (Burgat-Sacaze 1981). Fortunately symptoms are not usually severe. It is unlikely that antibiotic residues are involved in primary sensitization, which probably occurs after therapeutic doses, but they could be responsible for triggering a response in previously sensitized individuals. Allergic responses may be more common than is generally realized, due to failure to identify the cause, or attributing allergic reactions to the food itself. There is also the possibility that metabolic products of antibiotics, no longer microbiologically active, may persist in tissues and milk and provoke immunological response (Malten 1968; Wal 1979). Release of penicilloyl derivatives, which can be assayed by immunological methods but not by their antimicrobial effect, has been observed after heat or enzyme treatment of milk, serum and tissue proteins (Wal 1979). There is also the possibility of microbial β-lactamases converting penicillin to derivatives that are immunologically active but without antimicrobial activity (Guay *et al.* 1981).

Direct toxic effects due to antibiotic residues are very unlikely because of the low levels involved. There have been reports, however, of toxic effects from ingesting low levels of chloramphenicol (Milhaud & Person 1981).

Selection of antibiotic-resistant organisms resulting directly from the consumption of antibiotic residues in food seems rather unlikely because the levels of antibiotics would be low and the food would be diluted by other foods, gastric secretion, etc. However, very low levels of antibiotics in feedingstuffs (5 parts/10^6: Report 1969) affect weight gain in animals. The mechanism by which this occurs is still not clear, but alteration of intestinal flora appears to be involved. In humans, any antibiotics not denatured or absorbed in the upper part of the intestinal tract would be concentrated in the hind gut, due to water absorption, and might affect the intestinal flora and hence select resistant strains (Milhaud & Person 1981). Smith &

Tucker (1975, 1978) reported that avoparcin, lincomycin, nitrovin, tylosin and flavomycin fed to chickens at growth-promoting concentrations, increased salmonella carriage.

A more important reason for monitoring antibiotic residues in foods forms part of a general policy to prevent unnecessary and indiscriminate use of therapeutic or 'prophylactic' doses of antibiotics as a substitute for good animal husbandry. In particular this contributes to the selection of multiple-resistant strains of bacteria, which can be acquired via food and cause serious infections in both man and animals (Report 1969; WHO 1978).

Antibiotic residues can also interfere with assays such as the methylene blue test, which are intended to estimate the total microbial load in milk. The time taken for reduction of the dye will be increased, thereby causing under-estimation of the microbial load.

This chapter reviews methods (mainly microbiological) for screening milk and animal tissues for the presence of antibiotic residues. For convenience, sulphonamides and nitrofurans are included.

General Principles

Bioassay methods for detecting antibiotics cannot compete in terms of specificity with physicochemical assays, but they have the advantages of rapidity and simplicity and are more sensitive to some agents. Their low specificity allows one test to be used to assay for compounds with widely different chemical structures. This enables large numbers of samples to be screened by relatively untrained staff. 'Positive' samples should be further examined using semi-specific techniques such as electrophoresis (see Lott & Vaughan, this volume, pp. 331–338), thin layer chromatography (Zuidweg *et al.* 1969; Bossuyt *et al.* 1976; Woolley *et al.* 1978), or specific chemical assays. Alternatively, presumptive identification of the antibiotics can sometimes be achieved by use of a specific antagonist (see pp. 364–365).

Bioassays for antibiotic residues have been developed along two principal lines. These involve inhibition of the growth of a sensitive organism as measured by (i) failure to form colonies or (ii) failure to produce an effect due to metabolism, e.g. acid production (van Os *et al.* 1975), reduction of a redox indicator (Neal & Calbert 1955; Kraak & Tolle 1967) or even production of gas (Mossel *et al.* 1955). Methods for the examination of milk will be reviewed first since these were developed earlier.

Methods for Assaying Milk

The earliest methods for antibiotic detection were based either on the classical methods developed by assaying antibiotics used in clinical medicine (e.g. well, cylinder or disc plate assays) or an inhibition of acid production by lactic starter organisms. These methods are excellently reviewed by Myers (1964). Advances since 1964 have been aimed mainly at speeding up the test, simplifying it and increasing the sensitivity.

Table 1 lists various methods and their sensitivity. β-Lactams are still the most common antibiotics detected in milk, so frequently the sensitivity is quoted only for penicillin. Tests are sometimes very insensitive to other antibiotics; for instance, the tests of Igarashi *et al.* (1961), van Os *et al.* (1975) and Kraak & Tolle (1967, 1969) using different strains of *Bacillus stearothermophilus* were very sensitive to penicillin, but quite insensitive to streptomycin or dihydrostreptomycin. Hamann *et al.* (1975, 1980) claim that their test using lactic acid bacteria is much more sensitive to non-penicillin antibiotics.

Many countries stipulate that milk should not contain antibiotics, although in practice there is usually an upper limit enforced by using financial penalties. For instance the limit in the UK is set by the Milk Marketing Board and is currently 0·02 u penicillin/ml. In France a ministerial decree was passed in 1971 that all penicillin-containing preparations for intra-mammary injection should include a dye that would cause a visible colour change at concentrations of penicillin down to 0·04 u/ml of milk. This has been found in France and other countries to be ineffective (Labie 1981; van Os 1978). The reasons for this include illegal use of preparations without dye, as well as the fact that antibiotics not injected by the intra-mammary route are not marked.

Most methods require that the milk is heated for about 5 min at 80–100°C to eliminate 'non-specific' inhibition, although Galesloot & Hassing (1962) considered this unnecessary. Some methods suggest that only samples showing positive reaction should be heated and then retested (Messer *et al.* 1978). Sensitivity of disc, cylinder and well methods depends on various factors which are discussed at length in standard texts on methods of antibiotic assay, e.g. volume of sample, depth of agar layer, concentration of inoculum, temperature of incubation, medium, time of diffusion, etc. (Davis & Stout 1971*a*, *b*; Acar 1980; Linton, this volume, pp. 19–30). The milk can be used neat or diluted, depending on the sensitivity required. Commercially produced materials or kits exist for most of these methods. All, except the Charm test which is specific for β-lactams, include a final confirmatory test for β-lactams, adding β-lactamase.

The most popular methods currently in use are described below.

Micrococcus luteus (Sarcina lutea) *cylinder plate method*

This is a standard method, described in various publications (Grove &

TABLE 1

Summary of methods of detecting penicillin and other antibiotics in milk

Principle	Organism	Incubation conditions: Time	Incubation conditions: Temperature (°C)	Lower limit of detection: Penicillin (u/ml*)	Lower limit of detection: Chlortetracycline (μg/ml)	Lower limit of detection: Streptomycin (μg/ml)	Reference
Morphological effect							
Microscopy	*Streptococcus cremoris*	5 h	30	0·05			Whitehead & Cox (1956)
	Strep. thermophilus	1–1½ h	37	0·015	0·15	0·75	Liska (1960)
Growth inhibition							
Cylinder plate	*Micrococcus luteus* ATCC 9341 (*Sarcina lutea*)	18 h	30	0·0125			Grove & Randall (1955); FDA (1968)
	Bacillus stearothermophilus var. *calidolactis*	4½ h	64	0·002			Vilim *et al.* (1979)
Disc plate	*B. subtilis* ATCC 6633	2½–3 h	37	0·05			Messer *et al.* (1978)
	B. stearothermophilus var. *calidolactis*	2½–5 h	55	0·0025			Arret & Kirshbaum (1959) Galesloot & Hassing (1962) IDF (1970)
Reversed phase disc (dry disc impregnated with nutrient medium)	*B. subtilis*	4–6 h	37	0·05			Kosikowski & Ledford (1960)
Reduction of Redox Indicator							
TTC† or rezazurin in tubes	*B. stearothermophilus* ATCC 7954	40 min	61–62	0·002	0·2 (oxytetracycline)	8·4	Igarashi *et al.* (1961)
Brilliant black in microtitre plates	*B. stearothermophilus* var. *calidolactis*	2—2½ h	55	0·006	0·8	8	Kraak & Tolle (1967, 1969)
TTC	*Strep. thermophilus*	5 min 2 h	80 37	0·04	0·2	4	Neal & Calbert (1955)
Inhibition of acid production							
Bromocresol purple pH indicator colour change	*B. stearothermophilus* var. *calidolactis*	2½ h	63–66	0·006	0·4 (tetracycline)	13 (dihydrostreptomycin)	van Os *et al.* (1975) ('Delvotest')
Measure pH or lactate production	'yoghurt bacteria'	45 min	37	0·01	0·1	0·05	Hamann *et al.* (1975, 1980)
Lactate production	*Strep. thermophilus*	2½ h	44–45	0·01			Wright & Tramer (1961)
Bromocresol purple colour change	*Strep. thermophilus*	4 h	45	0·02–0·04			'Intertest' (Intervet) & 'Antibiotics in Milk' test (AIM: Oxoid)
Radio-labelled antibiotic	*B. stearothermophilus* ATCC 10149 or 15952	15 min	90	0·001			'Charm' test (US Patent 1980)

* One unit of penicillin is *ca.* 0·6 μg.
† 2,3,5-triphenyltetrazolium chloride.

Randall 1955; FDA 1968; FAO 1969; Messer *et al.* 1978). The method uses a standard strain of *Micrococcus luteus* (ATCC 9341). Seeded agar (4 ml) is overlayed onto unseeded agar (10 ml) in 10 cm Petri dishes. Six stainless steel cylinders (inside diameter 6 mm, length 10 mm) are placed on the agar and filled with appropriate standards and samples. Standards are prepared by diluting a solution of penicillin in antibiotic-free milk. The lower limit of detection is about 0·0125 u/ml. Plates are read after overnight incubation at 30°C.

Disc plate methods

These two methods are more rapid and convenient than the cylinder plate method described above because spores are used for the inoculum which can be prepared in advance and stored. Also it is possible to incubate at a higher temperature for a shorter time.

Bacillus subtilis (*ATCC 6633*)

This method (Messer *et al.* 1978) employs the same agar medium as used for the cylinder plate method above, seeded with *ca.* 10^6 spores/ml dispensed into standard 10 cm Petri dishes in 6 ml quantities. Standards are prepared as above, by adding penicillin to antibiotic-free milk. Half-inch filter paper discs are touched onto the milk and allowed to take it up by capillary action. The discs are laid on the surface of the seeded agar at least 20 mm apart. Plates are incubated for 14–25 h at 32°C or 5–7 h at 37°C. Using a higher inoculum ($2·5 \times 10^7$ spores/ml) it is possible to read the results after 3–4 h at 37°C. This method will detect down to 0·05 u penicillin/ml. Difco market the materials for this method, including a spore suspension.

Bacillus stearothermophilus

Various methods have been developed using this thermophilic organism which is more sensitive to penicillin than *B. subtilis*. Galesloot & Hassing (1962) described a procedure using a strain of *B. stearothermophilus* var. *calidolactis* which was developed from the tube method of Igarashi *et al.* (1961), using a different strain of *B. stearothermophilus*. The Galesloot & Hassing method was adopted as a standard by the International Dairy Federation (IDF 1970). The procedure is similar to that for the *B. subtilis* method above, except that plate count agar is used for the plating medium. The plates are incubated at 55°C for 2½–5 h and examined for zones of inhibition. It should detect down to 0·0025 u penicillin/ml. A disadvantage of this method is that it requires a fresh culture of the organism for preparation of the seeded agar. Suspensions of spores are available commercially which are more convenient to use. Difco market a modification of this method using a spore suspension of *B. stearothermophilus* ATCC 10149 and a more complex test medium containing a pH indicator (bromocresol purple). Incubation is for 160 min at 65°C or 210 min at 56°C. The indicator is stated to remain purple under the discs down to 0·002–0·003 u penicillin/ml if the results are read promptly, although no growth inhibition is visible below 0·005 u/ml. A further variation of this method is the Delvotest (described below).

Streptococcus thermophilus *tube test*

This is the test at present approved by the British Milk Marketing Board. Commercial kits are marketed by Oxoid ('Antibiotics in Milk' (AIM) test) and by Intervet (Science Park, Milton, Cambridge, UK: 'Intertest' and 'Accusphere'). Both kits provide a freeze-dried mixture of a culture of *Streptococcus thermophilus*, nutrients and bromocresol purple indicator. This is reconstituted and added to a standard volume of milk sample, which has been heated to 95°C. The samples are incubated in tubes at 45°C for 4 h. Tubes where the colour is unchanged (blue) contain inhibitor. When 2·5 ml of undiluted milk is tested 0·02 u penicillin/ml are detected.

B. stearothermophilus *var.* calidolactis *tube test*

Gist-Brocades (Delft, The Netherlands) market this test under the trade name 'Delvotest'. Like AIM and Intertest it relies on a bromocresol purple indicator but is carried out with a solid medium. Various versions of the test are available in ampoules using 0·3 ml of plain agar seeded with 10^6 *B. stearothermophilus* var. *calidolactis* spores or in a multititre plate system with cupules containing *ca.* 0·15 ml of the seeded agar (Delvotest P and Delvotest P multi, respectively). There is also a version called 'Delvotest sulpha-sensitive' which contains trimethoprim to enhance sensitivity to sulphonamides (Gudding 1976; see p. 359). To carry out the test, portions of milk and a nutrient tablet are added to the ampoules or cupules. The cupules are sealed and incubated by floating on a water bath at 64°C for $2\frac{1}{2}$–3 h. The sensitivity depends on the volume of milk added. Using 0·1 ml of milk, van Os & Beukers (1980) reported that 0·006 u/ml of penicillin gave a positive result (purple indicator). Similar sensitivity was shown to other β-lactams, but because the test was developed for β-lactams it is much less sensitive to other antibiotics such as chloramphenicol (7·5 μg/ml), dihydrostreptomycin (3 μg/ml) tetracycline (0·5 μg/ml) and kanamycin (10 μg/ml).

B. stearothermophilus *var.* calidolactis *brilliant black reductase test*

This method, developed by Kraak & Tolle (1967, 1969), uses a high concentration of spores (*ca.* 10^8/ml) in a medium containing brilliant black. Incubation is for 3 h at 55°C or 2½ h at 62·6°C. If antibiotics are present the brilliant black is not reduced. The test can be carried out in microtitre plates, enabling large numbers of samples to be screened. A kit of ready-prepared agar is available commercially, as well as an automatic system (Foss, York, England, a subsidiary of Foss, Hellerup, Denmark). The sensitivity of the test can be varied, depending on the volume of milk added, and is generally between 0·005 and 0·01 u penicillin/ml.

The Charm test (*US Patent 1980*)

This novel method is at present only used to detect β-lactams. The sample is incubated with sensitive cells of bacteria so that any antibiotic present is absorbed onto the receptor sites of the cells. Radio-labelled antibiotic is also added to the system. The amount of labelled antibiotic which absorbs to the cells is inversely proportional to the amount of antibiotic originally present. The system used at present employs a freeze-dried preparation of *B. stearothermophilus* var. *calidolactis* (ATCC 10149) because of its supersensitivity to β-lactams and its ability to withstand high temperatures. ^{14}C-labelled benzylpenicillin is used. The cells are incubated for 3 min at 90°C with the sample and ^{14}C-benzylpenicillin. The cells are separated by centrifugation, washed in phosphate buffer and the radioactivity determined using a scintillation counter. Numerous variations of this system are possible, e.g. using different bacteria or cell fractions such as walls, membranes, ribosomes, etc. and different labelled antibiotics or antibiotic derivatives (e.g. penicillanic acid). The main advantage is the speed, about 10 min, with which the test can be carried out, enabling for instance, a tanker of milk to be checked for antibiotics *before* being unloaded. The test is claimed to respond to as little as 0·001 u penicillin G/ml using 1 ml sample of milk.

Other methods

Other methods, which have not been used on a large scale, but which are also rapid, include an enzyme-linked immunosorbent assay method (ELISA: Brown *et al.* 1980), and a competitive binding colour test, using a colour conjugator to penicillin (Charm & Wong 1980), which is similar to, but less sensitive than, the Charm test (detecting down to 0·07 u/ml).

TABLE 2

Comparison of sensitivity of various tests for antibiotics in milk, compared with inhibitory levels for lactic acid starter bacteria and the lower limits recommended by WHO (1969)

Antibiotic	Delvotest*	Intertest Accuspheres†	Yoghurt culture‡	*Strep. thermophilus* inhibition§	Partial inhibition of starter culture‖: Butter	Partial inhibition of starter culture‖: Cheese	Tolerance limit (WHO 1969)
Penicillin G	0·006	0·04	0·01	0·03–0·05	0·017–0·17	0·05–0·20	0 006 (Penicillin G, Ampicillin, Cloxacillin, Cephaloridin)
Ampicillin	0·006	0·016					
Cloxacillin	0·03	0·08					
Cephaloridin		0·02					
(Dihydro)streptomycin	3	2	0·05	0·05–0·5	0·1–0·2	0·04	0·2
Neomycin	2	4		0·5			0·15
Kanamycin	10						
Spectinomycin		4					
Tetracycline	0·5	0·2		0·01			0·1
Oxytetracycline	0·4	0·2		0·001–0·005	0·01–0·1	0·01	
Chlortetracycline	1		0·12	0·001–0·01	0·01–0·1	0·02–0·25	0·02
Chloramphenicol	7·5	0·2	0·1	0·05–0·5	0·1–0·2	0·02	zero
Erythromycin	0·8	0·04		0·0005–0·05			0·03

Figures are u/ml for penicillin G and μg/ml for all other antibiotics.

* From van Os & Beckers (1980).

† Figures supplied by Intervet Laboratories Ltd (originally μg per test (2·5 ml)).

‡ From Hamann *et al.* 1980.

§ From Ziv *et al.* (1973).

‖ From Terplan & Zaadhof (1967).

Comparisons of methods

All these methods are quite sensitive to β-lactams. In general, the degree of sensitivity can be increased by increasing the volume of milk tested. However, sensitivity to other antibiotics or to sulphonamides is often quite low (Tables 1 and 2). Presence of β-lactams can be tested by repeating the test with added β-lactamase although not all β-lactams are inactivated (Gedek 1977). A number of surveys have indicated that a very high proportion of antibiotics in milk are β-lactams (Kelly & Collins 1967; Kraak & Tolle 1969; Ginn *et al.* 1978; Dr G. A. Prentice, pers. comm.). An alternative explanation, however, is that other antibiotics are not detected by the systems in use. It might be better, therefore, to judge systems by their sensitivity to other antibiotics as well as penicillin. From this point of view, and from the limited information available, systems using lactic acid bacteria are generally more sensitive to non-β-lactam antibiotics (Table 2). For instance, the lower limit for detection of chloramphenicol is 7·5 μg/ml using the Delvotest and *B. stearothermophilus* var. *calidolactis*, but 0·1 μg/ml when using the yoghurt bacteria of Hamann *et al.* (1975, 1980). In order to avoid inhibition of dairy starters it would also be logical to use lactic acid bacteria to screen for antibiotics.

Detection of Antibiotics in Animal Tissues

Most methods were developed from those designed for detecting antibiotics in milk. Lange & Madelung (1959) were among the first to investigate the problem, primarily from the point of view of carrying out post-mortem checks for bacterial infections, where the presence of antibiotics might prevent isolation of the causative organism. They used a strain of *Sarcina lutea* (*Micrococcus luteus*). They found that a method using extracts obtained by heating tissues (liver and lymph glands) in physiological saline at 73°C for 5 min before testing by the cylinder plate method, was better than putting the tissues directly onto seeded plates.

Methods have been published using almost all the bacteria commonly used for testing milk: *M. luteus* (e.g. Huber *et al.* 1969; Billon 1976; McCracken & O'Brien 1976; Bogaerts & Wolf 1980), *B. subtilis* (e.g. Huber *et al.* 1969; Billon 1976; Johnston *et al.* 1981), *B. stearothermophilus* (e.g. van Schothorst & Peelen-Knol 1970; Bielecka *et al.* 1981), *Escherichia coli* (Nouws *et al.* 1979) and *B. cereus* (Smither 1975). Some methods involve the use of urine (Kampelmacher *et al.* 1962; Huber *et al.* 1969) or cutting open kidneys and allowing filter discs (van Schothorst & Peelen-Knol 1970) or swabs (Johnston *et al.* 1981) to soak up the exudate. Others use tissue exudate from frozen and thawed samples (Billon 1976) or extract the tissue by means of solvents (Smither 1975; McCracken *et al.* 1976). Still others are made as simple as possible, and merely involve placing pieces of meat on the surface of seeded agar (Bogaerts & Wolf 1980).

In general, the methods which involve solvent extraction are the most sensitive because they normally involve a concentration step. However, they are obviously rather time-consuming, especially when different solvents are recommended for different antibiotics (e.g. McCracken *et al.* 1976).

Unlike milk, meat is not screened for antibiotics on a wide scale and, except for spore suspensions of *B. subtilis* and *B. stearothermophilus*, kits are not available commercially, although kits intended for use with milk could be adapted. Some systems that are widely used will be described in detail. It is not proposed to consider bioassays specific for single antibiotics, of which there are many.

Four plate test

This is a system which has been developed in the EEC countries intended for monitoring meat at national borders. It has evolved from an amalgamation of the German 'Hemmstofftest' and the Dutch kidney test, with some modifications (van Schothorst *et al.* 1978). The Dutch kidney test involved inserting 12·7 mm paper discs into the kidney cortex until soaked with exudate and testing the discs for inhibitory activity on antibiotic medium pH 6 with 0·2% KH_2PO_4, surface inoculated with *M. luteus* ATCC 9341 (van Schothorst & Peelen-Knol 1970). The Hemmstofftest (Levetsow & Weise 1974) employed 9 mm diam. by 2 mm thick discs of frozen kidney and muscle, which were allowed to thaw on the surface of plates of nutrient agar supplemented with 0·1% KH_2PO_4, seeded with *B. subtilis* BGA (Bundesgesundheitsamt, Federal Bureau of Health). Two plates were used, one at pH 6 and one at pH 8. The *M. luteus* kidney test is more sensitive to penicillin than the Hemmstofftest, but both are insensitive to sulphonamides and chloramphenicol (Table 3). The original four plate test (FPT), therefore, incorporated the two *B. subtilis* BGA plates from the Hemmstofftest, and an *M. luteus* plate (pH 6·0) from the Dutch kidney test, as well as a plate (pH 7·2) seeded with *E. coli*, which was more sensitive to sulphonamides. Discs of kidney and muscle were examined, as in the Hemmstofftest (Nouws *et al.* 1979).

Subsequently, the FPT was modified, replacing the *E. coli* plate with a third *B. subtilis* BGA plate at pH 7·2 with 0·05 μg trimethoprim/ml, which greatly enhances sensitivity to sulphonamides (Gudding 1976: Table 4). This method has been published in English (Bogaerts & Wolf 1980) and in

French (Billon & Tao 1980), and the version used in our laboratory is described below.

TABLE 3

Lower limits of sensitivity of the Four Plate Test to various antibiotics

Antibiotic	Lower limits of sensitivity (μg/g) in	
	Muscle*	Muscle homogenate†
Most β-lactams	0·03–0·06	
Cloxacillin	0·1	
(Dihydro)streptomycin	0·2–0·5	4
Neomycin	0·2–0·5	2
Spectinomycin		>40
Lincomycin	0·2–0·5	4
Kanamycin	0·2–0·5	4
Chloramphenicol	10	
Chlortetracycline	0·1	0·16
Oxytetracycline	0·5	
Erythromycin	0·1	
Spiramycin	0·3	
Tylosin	0·3	
Nystatin		>40
Griseofulvin		>40
Novobiocin	0·05	
Bacitracin	0·2–1·0	
Polymyxin		>40

* Nouws *et al.* (1979).
† Data from this laboratory.

Modified four plate test

In practice we have found (Ministry of Agriculture, Fisheries and Food, UK) that the use of two *B. subtilis* BGA plates (at pH 8 and 7·2) yields as many positive results as the four plates described for the test, and only two are used normally.

Preparation of agar media

For the basal medium, any well-known brand of nutrient agar can be used or a combination of nutrient broth plus agar, but it is wise to check that the agar has suitable diffusion characteristics for antibiotic assays. This is done as follows (Bechtle & Scherr 1958): the nutrient agar is prepared and sterilized as described below. It is tempered to 50°C, and 15 ml quantities poured into 10 cm plastic Petri dishes and allowed to gel. Six mm wells are made, using a cork borer and 3 drops of 1% w/v safranin added to fill the wells. The plates are left at room temperature for the dye to diffuse. Annular zones should be 10–12 mm diam. after 2 h and at least 14·5 mm diam. after 4 h (E. Y. Bridson, pers. comm.). The edge of the zone should be diffuse, not sharp.

The basic recipe consists of nutrient agar plus 0·1% w/v KH_2PO_4. The mixture is dissolved by boiling, cooled to 50°C and the pH is adjusted using 0·1 N NaOH, such that the pH after sterilization will be 6·0, 7·2 or 8·0. Sterilization is carried out at 121°C for 15 min.

TABLE 4

Lower limits of sensitivity for sulphonamides, nitrofurans and trimethoprim

Drug	*E. coli** (pH 7·2)	*B. subtilis*† (pH 7·2)	*B. subtilis*‡ (pH 7·0)
Sulphadoxine	20	0·5	
Sulphadimidine (sulphamethazine)	7	0·5	0·63
Sulphamerazine	3	0·5	0·63
Sulphathiazole	1	0·5	0·32
Sulphadiazine	2	0·5	1·25
Diphenylsulphone	30	0·5	
Nitrofurazone		40	
Furazolidone		50–100	
Trimethoprim	2		

* From Nouws *et al.* (1979): μg/g muscle homogenate.
† Our data: μg/g derived from standard solutions applied to filter paper discs; medium was nutrient agar plus 0·05 μg trimethoprim/ml.
‡ From Nouws (1981): μg/g muscle homogenate; medium was nutrient agar plus 0·4% glucose, 1% NaCl and 0·15 μg trimethoprim/ml.

Preparation of inocula

(a) B. subtilis *BGA*. Nutrient agar plates are heavily surface-inoculated and incubated at 30°C for 10 days. The spores and vegetative cells are harvested by washing off into 0·85% sterile saline, washed twice by centrifuging and resuspended in fresh saline solution. Finally the cells are resuspended in a third portion of saline and heated at 70°C for 30 min to destroy vegetative cells.

The concentration of spores is determined using a conventional viable colony-counting method and is adjusted so that a final concentration of 10^4 c.f.u./ml of medium can conveniently be attained. In practice a suspension containing 10^6 c.f.u./ml is usually used. The suspension will keep at 4°C for several months. Stock cultures are maintained on nutrient agar slopes and stored at 4°C.

(b) M. luteus *ATCC 9341*. Brain heart infusion broth is inoculated and incubated for 24 h at 37°C. A fresh culture is required for each day. The suspension is diluted with sterile medium without prior washing and added to molten nutrient agar pH 8·0, tempered to 45°C, again to give a final concentration of about 10^4 c.f.u./ml.

Stock cultures are subcultured monthly onto brain heart infusion agar slopes, and stored at 4°C.

Trimethoprim solution

Ten mg trimethoprim is dissolved in 10 ml ethanol and the solution diluted with distilled water to a concentration of 5 μg/ml. The solution is stored at 4°C and made up each week. One ml of trimethoprim solution is added per 100 ml of medium.

Standard solutions of antibiotics

Standard solutions of benzylpenicillin, streptomycin, chloramphenicol, chlortetracycline and sulphadimidine are prepared, such that 10 μl contains 30 ng, 1 μg, 2 μg, 50 ng and 2 μg respectively. The 10 μl volumes are dispensed onto 8 mm diam. filter paper discs as standards on the agar plates. Fresh solutions are made up each week and stored at 4°C.

Preparation of plates

The sterile molten media are tempered to 45°C in a water bath, the bacterial suspensions added, and the trimethoprim solution added to medium at pH 7·2. After thorough mixing the agar is poured to a depth of 2 mm in levelled sterile dishes. We use 25 cm square plastic bioassay plates (Nunc: Gibco Ltd, Uxbridge, Middx, UK), adding 100 ml of medium per plate, but other size plates can be used, provided they have flat bottoms and are used with the required depth of agar. A level area is vital for pouring. We use a levelling table with adjustable screws at each corner and a spirit level.

The surface of the plates is dried by leaving them uncovered in a laminar flow cabinet for about 30 min. The *B. subtilis* plates can be stored for up to a week at 4°C before use.

Application of samples

The tissue samples should have as low a microbial count as possible in order to minimize interference in the test by contaminating microflora. Ideally the samples should be tested immediately after slaughter. In practice our samples are usually received deep-frozen. It is normal to use the diaphragm for the muscle sample because of its low commercial value. Deep frozen tissues have the added advantage that it is relatively easy to take a sample. This is done using a power drill fitted with a modified 8 mm i.d. stainless steel cork borer. Cores are drilled out, the outside layers and fat are discarded and discs *ca.* 2 mm thick are cut. The instruments, including the cork borer, are sterilized between each sample by flaming with 70% w/v industrial methylated spirits. Two discs of each tissue-type from each animal are placed on each plate, such that each disc is not less than 4 cm from the next. Twenty-five samples or standard filter-paper discs can be placed on each 25 cm square dish. Two standard paper discs are normally included on each plate. The sulphadimidine disc only gives a positive result on the trimethoprim-containing plate.

The plates with samples are left for 3 h at 4°C to allow any antibiotic residues to diffuse into the agar. The plates are then incubated for 18–24 h at 37°C and examined for zones of inhibition.

An annular zone (measured from the edge of the meat or paper disc) less than 2 mm wide, is considered negative. When one of a pair of samples gives a zone (e.g. one of two samples from the same kidney) the test is repeated. If the result is again unclear the test is considered negative. Positive results are examined further. We use an electrophoretic method. Only samples giving a positive result by electrophoresis as well as a positive FPT results on at least one plate are considered positive.

Swab test on premises (STOP) test

An alternative simple method is that used by the US Department of Agriculture (Johnston *et al.* 1981). This employs *B. subtilis* ATCC 6633 seeded in double layer plates, and is specifically designed to be used by non-specialist personnel in the slaughterhouse. Slits are made in the meat (near a suspected site of injection, if any) and sterile cotton-wool swabs inserted in the meat for about 30 min, so that they soak up exudate. The swabs are then laid on the seeded agar and incubated for 16–20 h at 29°C. Ready-poured plates are supplied by the USDA directly to the inspectors at the slaughterhouse.

Premature growth of the organism can be avoided by surface inoculating the plates immediately prior to use with a spore suspension in 50% ethanol. The ethanol guards against contamination of the suspension by the inexperienced worker (Dr R. W. Johnston, pers. comm.). The advantage of the USDA method and the Dutch kidney method is that they are simple and can be applied as a control method in the slaughterhouse, either to random samples or to specific carcases, where there is reason to suspect that antibiotics may have been used. Suspect carcases can be retained until the results of the test are known. The FPT test is generally more sensitive, but needs to be carried out by more skilled personnel and is more suitable for monitoring purposes. Whichever method is used, it is necessary to carry out further confirmatory tests.

Chloramphenicol in kidneys: see Note Added in Proof, p. 370

Identification of inhibitory substance

An inhibitory zone on a test plate is not sufficient to conclude that antibiotics are present. A number of workers have reported that meat and other tissues can contain non-antibiotic inhibitors. Substances tentatively identified include C_{14}–C_{20} saturated and unsaturated fatty acids, long chain aliphatic and cholesterol-like compounds and lactic acid (Smither 1978) and lysozyme in kidneys (van der Waal 1978). Kundrat (1973) demonstrated that many *Bacillus* spp., including *B. subtilis* BGA, are inhibited by *Pseudomonas* spp. which are common meat spoilage organisms, and observed that *B. subtilis* BGA is particularly inhibited by pig kidneys and liver. Suggestions for reducing the incidence of non-specific inhibition include the examination of fresh and not frozen material, and especially taking precautions to prevent any microbial spoilage or even multiplication which can be responsible for the presence of lactic and fatty acids. Use of a suitable dialysis membrane placed between the sample and the seeded agar can exclude large molecular weight inhibitors like lysozyme (Schmidt & Cremmling (1975). This can be done by putting the membrane under one half of the tissue disc only (Forschner & Seidler 1976).

Our experience confirms that frozen (but not fresh) pig kidneys are especially prone to give 'false positive' reactions, for reasons that are not clear. Many non-specific reactions give quite small zones, hence we disregard annular zones of less than 2 mm when carrying out the FPT.

Identification of antibiotics present

An indication of the antibiotic present can occasionally be obtained by observing which plate(s) in the FPT give positive reactions, e.g. samples only giving zones on the plate at pH 7·2 with trimethoprim are likely to contain sulphonamides. A better, but more time-consuming, indication can be obtained by using various combinations of sensitive organisms and extraction solvents (Frères & Valdebouze 1969*a*, *b*; Billon 1981).

Use of antagonists

This is a potentially useful method, but except for identifying β-lactams in milk, has been little applied. Read *et al.* (1971) reported that 50 μg of *p*-aminobenzoic acid in a paper disc successfully neutralized the activity of sulphonamides in milk. Antagonists exist for many antibiotics (Russell *et al.* 1979) and the test could be repeated incorporating suitable antagonists, e.g. an appropriate β-lactamase for β-lactams, chloramphenicol acetyltransferase for chloramphenicol and thymidine for trimethoprim.

Other methods

Most workers examining meat appear to favour use of gel electrophoresis (Lott & Vaughan, this volume) or thin layer chromatography (TLC) (e.g. Frères & Valdebouze 1973; Langner *et al.* 1973; Bossuyt *et al.* 1976) with bio-autography to examine samples giving inhibitory zones. Confirmatory electrophoresis or TLC is rarely used for milk, although there is no reason why systems developed for meat should not be adapted for milk (e.g. Stadhouders *et al.* 1981).

Incidence of Residues in Meat

Rieve *et al.* (1974) reported a very high incidence of antibiotics in kidneys in Germany, 23% of 17,419 examined, and of these 47% contained penicillin. Tetracyclines, chloramphenicol and streptomycin were also found quite frequently, as well as various combinations of antibiotics. The incidence appears to have dropped since then; Smither *et al.* (1980) in the UK found that only 34 of 5442 samples were positive by FPT, and only two of these (0·037%) were confirmed positive using electrophoresis. More recent MAFF surveys (unpublished) have yielded slightly higher proportions of confirmed positive samples. Tentative identification indicates that sulphonamides, chloramphenicol and streptomycin occur most commonly.

Surveys in 1979–80 revealed sulphonamide residues in over 20% of pig carcases in some parts of the United States, necessitating corrective action (Anon 1980). Recent reports indicate that high levels of sulphonamides are present in many calves slaughtered within a week of birth, due to the administration of 'boluses' which remain in the stomach and release antimicrobials over a period of time (Anon 1982*b*). There is also concern about possible illegal use of chloramphenicol (Anon 1982*a*).

We are grateful to Dr D. H. Watson, MAFF, Food Science Division, for useful comments during the preparation of this paper, and for permission to use the data prepared for the MAFF Veterinary Drug Residues Working Party.

References

ACAR, J. F. 1980 The disc susceptibility test. In *Antibiotics in Laboratory Medicine* ed. Lorian, V. pp. 24–54. Baltimore: Williams and Wilkins.

ANON 1980 Targeted sulfa-testing in swine expanded to four more states. *Food Chemical News* December 22, p. 4.

ANON 1982*a* Import alert issued on chloramphenicol. *Food Chemical News* March 22, p. 23.

ANON 1982*b* USDA/FDA/Industry task force to work on drug residue in calves problem. *Food Chemical News* April **12,** 36–37.

ARRET, B. & KIRSHBAUM, A. 1959 A rapid assay method for detecting penicillin in milk. *Journal of Milk and Food Technology* **22,** 329–331.

BECHTLE, R. M. & SCHERR, G. H. 1958 A new agar for *in vitro* antimicrobial sensitivity testing. *Antibiotics and Chemotherapy* **8,** 599–606.

BIELECKA, M., BALDOCK, J. D. & KOTULA, A. W. 1981 Determination of antibiotics in meat using *Bacillus stearothermophilus* spores. *Journal of Food Protection* **44,** 194–200.

BILLON, J. 1976 Recherche des résidus d'antibiotiques dans les viandes. *Bulletin de l'Académie Vétérinaire de France* **49,** 137–142.

BILLON, J. 1981 Recherche, identification et dosage des résidus d'antibiotiques dans le lait. *Recueil de Médecine Vétérinaire* **157,** 169–174.

BILLON, J. & TAO, S. H. 1980 Recherche des antibiotiques et des résidus de substances à activité antimicrobienne dans les aliments. *Revue Technique Vétérinaire de l'Alimentation* **164,** 9–17.

BOGAERTS, R. & WOLF, F. 1980 A standardized method for the detection of residues of anti-bacterial substances in fresh meat. *Fleischwirtschaft* **60,** 672–673.

BOSSUYT, R., VAN RENTERGHEM, R. & WAES, G. 1976 Identification of antibiotic residues in milk by thin-layer chromatography. *Journal of Chromatography* **124,** 37–42.

BROWN, R. J., WILCHEK, M. & SWAISGOOD, H. E. 1980 Detection and measurement of antibiotics in biological fluids by enzyme immunoassay. *Journal of Dairy Science* **63** (Supplement 1), 54–55.

BURGAT-SACAZE, V. 1981 Risque d'accidents allergiques dus aux résidus. *Recueil de Médecine Vétérinaire* **157,** 187–190.

CHARM, S. L. & WONG, B. L. 1980 The rapid quantitative assay and color test for penicillin by specific binding to cell wall enzyme. *Journal of Dairy Science* **63** (Supplement 1), 55.

DAVIS, W. W. & STOUT, T. R. 1971*a* Disc plate method of microbiological antibiotic assay. 1. Factors influencing variability and error. *Applied Microbiology* **22,** 659–665.

DAVIS, W. W. & STOUT, T. R. 1971*b* Disc plate method of microbiological antibiotic assay. II Novel procedure offering improved accuracy. *Applied Microbiology* **22,** 666–670.

FAO 1969 *Specifications for Identity and Purity of some Antibiotics*. FAO Nutrition Meeting Report Series No 45A, Food and Agriculture Organization.

FDA 1968 *Antibiotic Residues in Milk, Dairy Products, and Animal Tissues: Methods, Reports and Protocols*. National Center for Antibiotic and Insulin Analysis, Food and Drug Administration, Department of Health, Education and Welfare, Washington, DC, 20204.

FORSCHNER, E. & SEIDLER, M. 1976 Alternativvorschlage zum Hemmstofftest. Rationalisierung und Absicherung. *Fleischwirtschaft* **56,** 1008–1013.

FRÈRES, D. & VALDEBOUZE, P. 1969*a* Recherche des résidus à activité antibiotique dans les tissues animaux. 1. Mise au point d'une methode de detection des antibiotiques dans le muscle. *Bulletin de l'Académie Vétérinaire* **42,** 835–845.

FRÈRES, D. & VALDEBOUZE, P. 1969*b* Methode de detection des antibiotiques dans les tissues animaux. *Bulletin de l'Académie Vétérinaire* **42,** 847–853.

FRÈRES, D. & VALDEBOUZE, P. 1973 Methode d'identification des antibiotiques dans les aliments pour animaux par chromatographie en couche mince. *Journal of Chromatography* **87,** 300–304.

GALESLOOT, TH. E. & HASSING, F. 1962 A rapid and sensitive paper disc method for the detection of penicillin in milk. *Netherlands Milk and Dairy Journal* **16,** 89–95.

GEDEK, W. 1977 Erfassung von Cephalosporinen in Rohmilch durch *B. cereus*-Beta-Lactamase. *Deutsche Tierarztliche Wochenschrift* **84,** 333–372.

GINN, R. E., TATINI, S. & PACKARD, V. S. 1978 Comparative evaluation of the Difco disc assay method for detecting penicillin in milk and milk products. *Journal of Food Protection* **41,** 361–363.

GOUNELLE, H. & SZAKVARY, A. 1966 Antibiotiques et aliments. 1. Les accidents allergiques liés aux résidus. *Bulletin de l'Académie Nationale de Médecine* **150,** 76–82.

GROVE, D. C. & RANDALL, W. A. 1955 *Assay Methods of Antibiotics. A Laboratory Manual.* New York: Medical Encyclopedia, Inc.

GUAY, R., BRASSARD, N. & LACASSE, P. 1981 Significance of the presence of β-lactamases in milk. *Journal of Food Protection* **46,** 796–797.

GUDDING, R. 1976 An improved bacteriological method for the detection of sulphonamide residues in food. *Acta veterinaria Scandinavica* **17,** 458–464.

HAMANN, J., HEESCHEN, W., TOLLE, A. & HAHN, G. 1975 Untersuchungen über Nachweis, Isolierung und Identifizierung von Antibiotikaruckständen in der Milch. 3. Mitteilung: Nachweis von Hemmstoffen mit Hilfe der enzymatisch-fluorometrischen Milchsäurebestimming in der kontinuierlichen Durchflussanalyse. *Milchwissenschaft* **30,** 139–143.

HAMANN, J., HEESCHEN, W. & TOLLE, A. 1980 Untersuchungen über Nachweis, Isolierung und Identifizierung von Antibiotika-Ruckständen in der Milch. 6. Die Hemmung der Laktatbildung als Meeskiterium in Screening-Test zum Nachweis antibiotisch wirksamer Substanzen. *Milchwissenschaft* **35,** 544–546.

HUBER, W. G., CARLSON, M. B. & LEPPER, M. H. 1969 Penicillin and antimicrobial residues in domestic animals at slaughter. *Journal of the American Veterinary Medical Association* **154,** 1590–1595.

IDF 1970 International Standard FIL-IDF57, International Dairy Federation, Square Vergote 41, 1040 Brussels, Belgium.

IGARASHI, R. T., BAUGHMAN, R. W., NELSON, F. E. & HARTMAN, P. A. 1961 Rapid antibiotic assay methods using *Bacillus stearothermophilus*. *Journal of Milk and Food Technology* **24,** 143–146.

JACQUET, J. & AUXEPAULES, M. 1978 Le problème de la pollution du lait par les antibiotiques. Etat actuel de la question. *Bulletin de l'Académie Vétérinaire de France* **51**, 73–79.

JACQUET, J., DELACROIX, J., LETOURNEUR, G. & VILLETTE, O. 1959 Mise au point sur la sensibilité actuelle des ferments lactiques à la pénicilline en fromagerie de pâtes molles. *Comptes rendu des Séances—Académie d'agriculture de France* **45,** 849–854.

JOHNSTON, R. W., REAMER, R. H., HARRIS, E. W., FUGATE, H. G. & SCHWAB, B. 1981 A new screening method for the detection of antibiotic residues in meat and poultry tissues. *Journal of Food Protection* **44,** 828–831.

KAMPELMACHER, E. H., GUINEE, P. A. M. & VAN NOORLE JANSEN, L. M. 1962 Simple test for antibiotics in slaughtered animals treated with antibiotics during life. *Tijdschrift Diergeneeskunde* **87,** 16–29.

KELLY, W. R. & COLLINS, J. D. 1967 Chemotherapeutic residues in the Dublin milk supply: public health aspects. *Journal of the Irish Medical Association* **60,** 35–40.

KOSIKOWSKI, F. V. & LEDFORD, R. A. 1960 A reverse phase disk assay test for antibiotics in milk. *Journal of the American Veterinary Medical Association* **136,** 297–299.

KRAAK, J. & TOLLE, A. 1967 Brillantschwarz-Reduktionstest mit *Bac. stearothermophilus* var *calidolactis* zum Nachweis von Hemmstoffen in der Milch. *Milchwissenschaft* **22,** 669–67.

KRAAK, J. & TOLLE, A. 1969 Zum Nachweis von Hemmstoffen in Milch mit dem Brillantschwarz-Reduktionstest. I Teil: Verbesserte Methodik. *Archiv für Lebensmittelhygiene* **20,** 145–149.

KUNDRAT, W. 1973 Vergleichende Versuche und Gedanken zur Durchfuhrung von Hemmstofftestes. *Fleischwirtschaft* **53,** 1121–1125.

LABIE, C. 1981 Dispositions législatives destinées à éviter la présence de résidus d' antibiotiques dans le lait. *Recueil de Médecine Vétérinaire* **157,** 161–167.

LANGE, A. M. & MADELUNG, P. 1959 Antibiotica-behandling og bakteriologisk kødkontrol. *Medlemsblad for den danske Dyrlaegeforening* **42,** 727–735.

LANGNER, H. J., TEUFEL, U., PANTKE, G., SIEGERT, M. & FROMMHOLD, M. 1973 Chemical and microbiological determination of antibiotics. Microbiological determination of various antibiotics. *ChemieMikrobiologieTechnologie der Lebensmittel* **2,** 71–78.

LEVETSOW, R. & WEISE, E. 1974 Zur Ruckstandsuntersuchung im Rahmen der amtlichen Fleischuntersuchung. *Schlacht- und Viehhof-zeitung* **74,** 329–336.

LISKA, B. J. 1960 A direct microscopic method for detecting antibiotic activity in milk. *Journal of Milk and Food Technology* **23,** 117–121.

MCCRACKEN, A. & O'BRIEN, J. J. 1976 Detection of antibiotic residues in calf tissues. *Research in Veterinary Science* **21,** 240–241.

MCCRACKEN, A., O'BRIEN, J. J. & CAMPBELL, N. 1976 Antibiotic residues and their recovery from animal tissues. *Journal of Applied Bacteriology* **41,** 129–135.

MALTEN, K. E. 1968 Allergy to antibiotics in minute amounts in foods. In *Antibiotics in Agriculture*, Proceedings 5th Symposium, Group European Nutrition, Jouy-en-Josas 1966. Bibliotheca *Nutritio et Dieta* Vol. 10, pp. 184–194. Basel & New York: Karger.

MARTH, E. H. & ELLICKSON, B. E. 1959 Problems created by the presence of antibiotics in milk and milk products. *Journal of Milk and Food Technology* **22,** 266–272.

MESSER, J. W., CLAYPOOL, L. L., HOUGHTBY, G. A., MIKOLJCIK, E. M. & SING, E. L. 1978 Detection of antibiotic residues in milk and dairy products. In *Standard Methods for the examination of Dairy Products* ed. Marth, E. H., 14th Edn, pp. 141–150. Washington, D.C.: American Public Health Association.

MILHAUD, G. & PERSON, J. M. 1981 Evaluation de la toxicité des résidus d'antibiotiques dans le lait. *Recueil de Médecine Véterinaire* **157,** 179–185.

MOSSEL, D. A. A., MANDERSLOOT, J. G. & GENTIS, A. S. S. 1955 A simplified microbiological test for the selection of preservatives in milk and milk products. *Netherlands Milk and Dairy Journal* **9,** 63–71.

MYERS, R. P. 1964 Antibiotic residues in milk. *Residue Reviews* **7,** 9–36.

NEAL, C. E. & CALBERT, H. E. 1955 The use of 2,3,5 triphenyltetrazolium chloride as a test for antibiotic substances in milk. *Journal of Dairy Science* **38,** 629–633.

NOUWS, J. F. M. 1981 Microbiological assay methods for sulphonamides in animal tissues, serum and milk. *Veterinary Quarterly* **3,** 136–142.

NOUWS, J. F. M., VAN SCHOTHORST, M. & ZIV, G. 1979 A critical evaluation of several microbiological test methods for residues of antimicrobial drugs in ruminants. *Archiv für Lebensmittelhygiene* **30,** 1–40.

READ, R. B., BRADSHAW, J. G., SWARTZENTRUBER, A. A. & BRAZIS, A. R. 1971 Detection of sulfa drugs and antibiotics in milk. *Applied Microbiology* **21,** 806–808

REPORT 1969 *Joint Committee on the Use of Antibiotics in Animal Husbandry and Veterinary Medicine.* London: HMSO.

RIEVE, D., WERMERSSEN, H. & ZIMMERMANN, T. 1974 Untersuchungen zur Bestimmung von Antibiotika als Ergänzung zum biologischen Hemmstofftest. *Archiv für Lebensmittelhygiene* **25,** 264–267.

RUSSELL, A. D., AHONKAI, I. & ROGERS, D. T. 1979 Microbiological applications of the inactivation of antibiotics and other antimicrobial agents. *Journal of Applied Bacteriology* **46,** 207–245.

SCHMIDT, U. & CREMMLING, K. 1975 Untersuchungen uber unspezifische Reaktionen im Hemmstofftest beim Antibiotica-Nachweis in Schweinenieren. *Fleischwirtschaft* **55,** 1736–1737.

SMITH, H. W. & TUCKER, J. F. 1975 The effect of feeding diets containing permitted antibiotics on the faecal excretion of *Salmonella typhimurium* by experimentally infected chickens. *Journal of Hygiene, Cambridge* **75,** 293–301.

SMITH, H. W. & TUCKER, J. F. 1978 The effect of antimicrobial feed additives on the colonisation of the alimentary tract of chickens by *Salmonella typhimurium. Journal of Hygiene, Cambridge* **80,** 217–231.

SMITHER, R. 1975 Evaluation of two simple assay methods for detecting antibiotic residues in chicken and pig muscle. *Journal of Applied Bacteriology* **38,** 235–243.

SMITHER, R. 1978 Bacterial inhibitors formed during the adventitious growth of micro-organisms in chicken liver and pig kidney. *Journal of Applied Bacteriology* **45,** 267–277.

SMITHER, R., LOTT, A. F., DALZIEL, R. W. & OSTLER, D. C. 1980 Antibiotic residues in meat in the United Kingdom; an assessment of specific tests to detect and identify antibiotic residues. *Journal of Hygiene, Cambridge* **85,** 359–369.

STADHOUDERS, J., HASSING, F. & GALESLOOT, T. E. 1981 An electrophoretic method for the identification of antibiotic residues in small volumes of milk. *Netherlands Milk and Dairy Journal* **35,** 23–33.

TERPLAN, G. & ZAADHOF, K. J. 1967 Zum Vorkommen und Nachweis von Hemmstoffen in der Milch- eine kurze Obersicht. *Milchwissenschaft* **22,** 761–771.

TRAMER, J. 1964 Antibiotics in milk. *Journal of the Society of Dairy Technology* **17,** 95–100.

US PATENT 1980 No 4,239,852 Antibiotic detection method. S. E. Charm, December 16th 1980.

VAN DER WAAL, G. 1978 Weitere Erfahrungen mit der Abrenzung lysozymbedingter unspezifischer Reaktionen im allgemeinen Hemmstofftest. *Archiv für Lebensmittelhygiene* **29,** 235.

VAN OS, J. L. 1978 Antibiotic residues in milk: dye marking versus direct control. *Journal of Food Protection* **41,** 574–576.

VAN OS, J. L. & BEUKERS, R. 1980 A multitest system for detection of antibiotics in milk. *Journal of Food Protection* **43,** 510–511, 519.

VAN OS, J. L., LAMERIS, S. A., DOODEWAARD, J. & OOSTENDORP, J. G. 1975 Diffusion test for the determination of antibiotic residues in milk. *Netherlands Milk and Dairy Journal* **29,** 16–34.

VAN SCHOTHORST, M. & PEELEN-KNOL, G. 1970 Detection and identification of some antibiotics in slaughter animals. *Netherlands Journal of Veterinary Science* **3,** 85–91.

VAN SCHOTHORST, M., VAN LEUSDEN, F. M. & NOUWS, J. F. M. 1978 Antibiotic residues: regulations, tolerances and detection in the European Economic Community. *Journal of the Association of Official Analytical Chemists* **61,** 1209–1213.

VICKERS, H. R. 1964 Dermatological hazards of the presence of penicillin in milk *Proceedings of the Royal Society of Medicine* **57,** 1091–1092.

VILIM, A. B., MOORE, S. D. & LAROCQUE, L. 1979 Microbiological determination of penicillin G, ampicillin and cloxacillin residues in milk. *Journal of the Association of Official Analytical Chemists* **62,** 1247–1250.

WAL, J. M. 1979 Evolution du concept de résidu dans les produits animaux des antibiotiques utilisés en élevage. *Annales de la nutrition et de l'alimentation* **33,** 325–341.

WHITEHEAD, H. R. & COX, G. A. 1956 The detection of penicillin in milk. *Journal of Applied Bacteriology* **19,** 247–249.

WHO 1969 *Specifications for the Identity and Purity of Food Additives and their Toxicological Evaluation: some Antibiotics.* Technical Report Series 430, World Health Organization: Geneva.

WHO 1978 *Surveillance for the Prevention and Control of Health Hazards due to Antibiotic Resistant Enterobacteria.* Technical Report Series 624, World Health Organization: Geneva.

WOOLLEY, J. L., MURCH, O. & SIGEL, C. W. 1978 Thin layer chromatographic screening method for sulfadiazine residues in calf tissues, plasma and urine. *Journal of the Association of Official Analytical Chemists* **61,** 545–549.

WRIGHT, R. C. & TRAMER, J. 1961 The estimation of penicillin in milk. *Journal of the Society of Dairy Technology* **14,** 85–87.

ZIV, G., GORDIN, S., BACHAR, G. & BERSTEIN, S. 1973 Concentration and persistence of antibiotics in milk following intramammary infusion in cows. *Refuah Veterinarith* **30** (3/4), 85–100.

ZUIDWEG, M. H. J., OOSTENDORP, J. J. & BOS, C. J. K. 1969 Thin-layer chromatography on Sephadex for the identification of antibiotics. *Journal of Chromatography* **42,** 552–554.

Note Added in Proof

Chloramphenicol in kidneys

A recent report (Nouws 1981) indicates that chloramphenicol is rapidly reduced to arylamines in liver and kidney *post mortem.* These compounds are inactive microbiologically. In order to detect chloramphenicol by bioassay in kidneys it is necessary to sample the kidney pelvis, which can be expected to contain some urine. Chloramphenicol is excreted as the glucuronide metabolite in urine, which is also inactive microbiologically. Treatment with β-glucuronidase will restore its activity. Thus chloramphenicol in kidneys is best detected by extracting exudate from the kidney pelvis using a paper disc and treating with β-glucuronidase (see Nouws 1981 for details of the method).

NOUWS, J. F. M. 1981 Tolerances and detection of antimicrobial residues in slaughtered animals. *Archiv für Lebensmittelhygiene* **32,** 103–110.

Subject Index

Thienamycin, 6
Thymidine, 32, 33, 304, 345, 365
Thymidine phosphorylase, 32
Thymidylic acid, 345

THE SOCIETY FOR APPLIED BACTERIOLOGY TECHNICAL SERIES

General Editor: F. A. Skinner

1 Identification Methods for Microbiologists Part A *1966*
Edited by B. M. Gibbs and F. A. Skinner
Out of print

2 Identification Methods for Microbiologists Part B *1968*
Edited by B. M. Gibbs and D. A. Shapton
Out of Print

3 Isolation Methods for Microbiologists *1969*
Edited by D. A. Shapton and G. W. Gould

4 Automation, Mechanization and Data Handling in Microbiology *1970*
Edited by Ann Baillie and R. J. Gilbert

5 Isolation of Anaerobes *1971*
Edited by D. A. Shapton and R. G. Board

6 Safety in Microbiology *1972*
Edited by D. A. Shapton and R. G. Board

7 Sampling—Microbiological Monitoring of Environments *1973*
Edited by R. G. Board and D. W. Lovelock

8 Some Methods for Microbiological Assay *1975*
Edited by R. G. Board and D. W. Lovelock

9 Microbial Aspects of the Deterioration of Materials *1975*
Edited by R. J. Gilbert and D. W. Lovelock

10 Microbial Ultrastructure: The Use of the Electron Microscope *1976*
Edited by R. Fuller and D. W. Lovelock

11 Techniques for the Study of Mixed Populations *1978*
Edited by D. W. Lovelock and R. Davies

12 Plant Pathogens *1979*
Edited by D. W. Lovelock

13 Cold Tolerant Microbes in Spoilage and the Environment *1979*
Edited by A. D. Russell and R. Fuller

14 Identification Methods for Microbiologists (2nd Edn) *1979*
Edited by F. A. Skinner and D. W. Lovelock

15 Microbial Growth and Survival in Extremes of Environment *1980*
Edited by G. W. Gould and Janet E. L. Corry

16 Disinfectants: Their Use and Evaluation of Effectiveness *1981*
Edited by C. H. Collins, M. C. Allwood, Sally F. Bloomfield and A. Fox

17 Isolation and Identification Methods for Food Poisoning Organisms *1982*
Edited by Janet E. L. Corry, Diane Roberts and F. A. Skinner

18. Antibiotics: Assessment of Antimicrobial Activity and Resistance *1983*
Edited by A. D. Russell and L. B. Quesnel